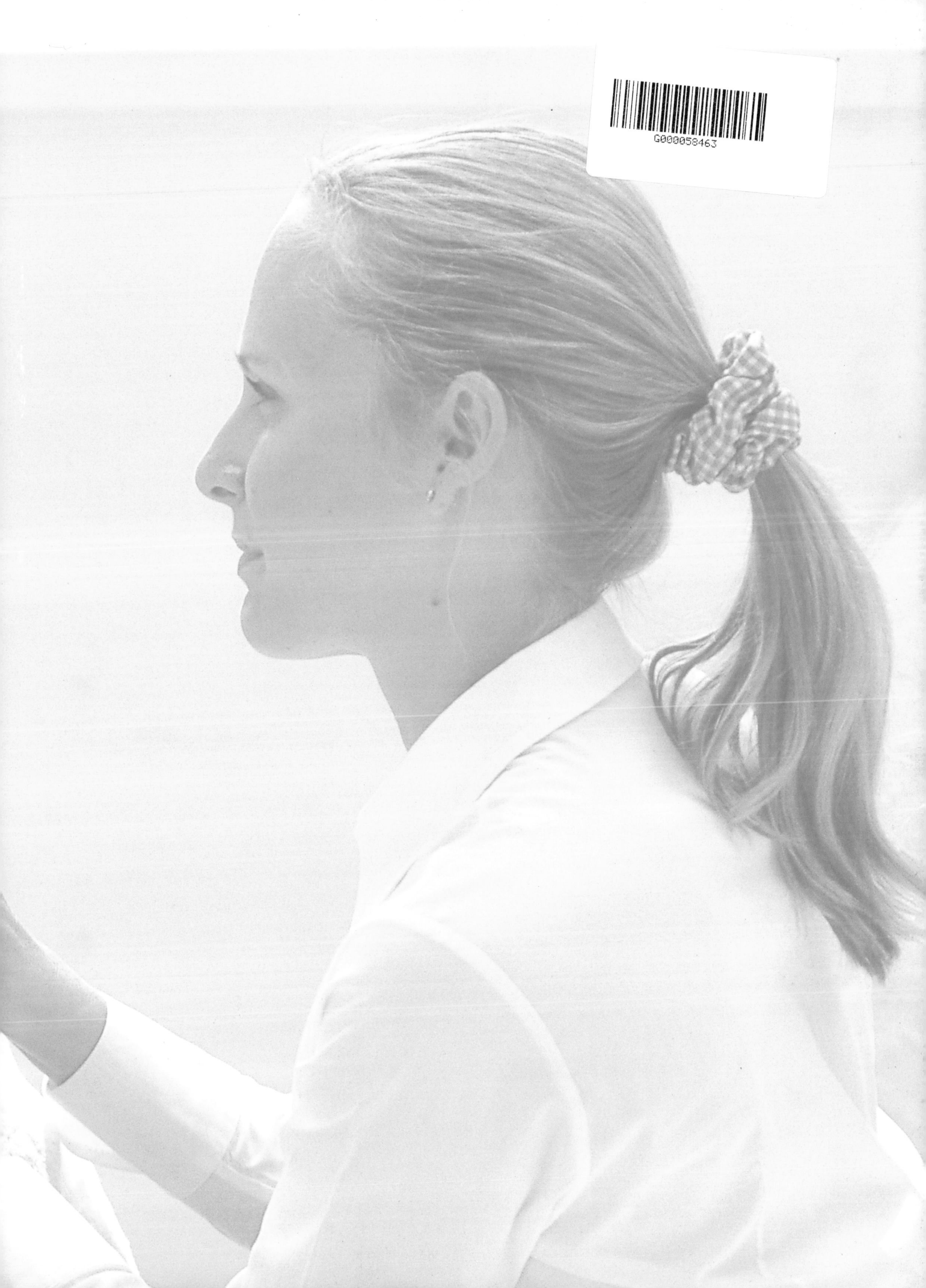

mind-blowing

FOOT MASSAGE

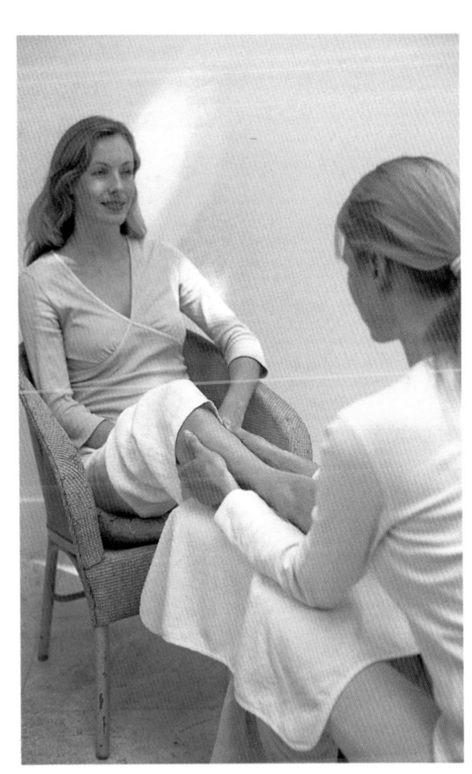

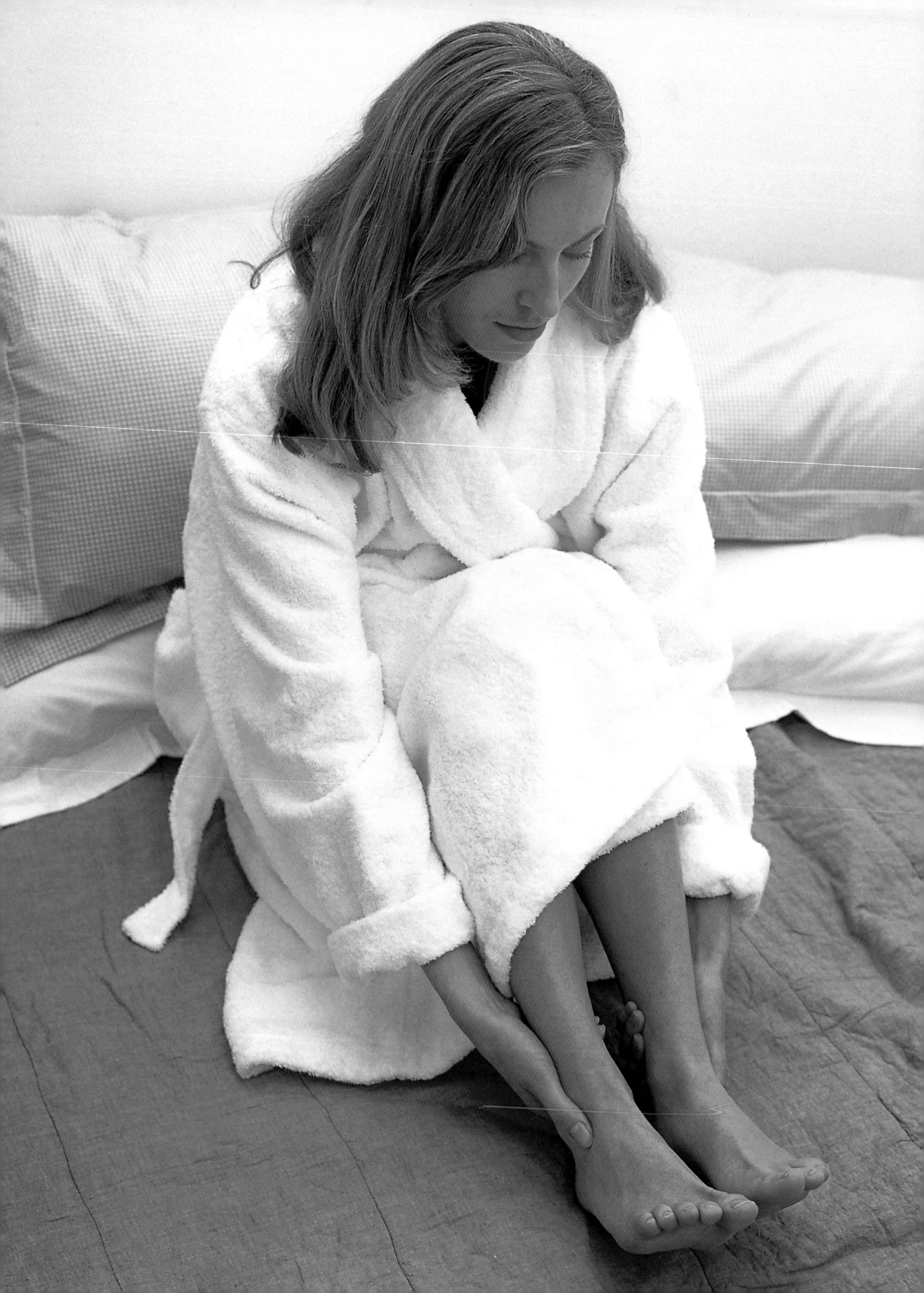

mind-blowing
FOOT MASSAGE

Use the power of massage and reflexology
to soothe, heal, energize and excite

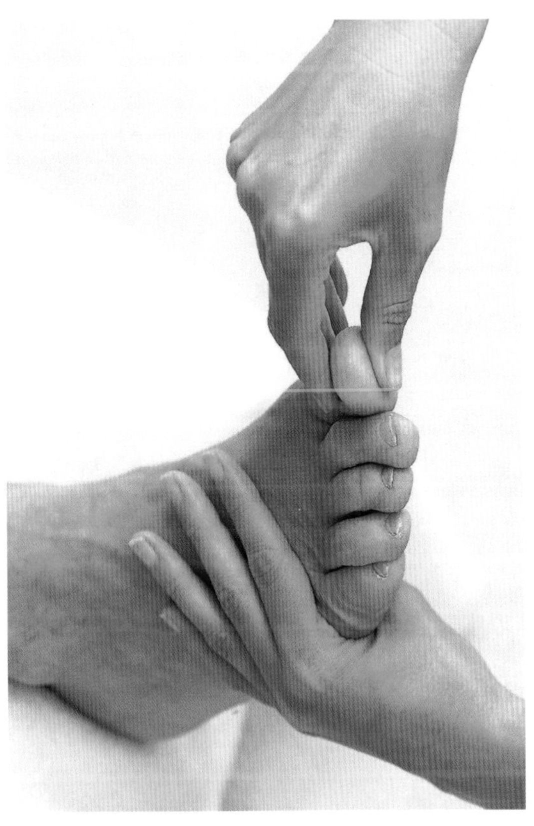

Renée Tanner

photography by Michelle Garrett

LORENZ BOOKS

This edition is published by Lorenz Books

Lorenz Books is an imprint of Anness Publishing Ltd
Hermes House, 88–89 Blackfriars Road, London SE1 8HA
tel. 020 7401 2077; fax 020 7633 9499
www.lorenzbooks.com info@anness.com

UK agent: The Manning Partnership Ltd, 6 The Old Dairy, Melcombe Road, Bath BA2 3LR; tel. 01225 478444; fax 01225 478440; sales@manning-partnership.co.uk

UK distributor: Grantham Book Services Ltd, Isaac Newton Way, Alma Park Industrial Estate, Grantham, Lincs NG31 9SD; tel. 01476 541080; fax 01476 541061; orders@gbs.tbs-ltd.co.uk

North American agent/distributor: National Book Network, 4501 Forbes Boulevard, Suite 200, Lanham, MD 20706; tel. 301 459 3366; fax 301 429 5746; www.nbnbooks.com

Australian agent/distributor: Pan Macmillan Australia, Level 18, St Martins Tower, 31 Market St, Sydney, NSW 2000; tel. 1300 135 113; fax 1300 135 103; customer.service@macmillan.com.au

New Zealand agent/distributor: David Bateman Ltd, 30 Tarndale Grove, Off Bush Road, Albany, Auckland; tel. (09) 415 7664; fax (09) 415 8892

A CIP catalogue record for this book is available from the British Library.

Publisher: Joanna Lorenz
Editorial Director: Helen Sudell
Project Editor: Ann Kay
Copy Editor/additional text: Kim Davies
Designer: Ann Samuel
Photographer: Michelle Garrett
Photographer's assistant: Lisa Shalet
Production Controller: Lee Sargent

10 9 8 7 6 5 4 3 2 1

Publisher's note
Always consult your doctor before commencing any health-related treatment or programme, especially if you have a medical condition or are pregnant. All guidelines and warnings published in this book should be read and noted with care. The publisher and author disclaim any liability or loss, personal or otherwise, arising from the procedures and information contained within this book.

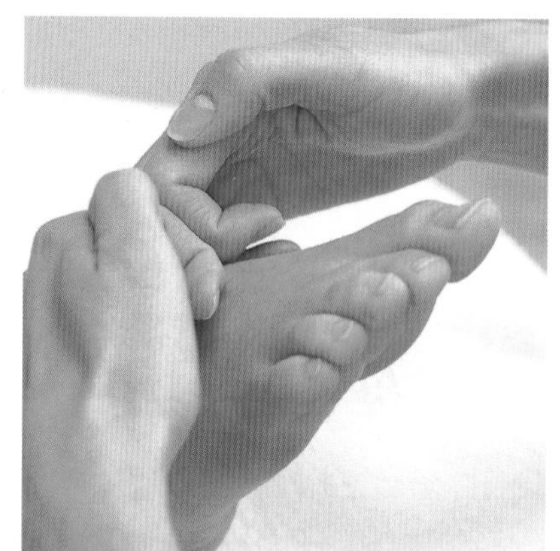

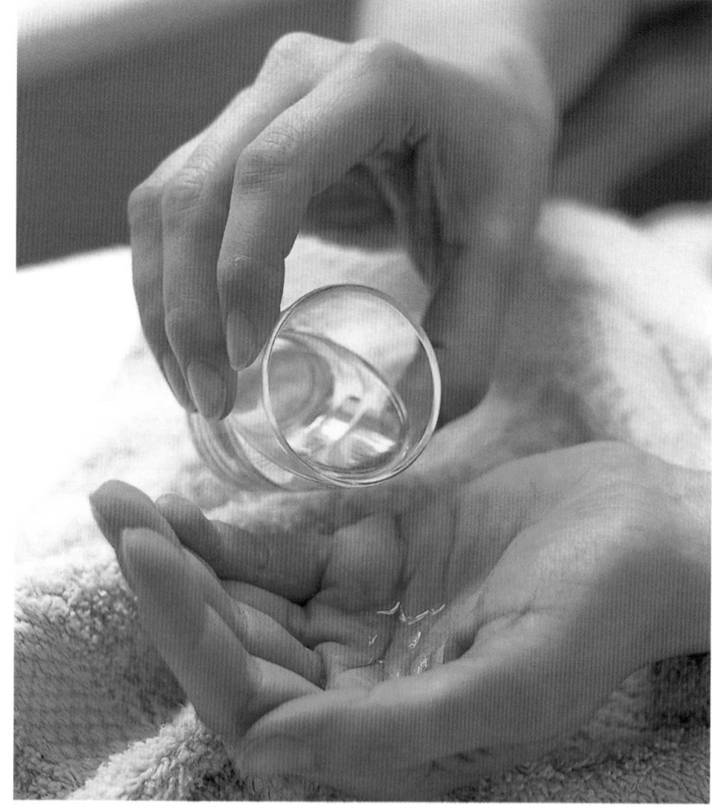

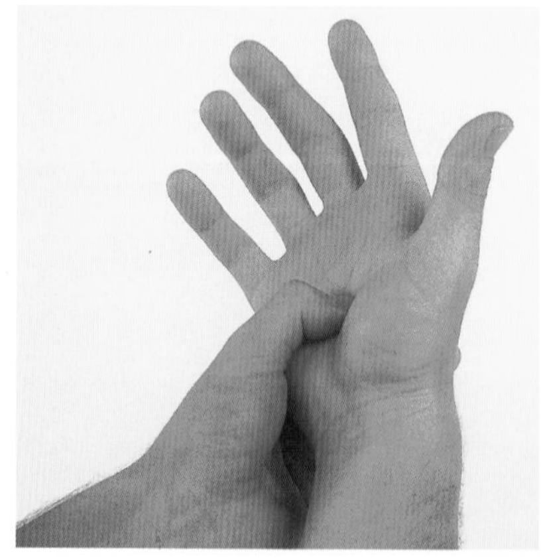

Contents

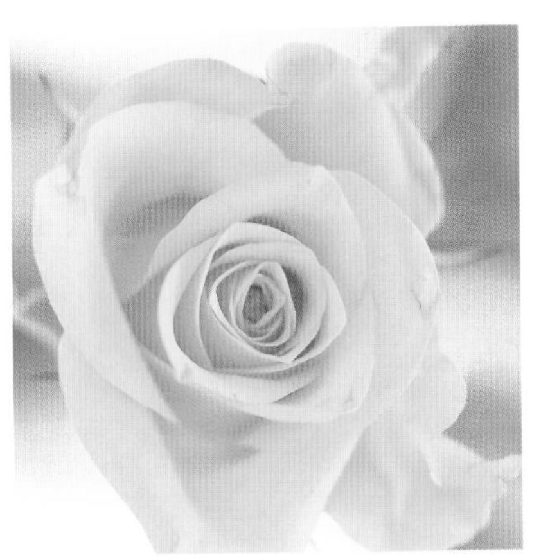

Introduction

Massage might be described as "therapeutic touch". It is a way of using the natural human instinct for touching and being touched as a means of healing illness and promoting well-being. There are many different kinds of therapeutic touch. This book explores three of them – massage, reflexology and acupressure – and looks at how they can be used on the feet to the benefit of your mind and body.

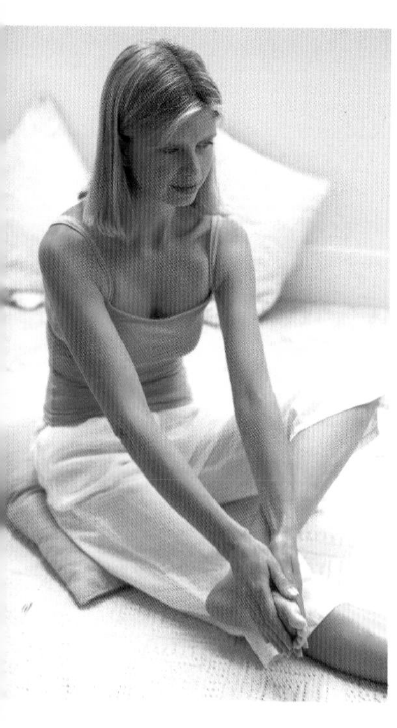

Our feet take a great deal of punishment in the course of a day, yet they are so often left out of our pampering regimes. This book sets out to show that there are all kinds of ways in which we can give our own feet a special treat. More than that, we can do it in a manner that can relax, stimulate, or nurture the whole body. So, for example, you could give your feet a vigorous rub to warm them up before a trip to the gym, and a soothing massage to help yourself relax and slow down afterwards. You might like to treat your feet to a long, luxurious soak in fragrant essential oils specially chosen for their health-giving properties. You could also use lymphatic massage to make ankles look trimmer, and to ease that aching so often felt in the legs at the end of a hard day.

This book will show you how to do these, and many other, invigorating and health-giving things for yourself. As well as providing step-by-step treatments that concentrate on a specific therapy, the book offers routines that combine several different therapies, in a fresh and effective way. For example, you may like to use a combination of reflexology and soothing massage to help you sleep at night.

The book also suggests a range of treatments that can be enjoyed between partners or friends, from a revitalizing routine to a sensual massage, and a special treatment for mothers-to-be. The feet, after all, are so much more than a means of transport. With the help of this book, you can make them a source of well-being and pleasure.

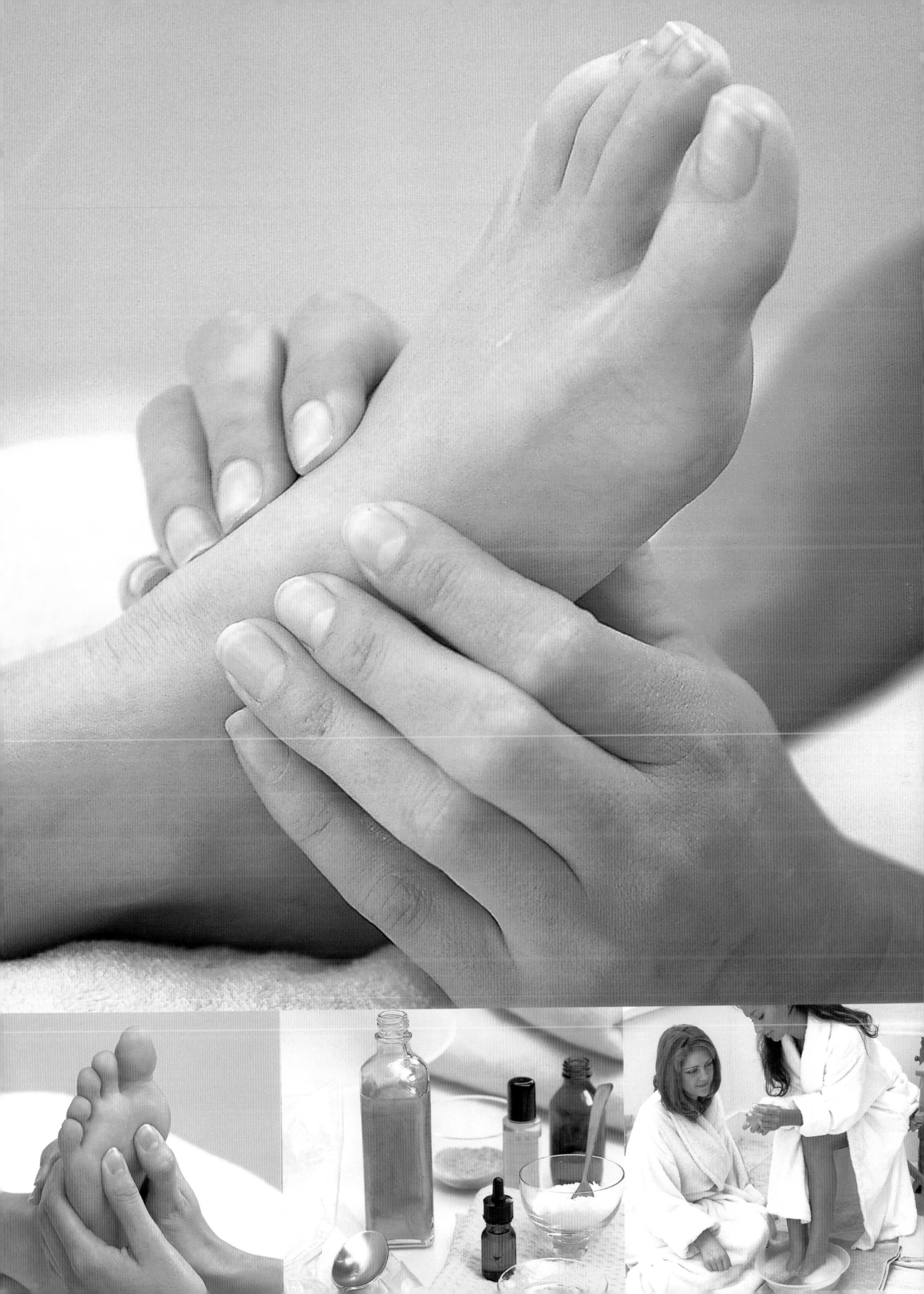

Treating the Feet

Our feet support us, and they take us wherever we want to go in life. They are also highly sensitive and responsive to touch. This section explains the importance of the feet, and suggests ways that we can care for them. There is also an overview of the many different therapies that we can use to treat our feet – and through them enhance the well-being of our mind and body.

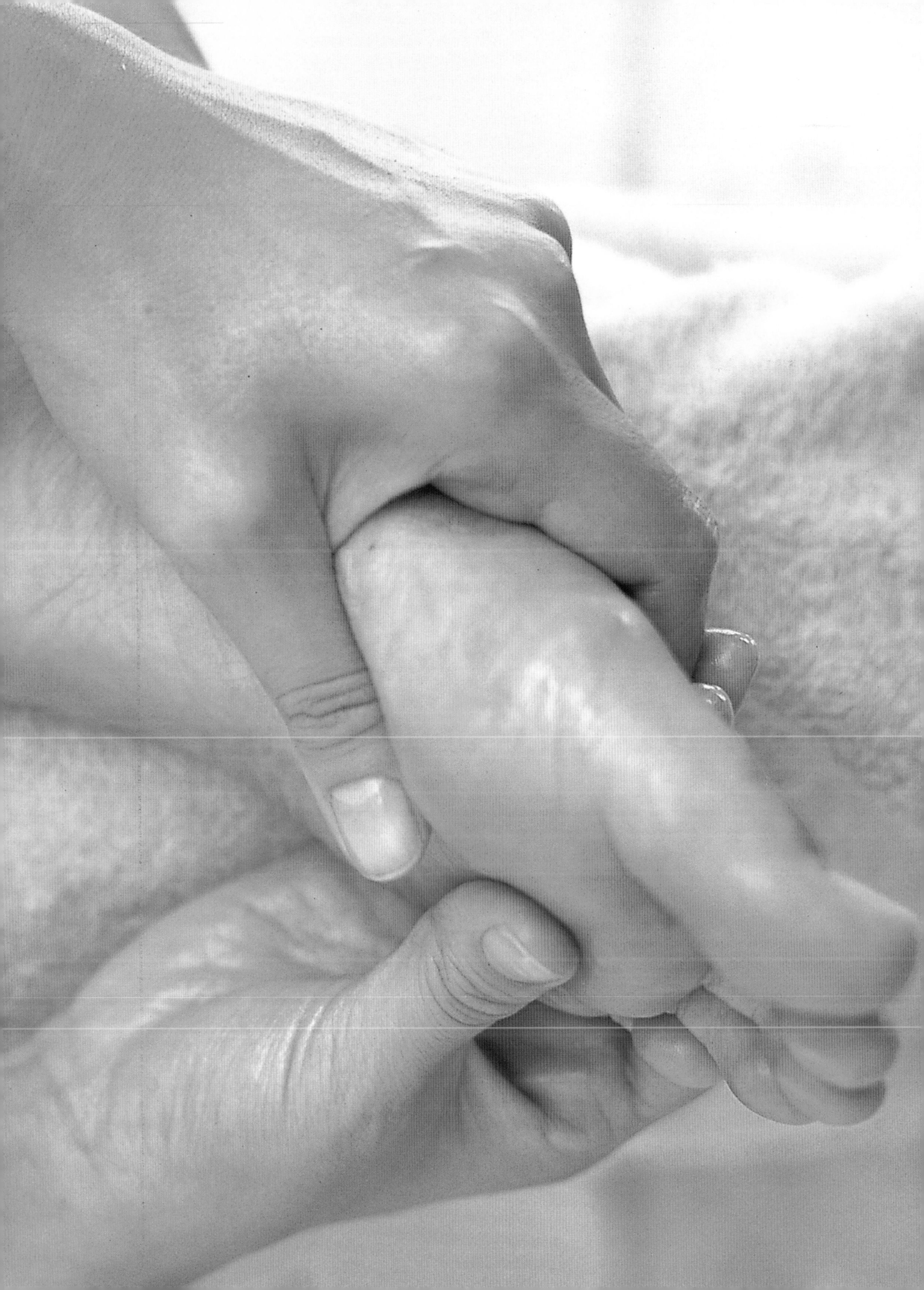

The power of touch

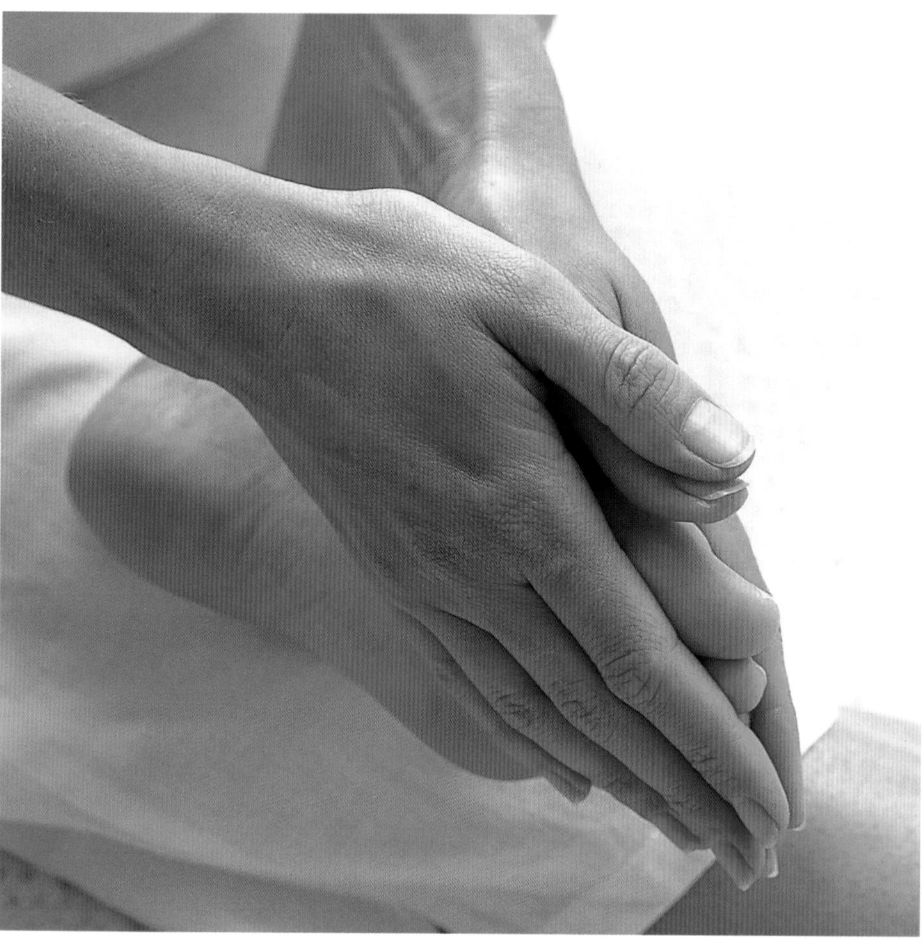

an ancient practice

For centuries massage has been seen as a way to help us maintain good health. Julius Caesar had daily massages for his neuralgia and headaches, and the renowned Roman writer Pliny had regular treatments to relieve his asthma. He felt so indebted to his foreign massage therapist that he persuaded the emperor to grant him the highest honour he could bestow, Roman citizenship.

◁ Follow your own natural instincts to touch and be touched, and give your inner self a boost by holding and massaging your feet.

▽ Even the simplest foot rub can be highly pleasurable, and it is easy to treat your own feet so long as you are flexible enough to reach them.

Touch is an essential element of a fulfilled and happy life. We draw warmth and comfort from physical contact with others, and we can offer it as a way of expressing love and care. Touch is a universal language that we all use instinctively – it allows us to convey sympathy, understanding and reassurance. Being deprived of touch can make us feel anxious and alone.

Massage and other touch therapies are wonderful ways of giving focused, healing touch, either to yourself or other people. Specific techniques can be used to create different effects, but technical skill alone will not give the desired result – the quality of the contact is much more important. The dexterity of your hands, the feeling of warmth and energy that they impart, and your ability to concentrate on what you are doing are intrinsic elements of a good massage.

focusing on the feet

Although all massage is beneficial, a treatment that concentrates on the feet is perhaps the most pleasurable and relaxing of all. Our feet are often neglected, and most of us fail to look after them properly: we cramp them into ill-fitting shoes and pay them little attention until they start to hurt. Yet our feet are vitally important - they support us through our lives, carrying us an average distance that is equivalent to going to the moon and back again twice over.

The feet are highly sensitive and very responsive to touch and massage: they contain more than 14,000 nerve endings between them. Stroking or rubbing the feet can have a soothing, relaxing effect on the entire body. As a result, foot massage is one of the most effective ways of lifting your mood and enhancing your general well-being in just a few minutes.

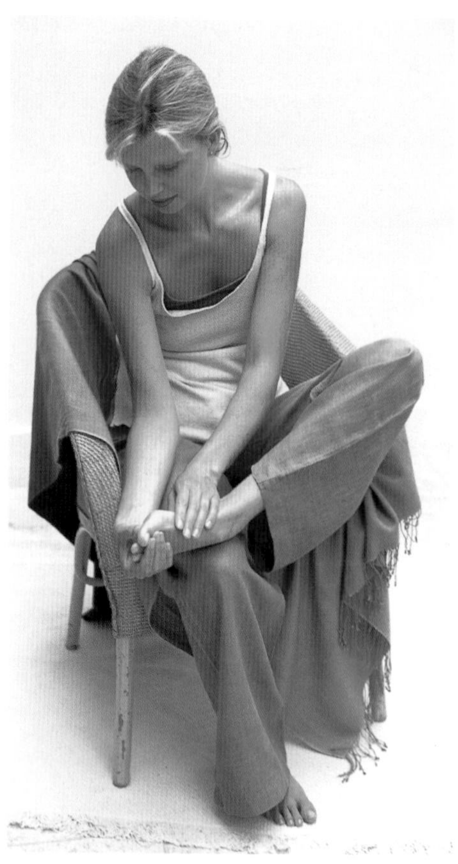

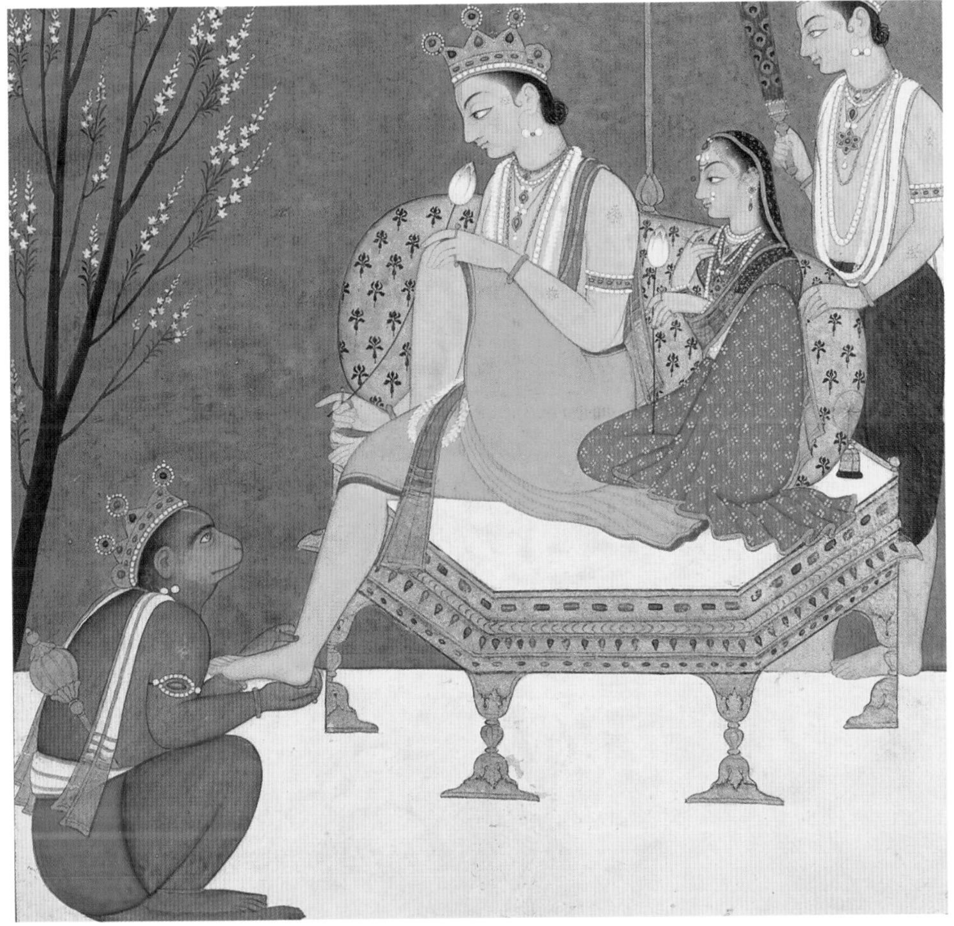

◁ **Depictions of the Hindu god Vishnu often show Sanskrit symbols on his feet. These seem to correspond to the reflex points used in modern-day reflexology.**

origins of foot massage

Throughout history, the feet have had symbolic importance. In ancient Egypt, they represented grounding to the earth's energies, while Greek legend teaches that the feet symbolize the soul.

Healers from many cultures have seen the feet as key to good health. In Japanese mythology, a great healer named Outo is said to have responded to a question about his therapeutic powers by saying: "See to the feet, my friend, and you will have seen to the body". The Chinese have been practising foot massage since 3000BC, and wall paintings discovered in Egypt show that a type of foot therapy was practised there about one thousand years later.

Foot massage has been used by the Native Americans for generations. There is also evidence that some kind of pressure work on the feet was known in middle Europe as far back as the fourteenth century.

approaches to massage

There are two main styles of massage – Eastern and Western. The Eastern techniques tend to be stimulating, and they use direct, focused pressure. Western practices usually incorporate stroking actions as well as kneading and more generalized pressure.

Most traditional systems of Eastern medicine are based on the idea that an invisible life force – known as *chi* in China – gives us health and happiness. Certain points in the body – including many on the feet and legs – act as gateways through which we can access and influence the flow of this energy. When these points are pressed, energy can be directed or increased, and any blockages in its path can be removed. This theory forms the basis of such techniques as acupressure.

In the West, massage techniques are aimed at relaxing the physical body. Massage is seen as an effective way to release tension from the muscles. It also improves the circulation, which helps to eliminate accumulated toxins and to increase the flow of nutrients to all areas of the body. Western massage techniques tend to be soothing and calming, and they incorporate smooth strokes and rhythmic pressure.

Western therapists are now increasingly using and adapting methods and theories from Eastern practices. The Eastern idea of energy flowing through the body, for example, is a key aspect of the Western therapy of reflexology. Many practitioners borrowing from both East and West, as we have done in this book, feel that this equips them better to tailor each treatment to meet the individual needs of the recipient.

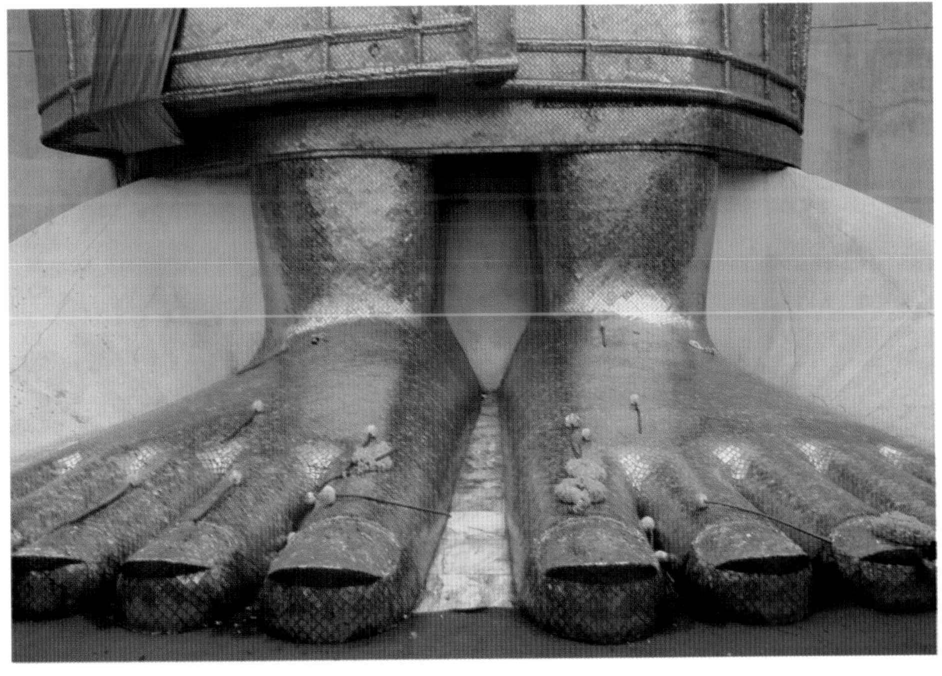

▷ **These feet belong to a giant statue of the Buddha in Bangkok, Thailand. In Buddhism, the feet are thought to symbolize the unity of the Universe, with all its elements represented by special signs on the soles of the feet.**

Ways of treating the feet

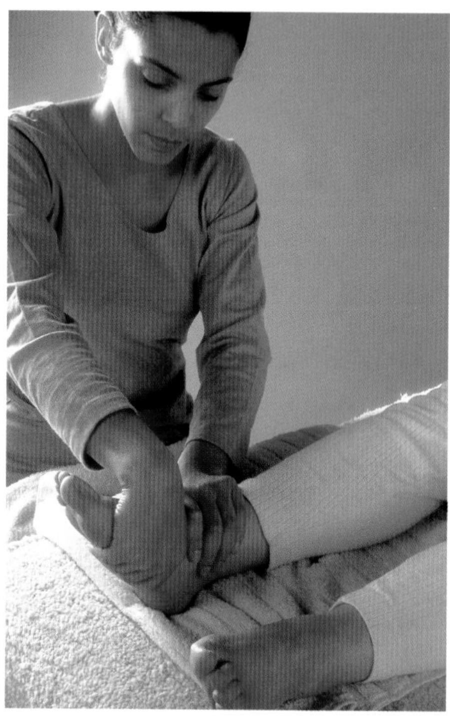

◁ **Foot massage techniques are broadly similar to those used on other areas of the body, with some minor adaptations.**

There are many different ways of working on the feet. It is worth spending the time to learn and assimilate fully the basic techniques of one method before going on to the next. That way, you will become adept at giving treatments.

therapeutic massage

Massage developed from our natural instinct to use touch to relieve pain: for example, we automatically rub an aching area, stroke a painful limb or hold an injured hand. Massage is highly relaxing to receive, making it an effective antidote to stress-related problems. For this reason, it has become very popular in recent years.

There are more than three thousand massage movements in common use, but you do not need to know more than three or four of them in order to give an effective foot treatment. The basic techniques are very easy to learn, and can be used at home to promote general well-being.

▷ **Essential oils can be added to foot creams for a healing and nourishing treat. Rose cream, for example, makes a superb moisturizer.**

Most massage practised in the West is Swedish massage. This was developed in the late 18th century by the Swedish gymnast, Per Henrik Ling. The therapy aims to bring about therapeutic results by manipulating the body's soft tissues: the muscles, skin, tendons and ligaments. A Swedish massage therapist will usually treat the whole body, but a treatment focusing on the feet and legs is also highly effective.

A variety of techniques are used, including stroking, kneading and fast rhythmic movements. These are delivered in a continuous flowing sequence. Oil is usually smoothed into the skin before and during the massage, to prevent pulling.

aromatherapy massage

In aromatherapy massage, oils extracted from plants are diluted in a carrier oil or cream, and then worked into the skin using Swedish massage techniques. The oils have delightful fragrances, which heighten the pleasure of the massage. They also have healing properties. Different oils can be used

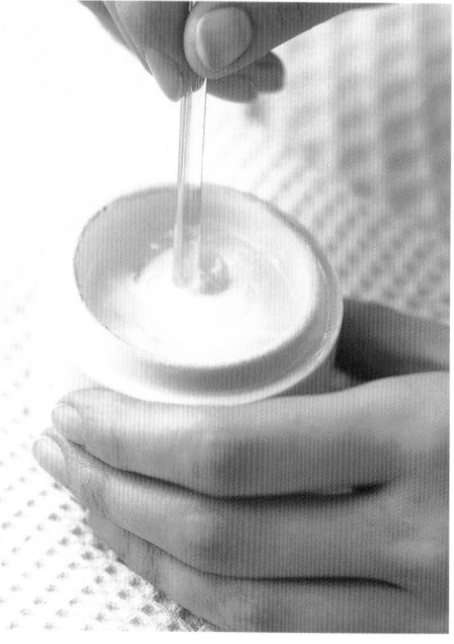

the birth of aromatherapy

Essential oils were originally used in cosmetics. In the early 20th century, a French chemist called Rene Maurice Gattefosse discovered by accident that the oils also had healing properties. While working in his laboratory he burned his hand. To ease the pain he plunged his hand into a bowl of cool lavender oil. He was impressed by the effect that it had in relieving pain, reducing redness and speeding up the skin's healing process. He went on to investigate the therapeutic properties of the oils, coining the term "aromatherapy" in 1928.

The use of essential oils combined with massage was developed by Margurite Maury, who worked with Gattefosse. She brought the idea of the everyday use of essential oils, to enhance health and well-being, to the wider world.

▽ **All kinds of plants yield essential oils with a wide range of healing properties. Roses are good for skin complaints.**

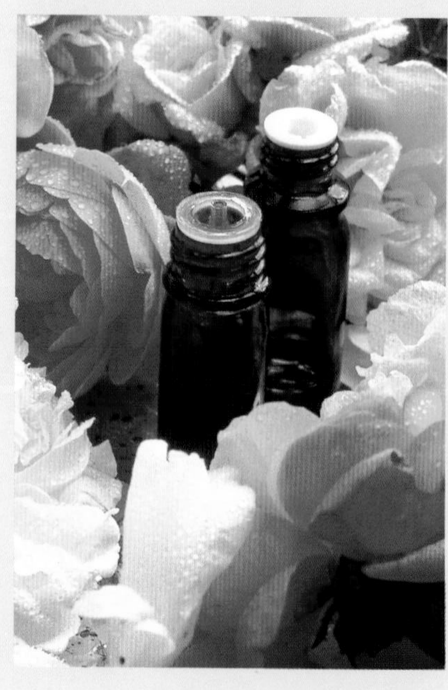

to induce feelings of calm, to boost energy or to treat minor ailments and relieve pain.

Aromatherapy foot massage is a highly enjoyable and easy way of using the therapy for self-help. You can also add the oils to baths and foot baths, incorporate them into nourishing creams for the feet and legs, or add them to compresses to help soothe away troublesome aches and pains. This book includes many suggestions for using essential oils, as well as recipes for luxurious or therapeutic aromatherapy home treatments.

reflexology

The therapy known as reflexology is a form of natural healing that focuses on the feet. It is based on the belief that there are specific reflex points on the feet which correspond to all the organs, systems and structures of the body. In reflexology, the points are stimulated by means of gentle finger-pressure. This helps to promote self-healing and good health in all kinds of ways.

Reflexology is a holistic therapy: it works on the whole person – the mind, body and spirit – rather than focusing on a specific condition or on a set of symptoms. Although reflexologists can detect specific problems, their main aim is to bring the whole body back to a natural state of balance and well-being. Over time, this can help to eliminate problems caused by specific disease.

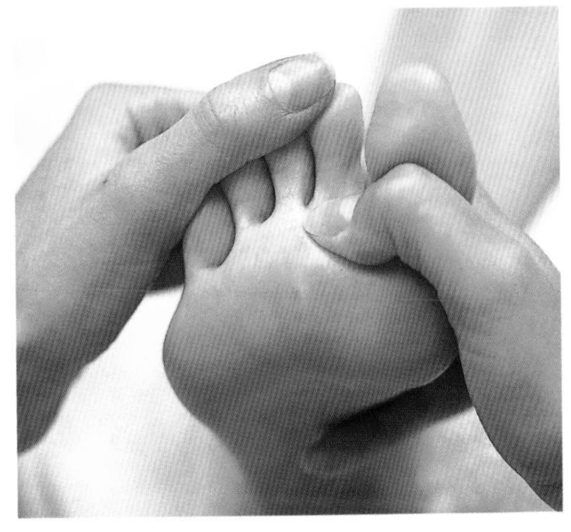

◁ **In both reflexology and acupressure, specific points on the foot are said to correspond to other parts of the body. Pressing these points stimulates healing, and can be used to treat anything from a sore throat to digestive problems and backache.**

acupressure

Like reflexology, acupressure is used to stimulate the body's own natural self-curative powers. Acupressure is similar to acupuncture in that they both use key energy points on the body – including many on the feet and legs – in order to bring about healing. However, while acupuncturists use special needles to stimulate the energy points, acupressure involves the use of finger or thumb pressure to work the points. Sometimes, the heels of the feet can be used for stimulation instead, or as well as, the fingers.

Acupressure can help to reduce tension, increase the circulation, and encourage the body and mind to relax. It helps to strengthen our resistance to disease, by relieving built-up stress and tension. One great advantage of the therapy is that it can be used as a quick fix, which can be done anywhere and at any time.

lymphatic drainage

One of gentlest forms of massage, lymphatic drainage massage works on the lymph system. Since lymph vessels are close to the surface, there is no need for heavy pressure. The body's lymphatic system is a secondary circulation system that supports the work of the blood circulation. The lymphatic system has no heart to help pump the fluid around the vessels, and therefore it must rely on the activity of the muscles to aid movement.

Lymphatic massage involves using sweeping, squeezing movements along the skin. The action is always directed towards the nearest lymph node: the main nodes used when treating the foot are located in the hollow behind the knee. Lymphatic drainage massage is hugely beneficial in helping to eliminate waste and strengthen the body's immune system.

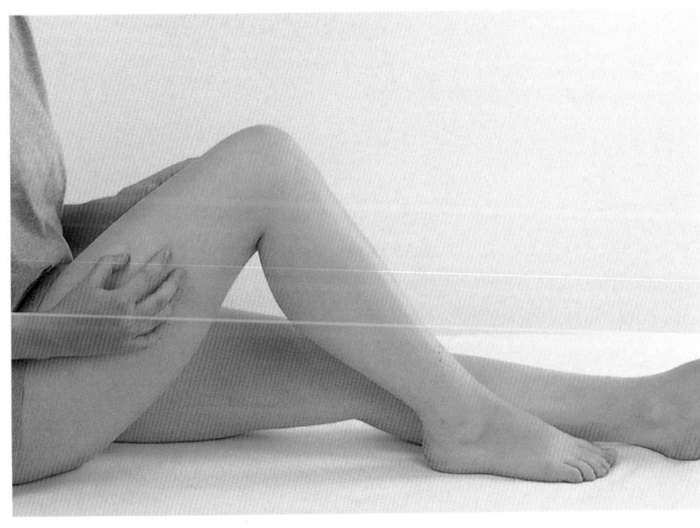

△ **1** To improve lymphatic drainage to the feet and legs, try a daily skin "brush", using your fingertips. Begin by working on the thigh. This clears the lymphatic channels ready to receive the lymph flood from the lower legs. Briskly brush all over the thigh from knee to top, three or four times.

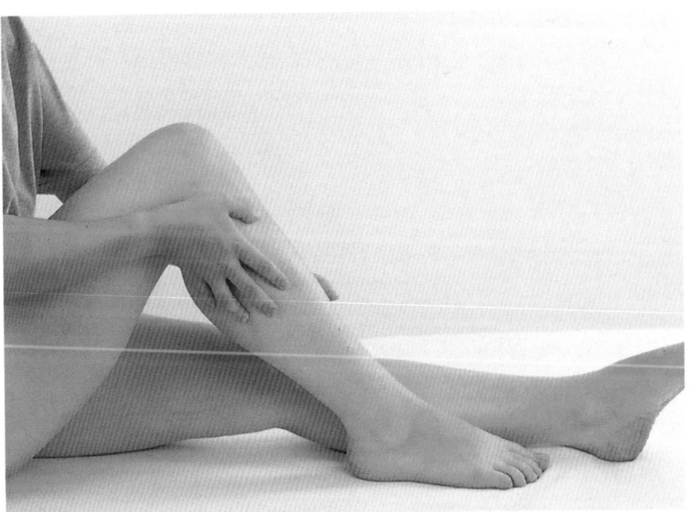

△ **2** Work on the lower leg in a similar way. Brush either side of the leg from ankle to knee, then treat the back of the leg. Follow this by brushing along the top of the foot, continuing up the front of the leg to the knee. Brush over each area twice more, making three times in total. Repeat on the other leg.

Caring for our feet

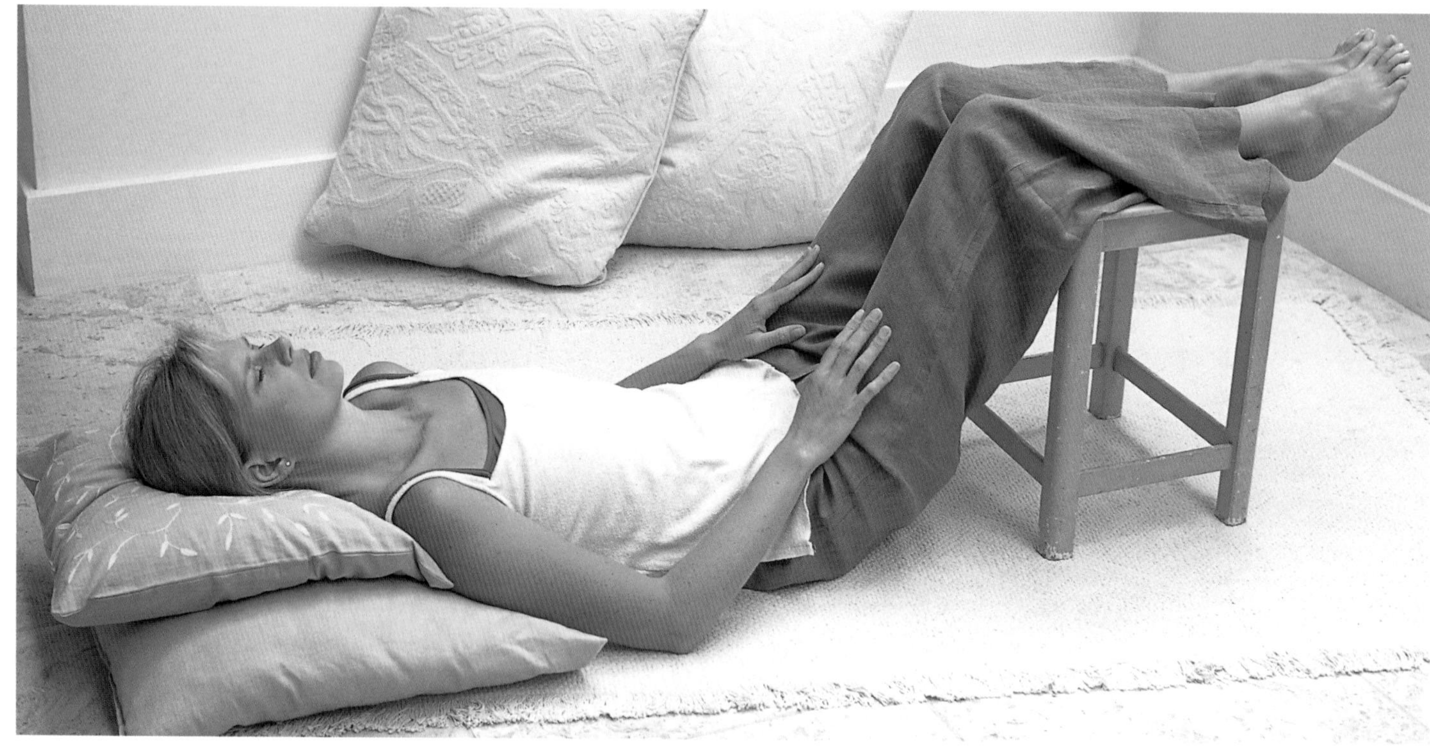

Our feet are an amazing construction. Twenty-six ingeniously shaped bones are bound together with bands of ligaments to form the basic structure of each foot. This structure is very strong – strong enough to bear the weight of our entire body – yet it is also remarkably supple. The foot is capable of making many intricate movements. Its dexterity is made possible through the actions of numerous small joints, as well as the 30 tiny muscles in the foot and by the leg muscles.

There are about 7200 nerve endings in each foot, making it highly sensitive to touch. The nerve supply comes from the sciatic nerve passing from the spinal nerve through the buttock and branching down the back and side of each leg to the foot.

helping the circulation

The foot is richly supplied with blood vessels. However, since it is at the end of the body and does not have its own pump, it depends on muscular activity of the foot and leg to keep a good return flow of blood to the heart. You can help the circulation in your feet by taking regular exercise – such as a daily walk – and by keeping your feet and toes moving whenever you are sitting down or standing up for long periods.

It is also beneficial to put your feet higher than your heart as often as possible – at least once a day. This will encourage any pooled blood to drain back down the legs. Regular massage will also keep the circulation of blood and lymph functioning well. This helps to remove any toxins from the feet, and also brings nutrients to them.

It is particularly important to put your feet up when you are pregnant, since you are particularly susceptible to varicose veins at this time.

pamper and protect

Our feet take a lot of punishment, and most of us take them for granted. Having a regular foot-care session can help to keep your feet healthy and prevent any problems

▷ **Pamper your feet on a regular basis; they take a great deal of punishment and richly deserve as much time and attention as you can manage.**

△ **Take time every so often to rest your feet above heart level. This helps to relax the muscles here and can be very soothing. It also lets blood drain away, which can help to prevent varicose veins and swollen ankles. Keeping fresh blood circulating will also help to nourish the skin.**

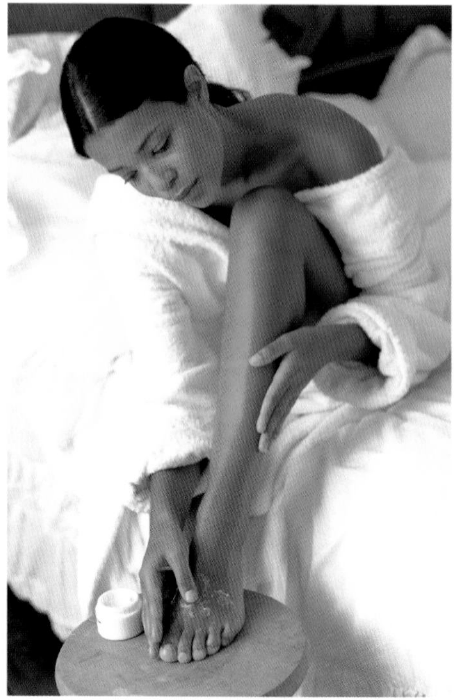

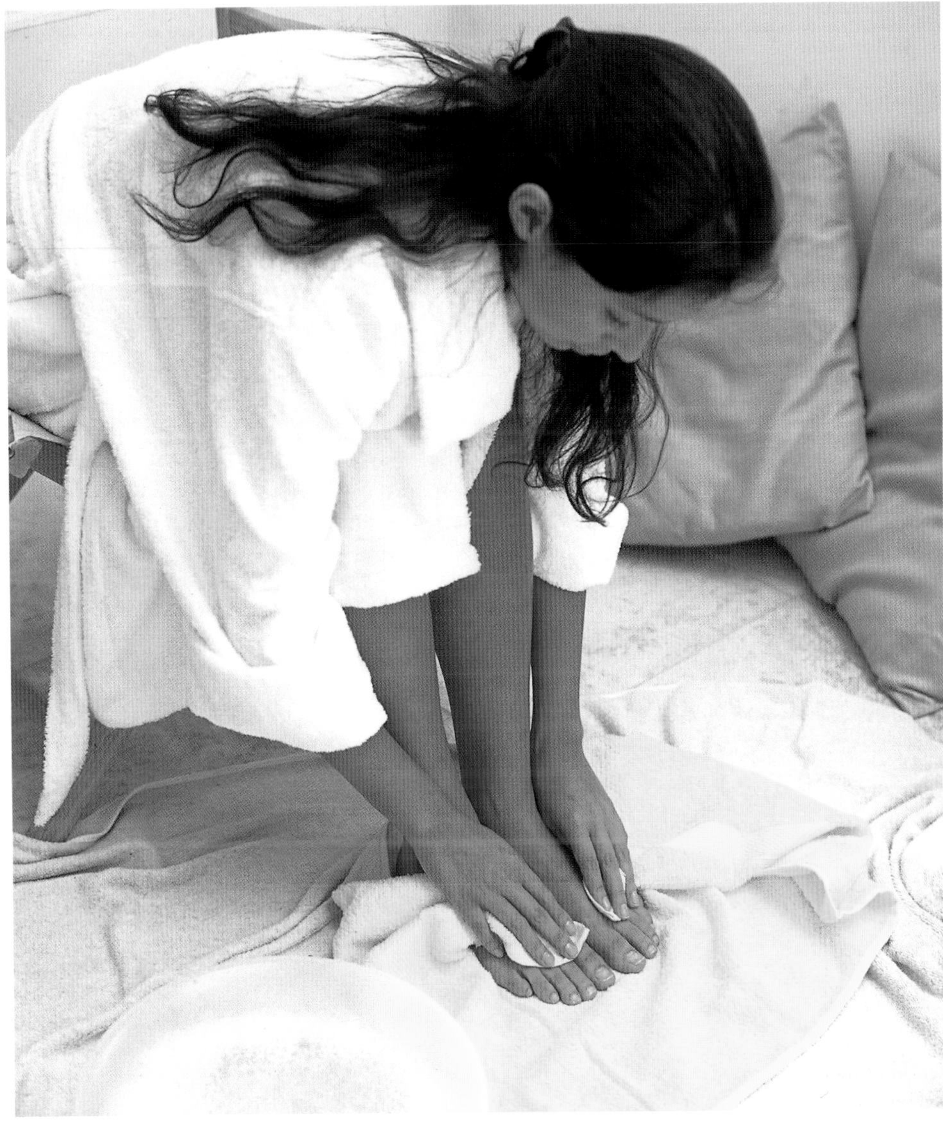

△ **Drying your feet thoroughly is an important part of good foot care and foot health. Special attention should be paid to drying the areas between the toes – allowing moisture to build up here can lead to problems such as athlete's foot.**

from arising. For a simple pamper, try soaking the feet for ten or fifteen minutes in warm water. Remove any hard skin with a pumice stone, then cut your toe nails. Always cut straight across rather than trying to shape the nail. This will help to prevent ingrowing toenails, which can be very painful. Moisturizing your feet daily will help to keep the skin soft and supple.

It is a good idea to visit a chiropodist for a professional pedicure at least twice a year. You should also act quickly if you notice flaking skin between the toes (athlete's foot), or a dark mark on the sole (a verucca) to prevent these problems from spreading. Seek medical advice if you develop any unusual symptoms on the feet.

the right shoe

You should avoid wearing high-heeled shoes since these distort the natural shape of the feet. The ideal shoe is not flat, but has a low heel.

Wearing badly fitting shoes puts unnecessary pressure on the feet, and it may lead to aching, blisters or bunions which are unsightly and can be painful. The idea that new shoes should hurt is a myth. Correctly fitting shoes should be comfortable from the first time of wear; they should not need to be "worn in".

Always try to buy new shoes in the afternoon. Our feet tend to swell slightly as the day progresses, and whenever they become hot. Shoes that you buy in the morning may feel tighter later in the day, and may restrict the blood and lymph flow to our feet and legs.

It is quite common for one foot to be slightly larger than the other. It is therefore important to try both shoes of the pair before making a purchase. Always buy the size that fits your larger foot, and buy foot pads or insoles, if necessary, to create a more comfortable fit for the smaller foot.

foot health

Do not massage anyone's feet if they have athlete's foot (tinea pedis) or a verucca, since they are both contagious. For self-massage of these problem areas, add 3 drops of essential oil of thyme to 5ml of carrier oil. Vitamin E oil is particularly good for these ailments.

▽ **The healthy foot is one that displays no signs of infection, skin breaks or ingrowing toe nails. Ideally the inner arch will be raised slightly off the ground as this is used as a shock absorber while walking and running.**

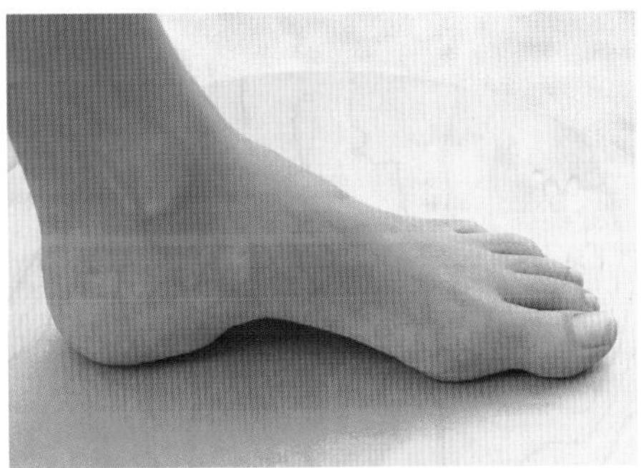

shoe-related allergies

Many chemicals are used in the adhesive, dye, rubber, tannins or metal commonly found in footwear. A small number of people suffer from allergic reactions to their shoes. It would be almost impossible to produce a shoe that is allergen-free because different people are allergic to different substances.

If you experience redness, itching or soreness in the feet, consult a doctor. He or she will be able to refer you to a dermatologist (skin specialist) if an allergy is suspected.

The dermatologist will usually perform a skin test to identify the substance or substances causing the allergy. You can then seek out footwear that is free of this particular chemical. If staff at the store cannot help, it is usually possible to check this information with the manufacturer.

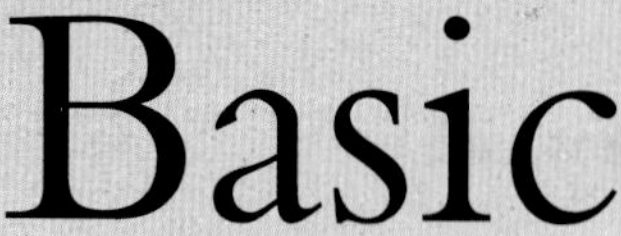

Basic Techniques

Anyone can learn to give pleasurable foot treatments to themselves and others. This chapter covers the basic techniques of massage, aromatherapy and reflexology, and offers some classic types of routine. There is also advice on how to prepare for a treatment – from warming up the hands to creating a healing atmosphere at home.

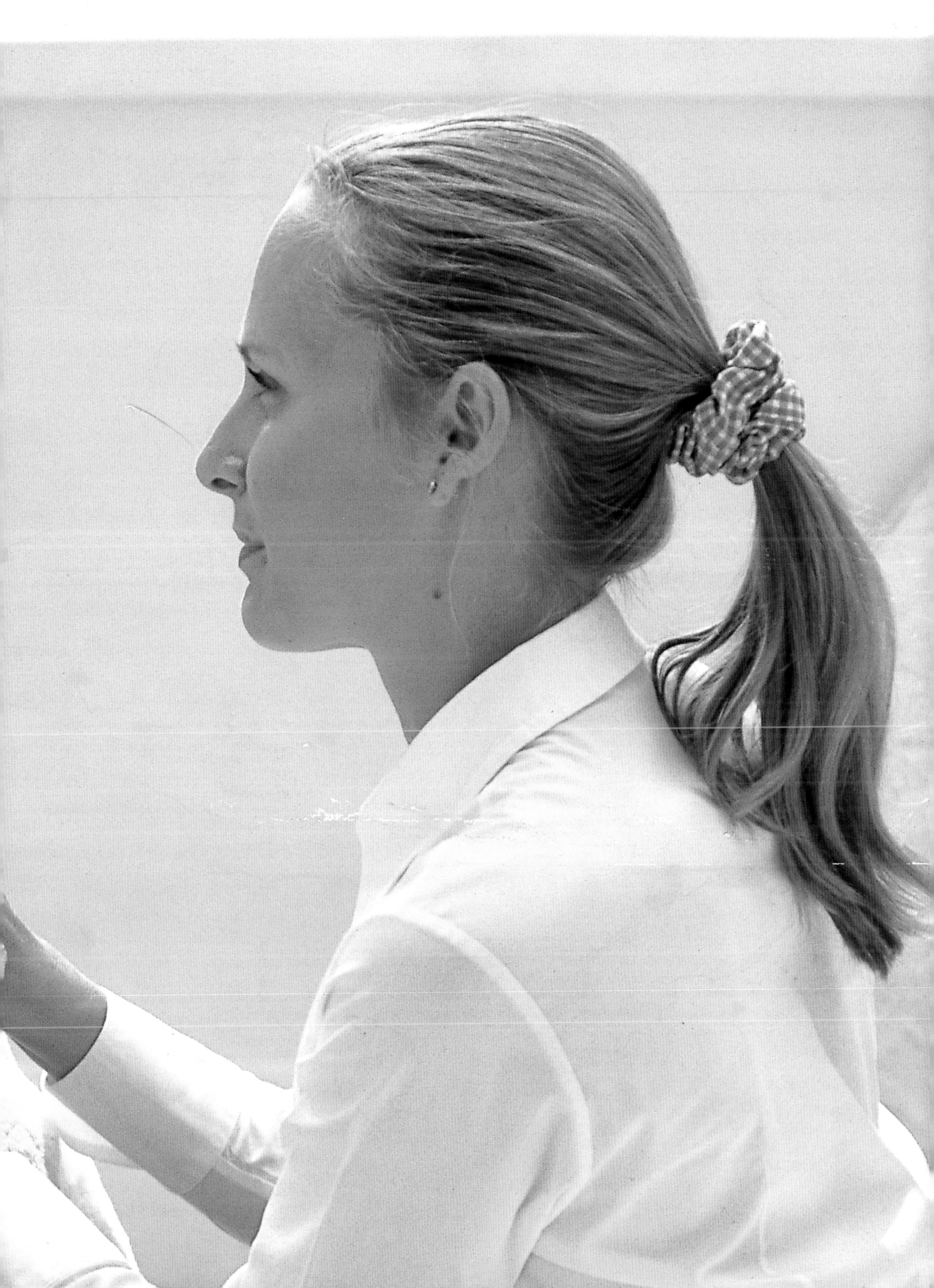

Setting the scene

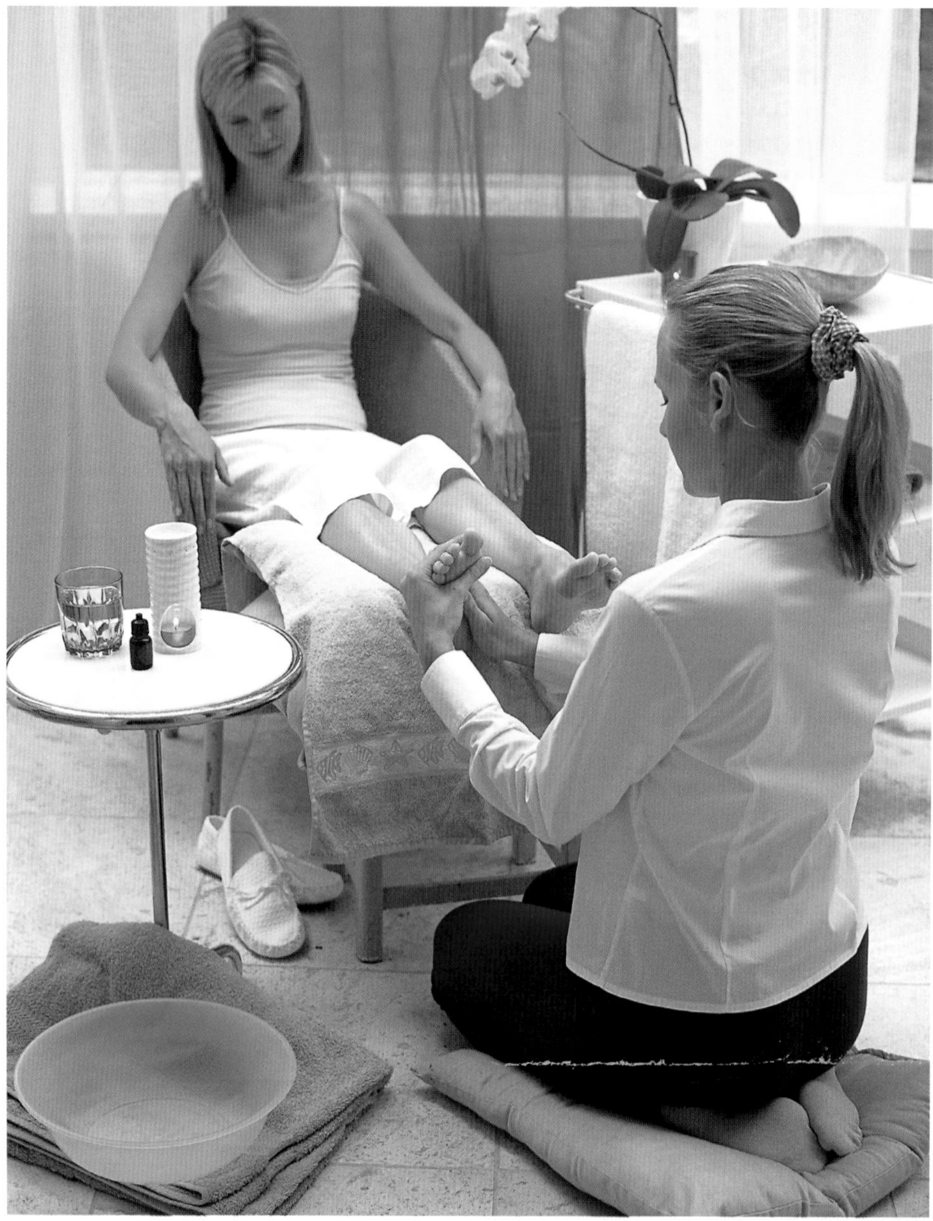

> **fragrant room spray**
> Try this sweet-smelling spray.
>
> **ingredients**
> - 5ml/1 tsp vodka
> - 20ml/4 tsp rosewater
> - 3 drops of your favourite oil
>
> Blend the ingredients in a 30ml (1fl oz) bottle. Shake well, then spray into the air. Don't spray on to furniture or fabrics.

◁ Keep your massage space clean and attractive. Using matching towels will help to create a luxurious and professional atmosphere. Be sure to get everything ready before you start massaging, so that you do not have to stop halfway through the treatment.

Always try to create a relaxing atmosphere in the room where you are treating, whether it is yours or someone else's. Ideally, the area should be warm, inviting and quiet. A few simple preparations will help to give any room a suitably supportive atmosphere for relaxing massage or reflexology work.

First of all, make sure that you are somewhere private, and that you won't be disturbed during the treatment or immediately afterwards. Turn off any phones, including mobiles, close the door and shut the windows if there is noise outside. Ignore the doorbell if it rings while you are treating, or make a previous arrangement with another family member to deal with any callers. Make sure that nobody else will come into the room while you are treating; interruptions will break your concentration as well as the relaxing flow of the massage.

clear away clutter

Tidy and clean the room, and clear away any clutter. You want as few distractions as possible when you are massaging.

Decide where you are going to massage. The floor is a good option because there is usually plenty of room to move about. It can be hard on your knees, so make sure that you have a few floor cushions to hand. The person you are massaging should sit in a comfortable arm chair with their legs supported on a small table or stool. You want to be able to reach their feet without bending or twisting in any way.

Have any massage oils and equipment that you will be using to hand. You'll want two or more towels; at least one to place under the foot being worked and another to keep the resting foot warm.

Sitting or lying down for any length of time can cause some loss of body heat, so make sure the room is warm. On cool days and evenings, you may like to offer the person a light blanket to keep him or her feeling warm and secure.

creating atmosphere

Where possible, have soft lighting. Turn off bright lights that are positioned directly overhead or in direct line with eye contact – either yours or the person you are treating. A couple of lamps will usually give

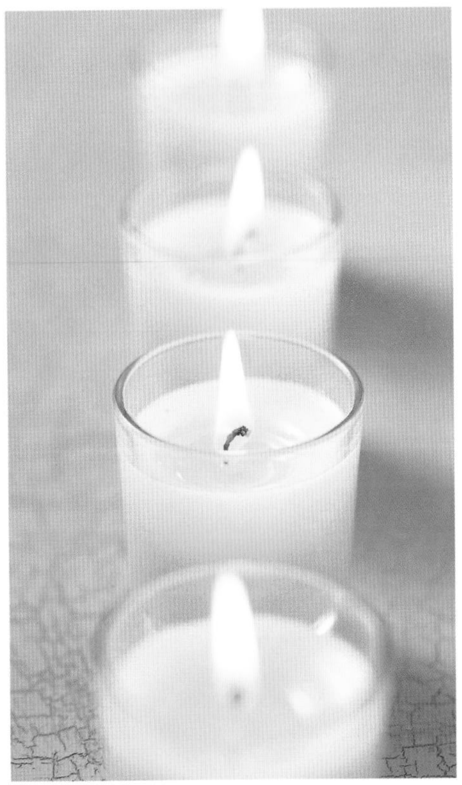

△ **A few candles will help to create soft relaxing lighting in the room. Scented candles will often help to lift the mood, too.**

enough light, and you may also like to light a few candles in the room. A flickering candle helps to create an atmosphere of calm and coziness.

Flowers always look attractive. If you have dried or fake flowers, try adding a drop of essential oil to three or four cotton buds and place them in the arrangement. Rose, jasmine, neroli, violet and ylang-ylang are good oils to try: they give appealing, slightly heady, floral aromas.

Other ways to introduce pleasant smells into the area are by using scented candles or by burning an essential oil in a vaporizer. You could also use an essential oil room spray half an hour before treatment. However, don't use a strong scent, since some people may find it off-putting.

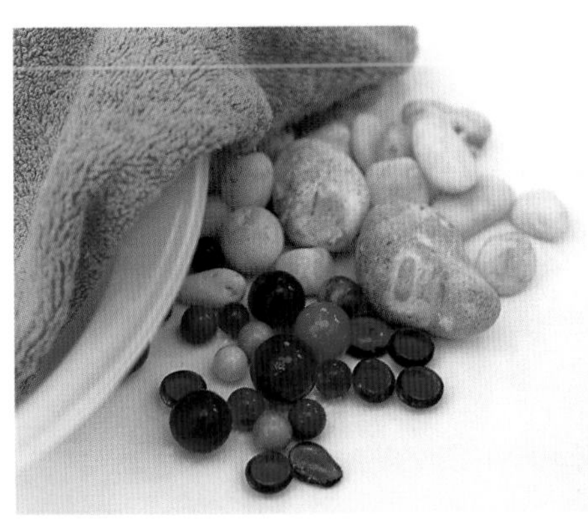

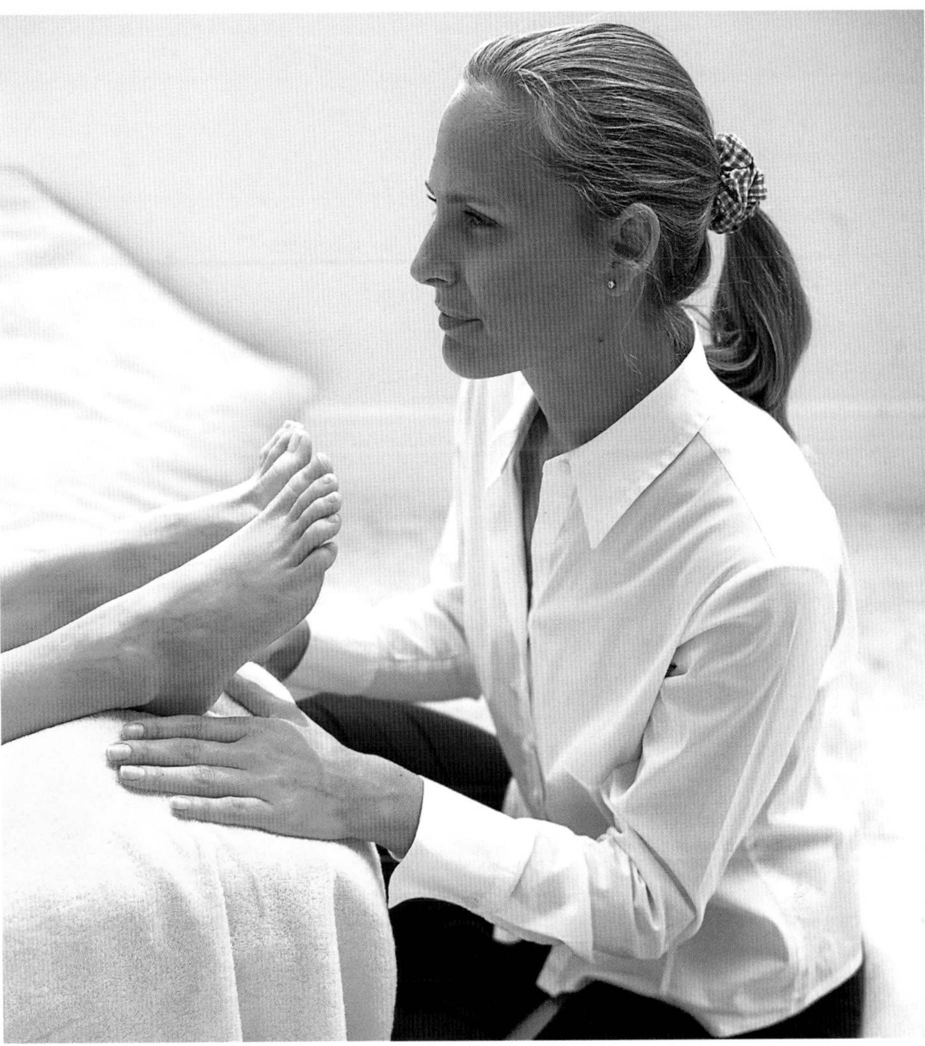

△ **Always make sure that you can reach the person's feet easily. You should be able to keep your back straight as you work.**

Most people like music, but tastes vary considerably. Choose soft instrumental music that is relaxing to mind and body, and keep the volume low so that it is not intrusive. Always ask the person if he or she would prefer to be treated in silence.

preparing yourself

Once the room is ready, prepare yourself. Wash your hands and check your nails. They should be well trimmed so that there is no danger of them catching the recipient's skin as you work.

Spend a few moments centring yourself before you start the massage. Sit comfortably with both feet flat on the floor. Relax your shoulders and face, then breathe slowly and deeply for a few moments. Warm up by rubbing your hands briskly together, or by practising the preparation exercises on the following pages.

◁ **Suggest that the receiver has a footbath before you treat them, particularly if he or she has come at the end of the day. Place a layer of marbles or pebbles in the footbowl. The receiver can roll their feet backwards and forwards over them for a relaxing mini-massage.**

When all is ready and you are about to start, see if you can feel the healing energy of your hands. Bring the hands together in a prayer-like position, but pull them apart just before they touch. You may feel a slightly pulling or tingling sensation as you do so – this is the energy of your hands. It is good to do this two or three times before starting the massage.

post-massage

After the massage or treatment, let the person relax for a few minutes. You may decide to leave the room for this, or simply to sit quietly beside him or her.

Drink a glass of water, and offer one to the receiver as well. Suggest that he or she spends the next hour or two quietly, in order to appreciate fully the relaxing effects of the foot treatment.

How to warm up

Practising massage should be a pleasure, not a chore. However, it is easy to become tired when you first start. The most important things to remember are your posture and your breathing; most people concentrate so hard that they tense up and forget to breathe normally. Practising deep breathing and doing a few warm-up exercises before you start will help. Then, keep checking your posture and your breathing at regular intervals during the massage.

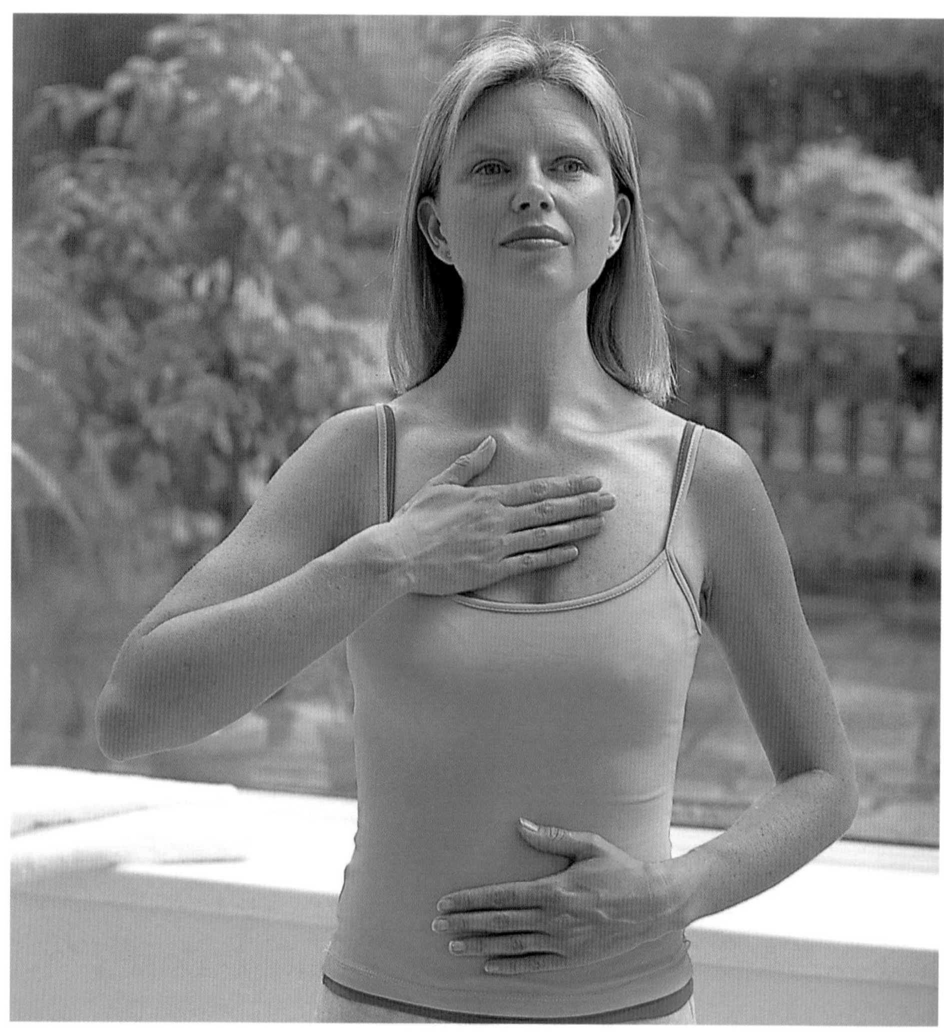

▷ **Try this deep-breathing exercise. Place one hand on your chest and the other on your abdomen. Breathe in for a count of three, feeling your abdomen expand. Breathe out to a count of four, and feel your abdomen relax.**

limbering up

These simple warm-up exercises enhance the flexibility of the arms, wrists and hands. They also encourage deep breathing, which will help you to massage in a comfortable way. You can do the exercises standing up, as shown here, or sitting down. Make sure that your posture is relaxed while you do them. They can all be practised individually as well as in a sequence.

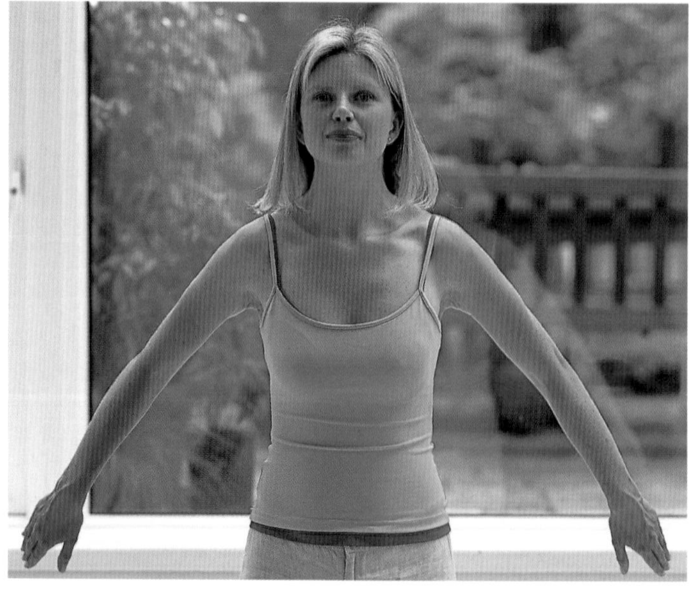

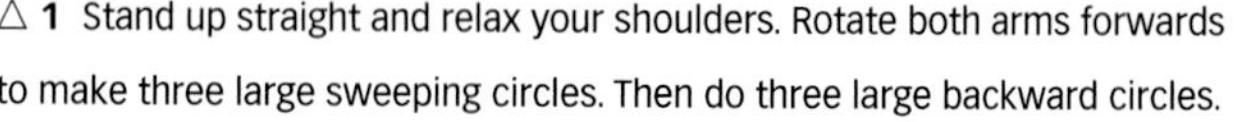

△ **1** Stand up straight and relax your shoulders. Rotate both arms forwards to make three large sweeping circles. Then do three large backward circles.

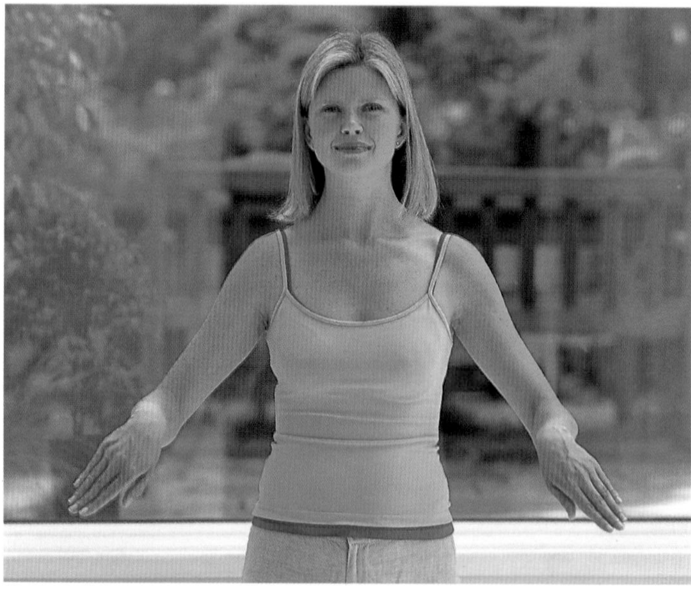

△ **2** Stretch both arms out from your sides, keeping your shoulders relaxed, Rotate your wrists five times in a clockwise motion, then five times anticlockwise.

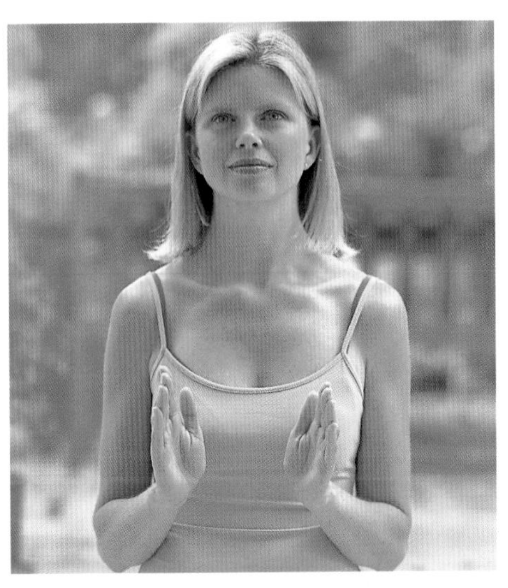

△ **3** Bring the hands up, palms facing. Move them up and down from the wrist to make a chopping motion.

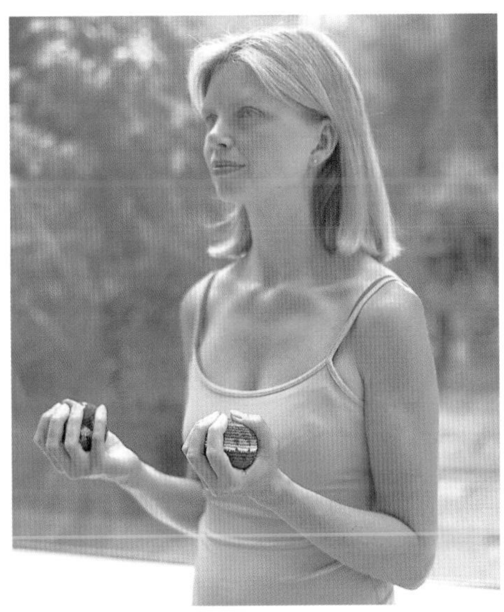

△ **4** Take a flexible ball in each hand. Gently squeeze each ball, then relax your hands. Repeat a few times.

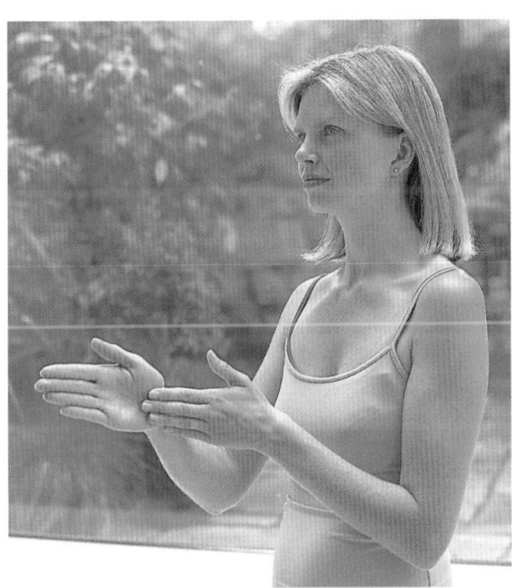

△ **5** Place the fingertips of one hand on the heel of the other. Brush forwards firmly. Do on the other side.

hand massage

You use a full range of hand movements when you massage. Giving your hands a quick self-treatment before you start will relax any tension here, helping you to massage effectively. It is also a good way of focusing your attention so you feel ready to treat. Do the left hand first, then the right.

▷ **1** Hold your right hand over the left one. Slide the right palm gently over the left palm in a circular motion – as though you are washing your hands.

▽ **2** Interlock your fingers, pushing them as close together as you can. Then pull them apart, maintaining firm pressure. Repeat three times.

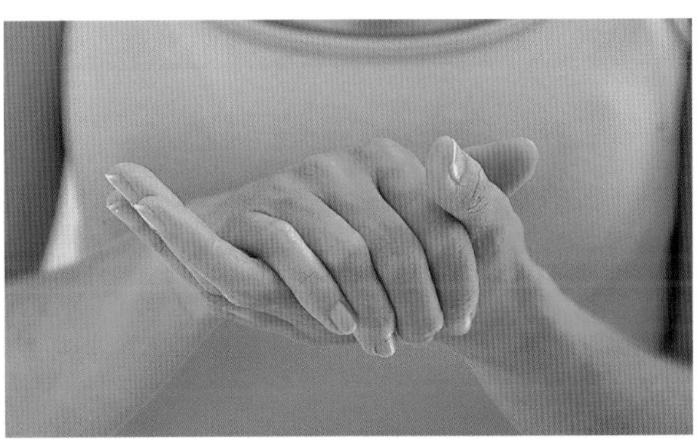

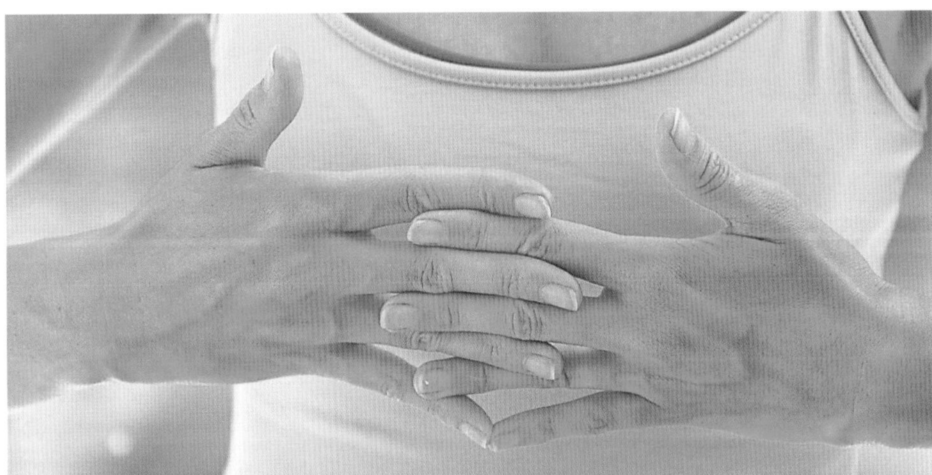

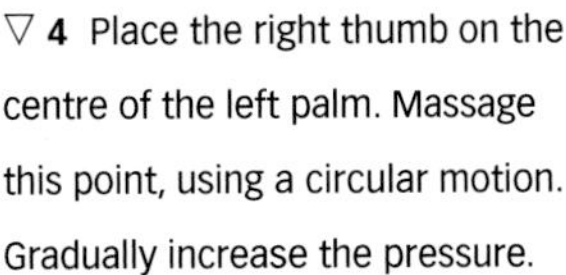

▷ **3** Stroke the fingertips of your right hand down the fingers and palm of the left. Pause, then repeat the movement using a slightly deeper pressure.

▽ **4** Place the right thumb on the centre of the left palm. Massage this point, using a circular motion. Gradually increase the pressure.

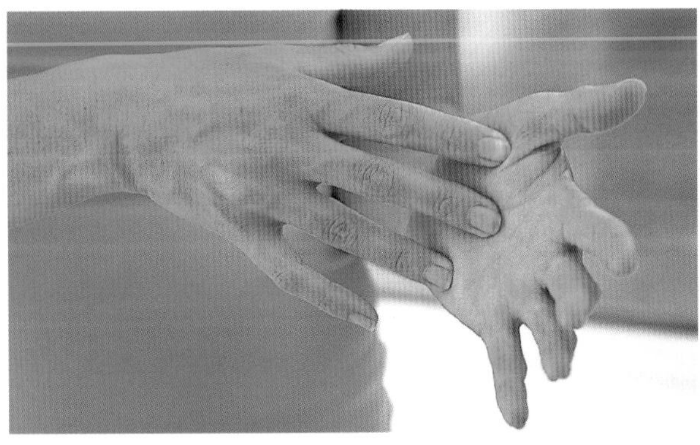

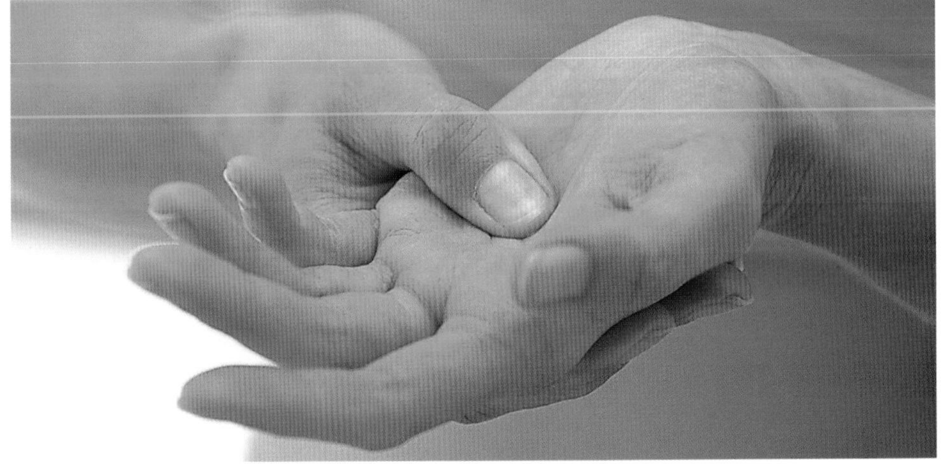

Massage techniques

You can give an excellent massage using just a few simple actions. Each movement can be performed twice or more, and your favourite few movements could be done three, even four times.

When you are learning new massage techniques, it is a good idea to try them out on yourself first. Practise until you become familiar with the different actions involved, and see how the movement feels when you vary the pressure. Always pay full attention to what you are doing. You will find that, if your attention wanders, your touch is unlikely to feel good. Feel your way into your hands and focus on the sensations here.

It is often helpful to massage without talking, except for when you are asking for or giving feedback. It is also much easier to concentrate on exactly what you are doing if you are quiet, and this will also help both you and the recipient to relax.

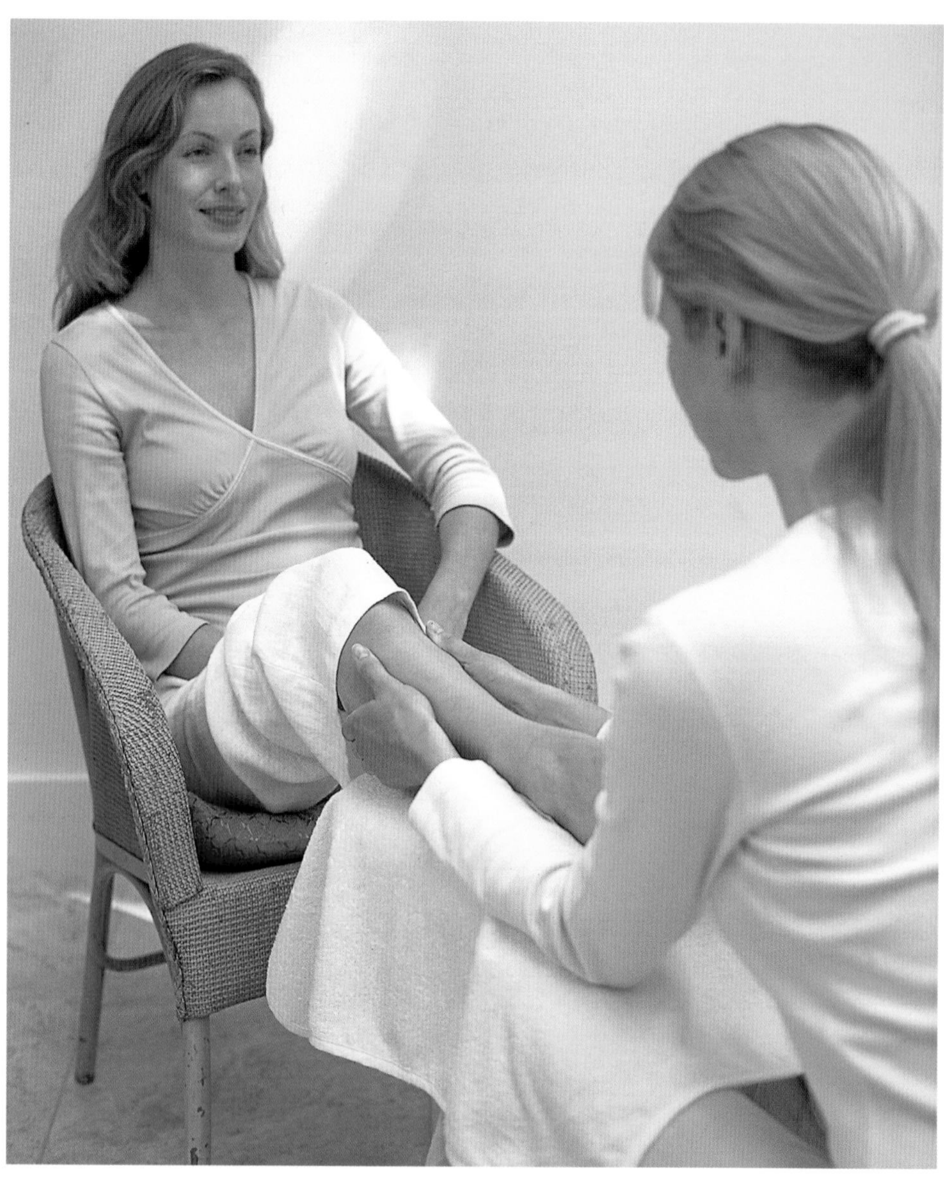

▷ If you are massaging someone else, make sure that he or she is comfortable, and that you are too. You will find it easier to concentrate if you maintain a good posture. Keep your back straight and your head balanced throughout the massage; imagine your head is connected to the ceiling and being pulled upwards. This posture will help you to use your body weight, giving depth to your movements.

getting feedback

People like different pressure. When you work on yourself, you get instant feedback about whether you are working at the correct level of firmness. When you work on other people, you have to monitor their reactions. Ask for feedback, but don't assume that you are getting it right just because the person doesn't tell you otherwise. Be aware of the person's general posture – if he or she is tense, you may be pressing too hard.

Always keep the pressure lighter on the top of the foot. The bones are closer to the surface than those on the sole, so it is easier to cause bruising and pain in this area.

massage aids

There are many aids now available for massage in general, and some can be suitable for use on the feet. Most masseurs say that it is better to use your hands if you are treating another person. However, some gadgets may help with self-treatment.

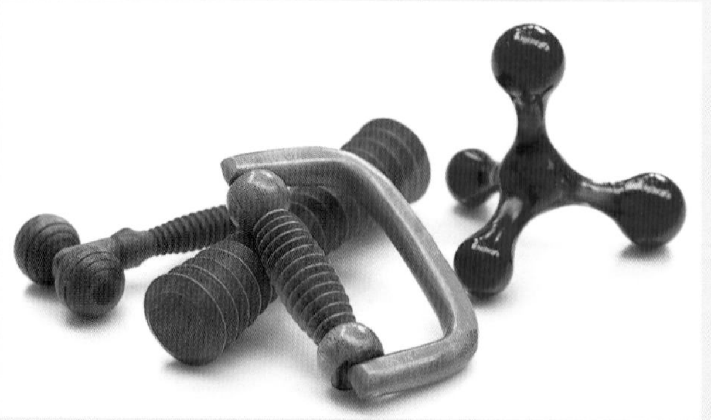

△ You may need to experiment with a few different massage aids to see what suits you best.

basic strokes

Always pay equal attention to both feet when you are massaging. You should start on the right foot, then move on to the left. The right side of the body is said to relate to your physical self; treating this one first will begin to relax muscle tension throughout the body, and will also boost the circulation and elimination processes. Treating the left foot will work on a physical level, too, but it will also help to release built-up tension in the sensitive emotional inner being.

▽ **Thumb circling**

Place the thumbs on the foot, one slightly higher than the other. Then, use the pad of alternate thumbs to massage the area all over, making small rotational movements. This movement is used for fleshy areas. It is good for the circulation and for warming the muscles of smaller areas.

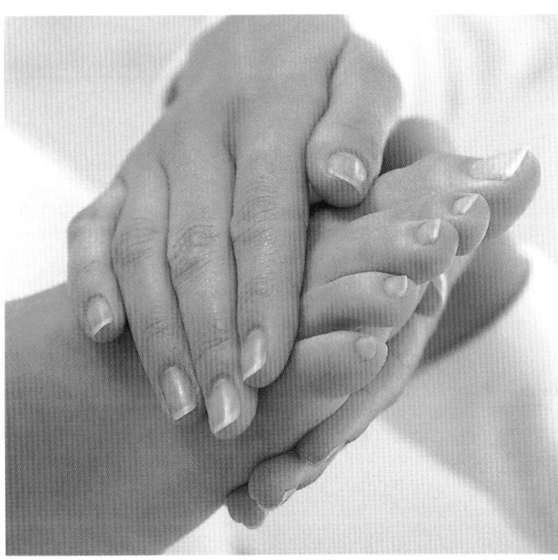

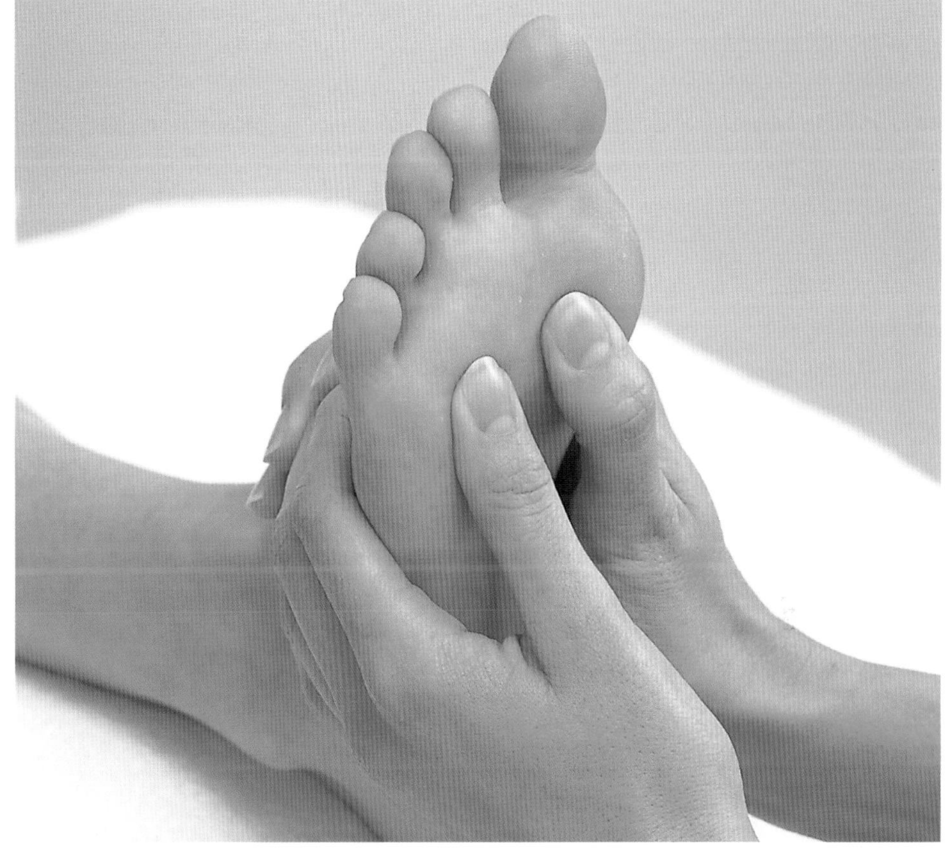

△ **Effleurage (stroking)**

Place your hands across the foot at the base of the toes. One hand should be on top and one below so the foot is sandwiched in-between them (sandwich hold). Slide your hands down the foot from the toes to the heel, then up from the heel to the toes. Repeat this movement twice more, or until the person feels relaxed. Use light pressure to start with, increasing it as you go. You usually start and finish a routine with effleurage, and it is also a good linking technique.

▷ **Knuckling (kneading)**

Make your hand into a fist. Press into the sole of the foot, using the flat part of the fingers from the knuckle to middle joint. Turn the fist as you press, so that you make a slight rotational movement. Cover the whole area from heel to toe. This movement is good for warming up the muscles, opening up the foot and releasing tension.

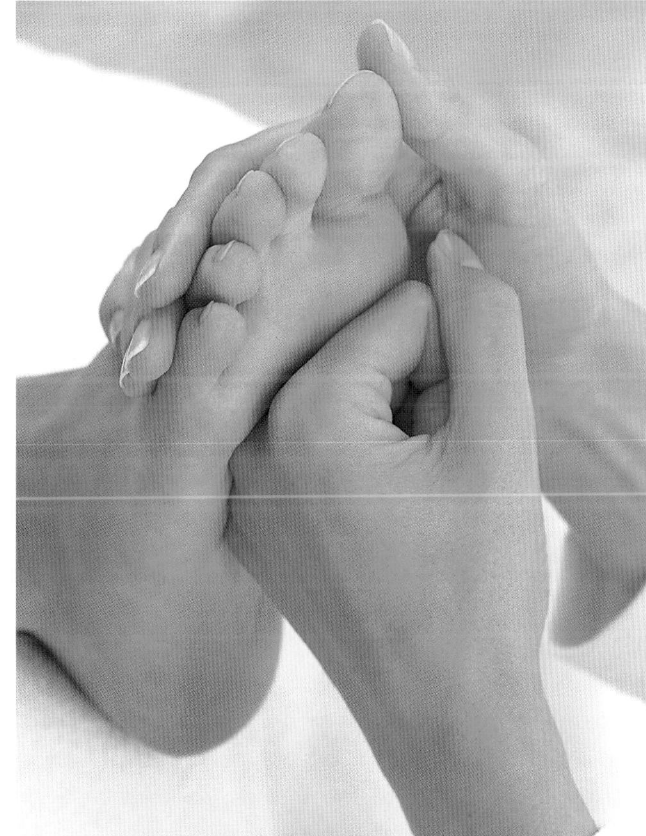

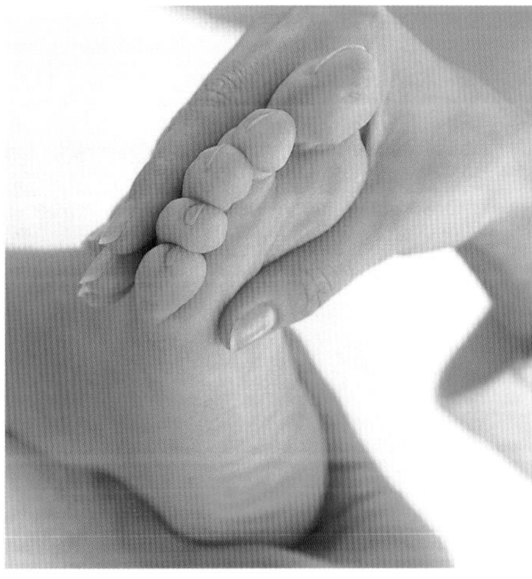

△ **Foot rotation**

Wrap your fingers around the top of the foot near the toes, and use your other hand to cup the heel. Slowly rotate the foot clockwise, then anticlockwise. Repeat, so you have rotated the foot in each direction twice. This movement loosens the ankle joint. It is important that you do not push the ankle further than its limits. Take particular care if treating someone with arthritis, diabetes or a foot disorder.

Spreading

▽ **1** To spread the top of the foot: place the thumbs and the heels of your hands on top of the foot, letting your fingers curl round to hold the sole. Pull the thumbs across the top of the foot towards the edges, keeping your fingers in position. Then return your thumbs to the starting position.

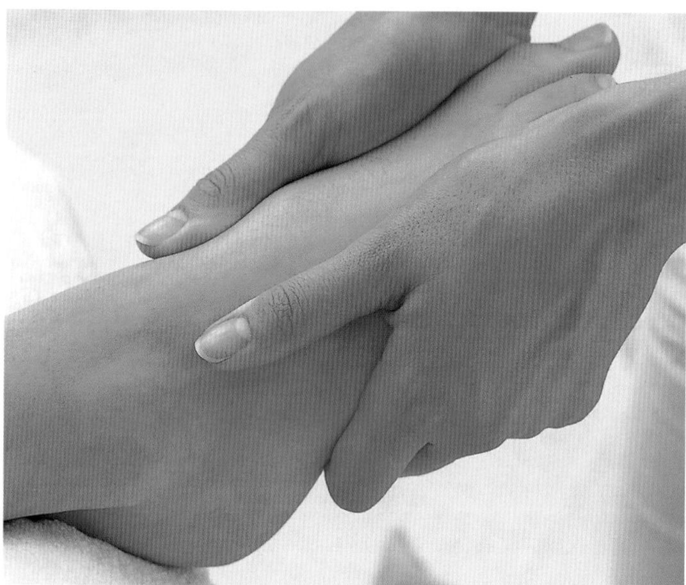

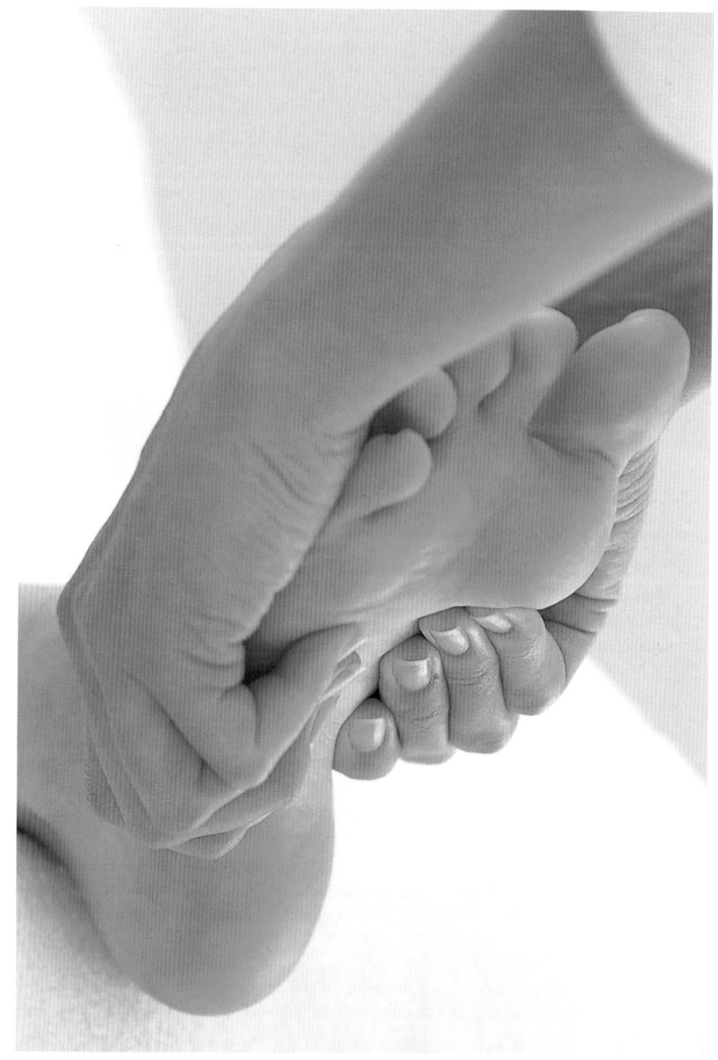

▷ **2** To spread the sole of the foot: keep your hands in the same position as before but reverse the action, so that you pull your fingers to the edges of the sole, leaving the thumbs in position. Start near the toes and work down the foot to the heel. This action works in a similar way to knuckling. It stretches the muscles and brings oxygen and nutrients to the area by improving blood flow.

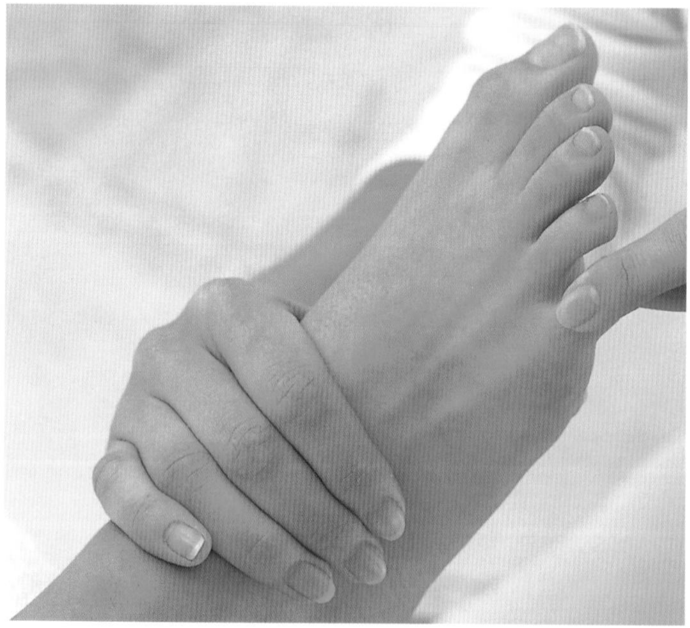

△ **Toe rotation**

Support the foot by placing your fingers across the top of it and curling your thumb underneath. Use your thumb and forefinger to grasp the base of the big toe. Gently rotate the toe in a clockwise direction, then anticlockwise. Work each toe in turn, ending with the little toe. This action helps to mobilize the joints and also improves the supply of nutrients and oxygen to the toes. Work gently, and take extra care if treating someone with arthritis.

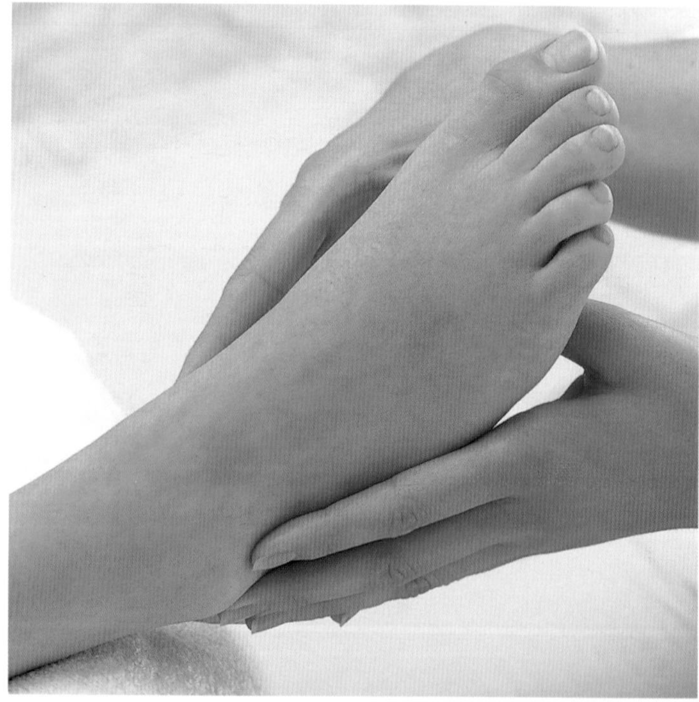

△ **Circling the ankle**

Circle around the inside and outside of the ankle bone at the same time, using the pads of your fingers. You can work quite strongly, provided that the person has no problems in this area. Work in a clockwise direction, then in an anticlockwise one. This movement helps to relax the ankles and improve mobility.

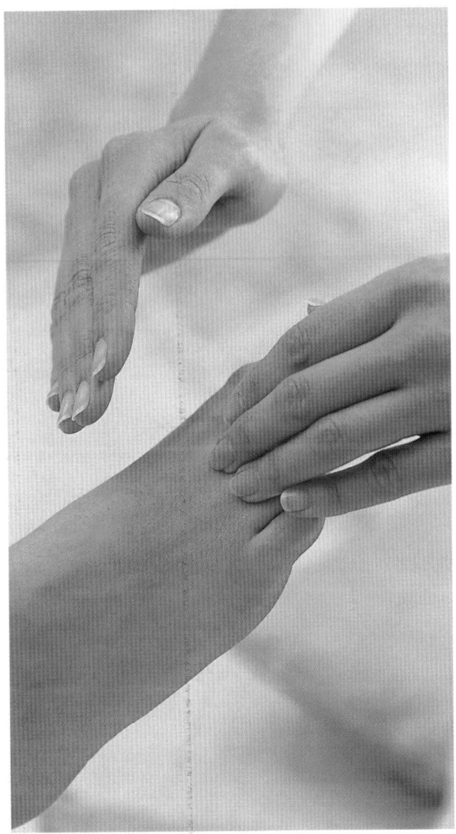

△ **Percussion (tapping)**

1 Use the tips of your fingers to tap all over the top of the foot. Work using alternate fingers. Do not tap too hard: the action should be pleasurable, and not a shock to the system. You can also use this movement on the sole of the foot.

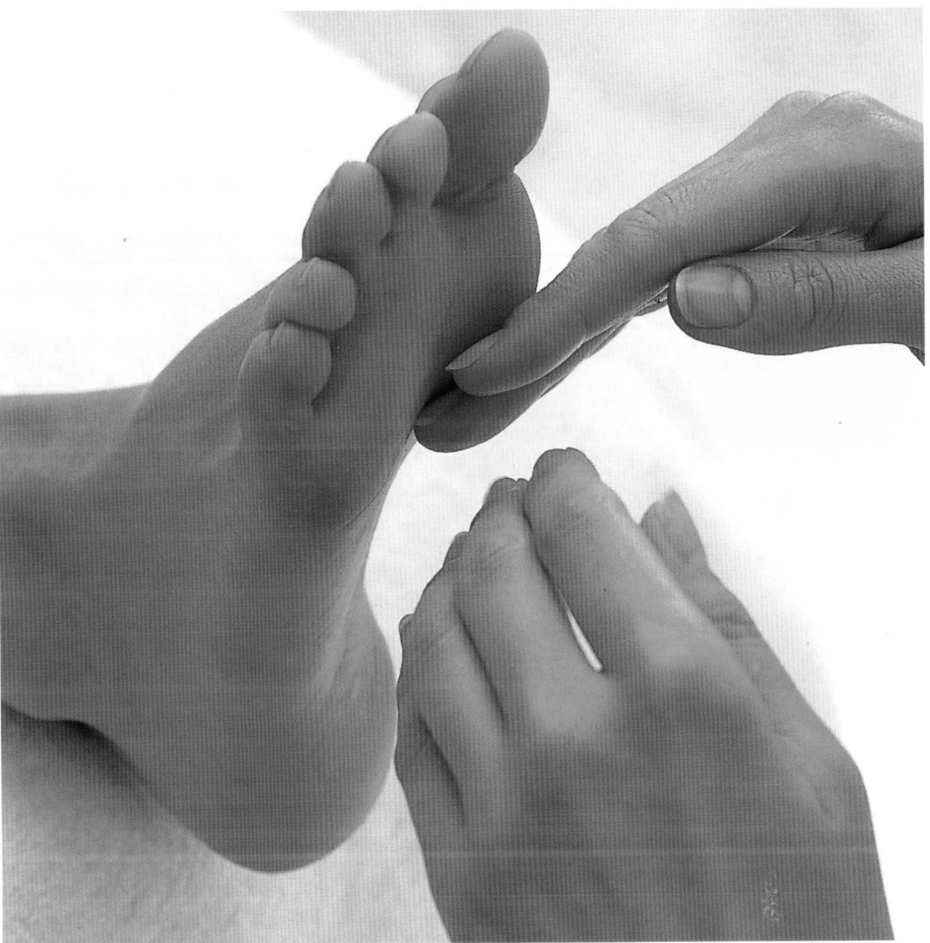

△ **2** To perform percussion on the sole: use the back of the hands to strike the sole lightly all over. This action is stimulating; it helps wake up the foot and increases the circulation. It is a good movement to do if the foot is cold. Be gentle if the person has arthritis, diabetes or a foot disorder.

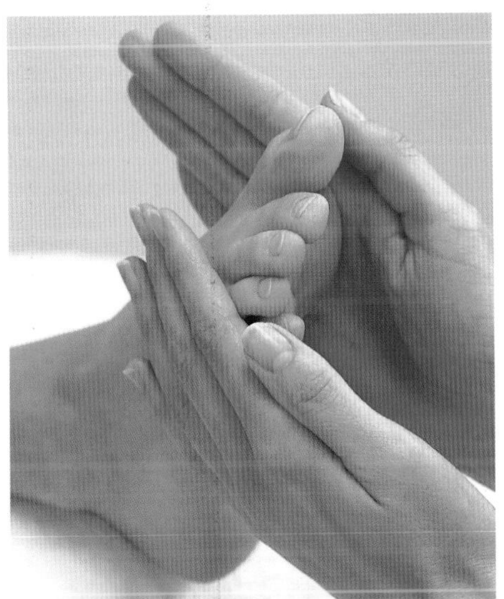

△ **Push-pull**

Place one hand on the outside of the foot and the other on the inside, so that the foot is gently wedged in-between them. Using the heel of the hands, pull one side towards you and push the other side away. Repeat, but this time reverse the action. Do this push-pull action twice more. This is a general movement which helps to open and relax the foot.

baby massage

Foot massage is a wonderful way to soothe and give pleasure to your baby. Always work very gently, massaging one foot at a time. As with adults, do the right foot first, then go on to the left. Try the following routine, or make up your own variation.

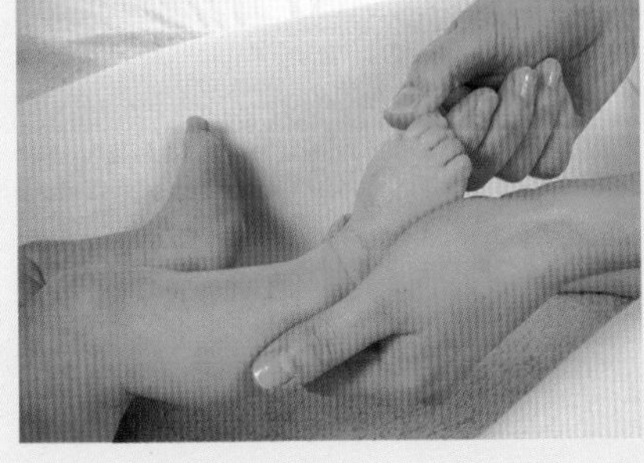

△ **Babies love to be touched – in fact, they cannot thrive without it.**

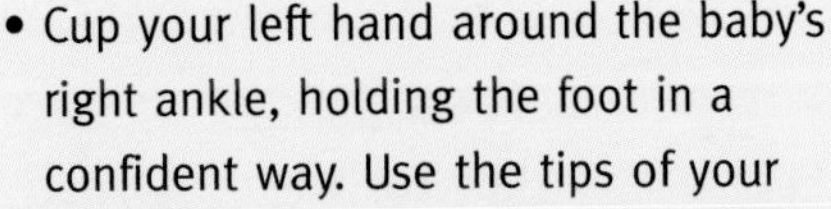

- Cup your left hand around the baby's right ankle, holding the foot in a confident way. Use the tips of your fingers to stroke the sole from heel to toe. Then stroke the top of the foot from toes to ankle. Do as many strokes as are needed to cover the area.
- Use two fingers to stroke the inner side of the foot, working from the big toe to the heel.
- Use two fingers to stroke down the outside edge of the foot in the same way.
- Use your right thumb to stroke across the sole, just below the ball. Start from the big toe side and stroke to the outer edge. Do this three times.
- To finish, gently hold the base of the big toe between your thumb and first finger. Gently stroke down to the tip of the toe. Repeat on the rest of the toes, ending with the little one. Then do the whole routine on the left foot.

Using oils

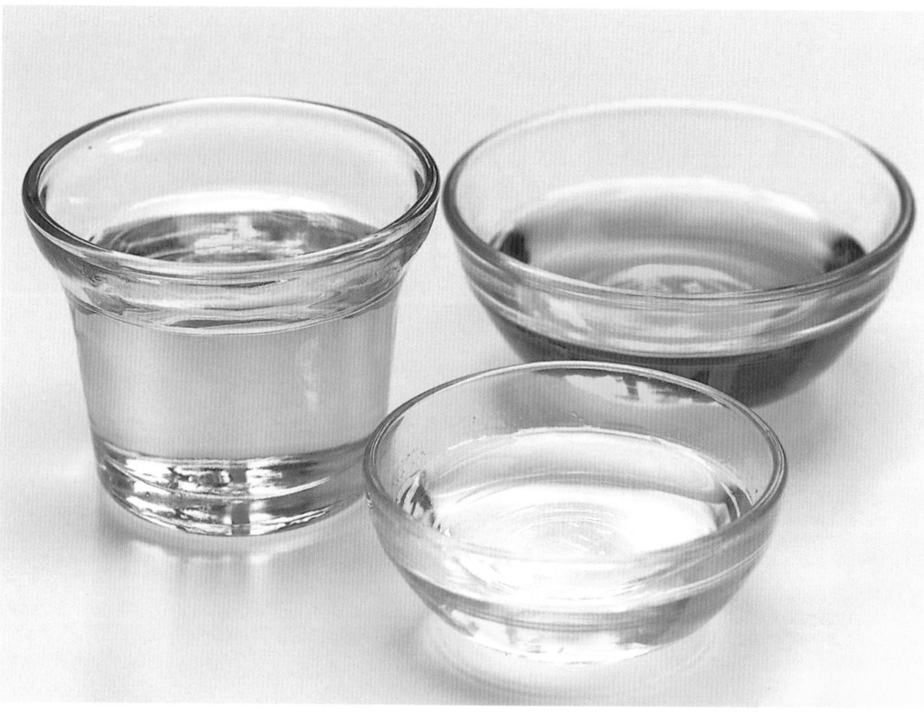

△ **Almond oil (front) is very gentle and is suitable for most skin types, including dry or dehydrated skin. Grapeseed (left) has almost no smell, so it is great for blending with essential oils. Olive oil (back right) is easy to get hold of – most of us have it in our kitchens. However, it has a strong smell that is difficult to disguise.**

Using oils and creams can make massaging much easier. They help to give your hands "slip", so that they glide over the feet rather than dragging and stretching the skin. Oils and creams also bring health benefits: they help keep the skin supple and moisturized, and prevent the build-up of hard skin. They also give you the chance to incorporate healing essential oils into the treatment – a few drops are added to the base cream or oil, then blended in well.

Several different oils can be used for massage. Almond, grapeseed or olive oils all work well, and are widely available. Avocado oil has good moisturizing properties, but is usually combined with almond or grapeseed, which give better slip.

If your skin is dry, dehydrated or mature, it is best to use a massage cream rather than an oil. The creams are heavier, take longer to be absorbed and leave a protective film on the skin, which helps to trap in moisture, preventing further dehydration. Good massage base creams are available from most drugstores and natural health stores, or you can use one of the recipes in this book to make your own.

getting started

Begin by pouring a little oil into the palm of one hand. You need only a drop or two; if you are using cream, just one or two small blobs will be sufficient.

Rub your palms together, then move your hands, one over the other, in a hand-washing motion. This distributes the oil all over the back of your hands, your fingers and cuticles, which has the extra benefit of making them soft and supple.

Add a little more of the massage medium into one palm, then gently bring your palms together, so you evenly cover both hands. The medium should not run all over the area but be just enough to give slip and shine. You are now ready to massage.

While working, observe the skin for changes in texture (from slippery to dry) and a gradual reduction in shine. At this point, add a little massage oil or cream in the same way described above.

If you are using a blend of different oils, it is worth making up enough to last for a few treatments and storing it in a clean, screwtop container. For an average-sized person, you will use about 10ml/2 tsp of oil or cream for each massage involving the feet, and a little more when you are also massaging the lower legs.

patch testing

Always test oils containing essential extracts on a small patch of skin before using. To patch test, add 2 drops of the proposed essential oil to 2 drops carrier oil. Apply to the delicate skin on the inside of your arm or in the crook of your elbow. Massage into the skin and cover with a band aid if necessary to protect clothes. Leave for six hours; if no reaction occurs it is probably (but not certainly) safe to use the oil. Should a reaction occur, apply lots of carrier oil to the area. This will help neutralize the effects. Do not rub.

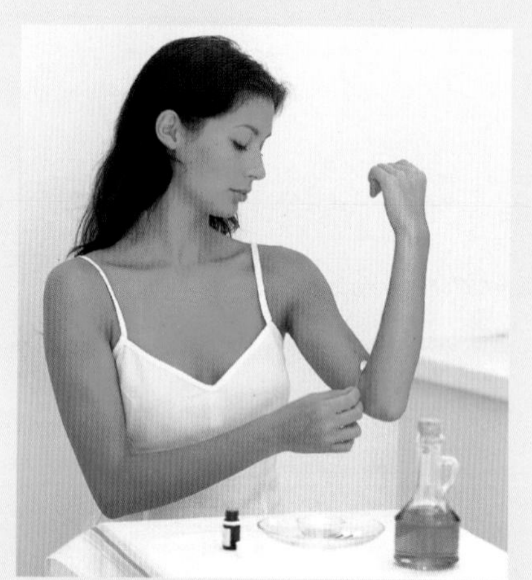

△ **Do a patch test to check for sensitivity before you use any new oil.**

blending oils

Essential oils should be well-diluted in an oil or massage cream (a carrier) before being applied to the skin. Blend one or two drops essential oil to 5ml/1 tsp of carrier oil. Do not be tempted to add more than the suggested amount of oil when following a recipe. If making a larger quantity, keep the ratio of essential oil to carrier constant.

You should use less essential oil (1 drop per 10ml/2 tsp carrier) if:

- your skin is sensitive
- you are allergy prone
- you are on high-dose medication
- you are pregnant
- you are treating a child

If blending in a bottle, shake well to mix. If blending in a dish, stir well using a clean spoon. When adding oil to an aqueous cream, put the essential oil into a spoonful of carrier oil or vodka first, and then blend this mixture with the cream.

Pregnant women and babies

Many essential oils should not be used during pregnancy. Avoid all oils, other than mandarin or tangerine, during the first three months. After that you can use gentle florals – camomile, geranium and lavender – as well as sandalwood. Take similar care when treating babies: always use low dilutions. Camomile and lavender are good oils to try.

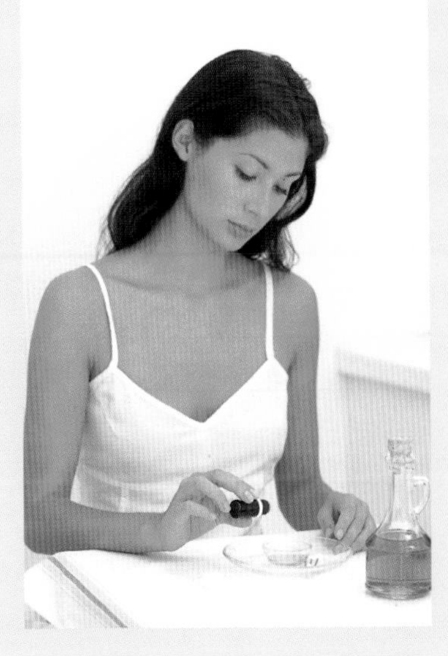

△ **Always dilute an essential oil in a carrier before applying to the skin.**

▷ **Essential oils are derived from all kinds of plants – citrus fruits, rose petals, camomile flowers, and herbs such as rosemary, bay and sage are just a few examples. The oil is distilled from whichever part of the plant contains the most natural oil. Always use pure oils, which have no added ingredients.**

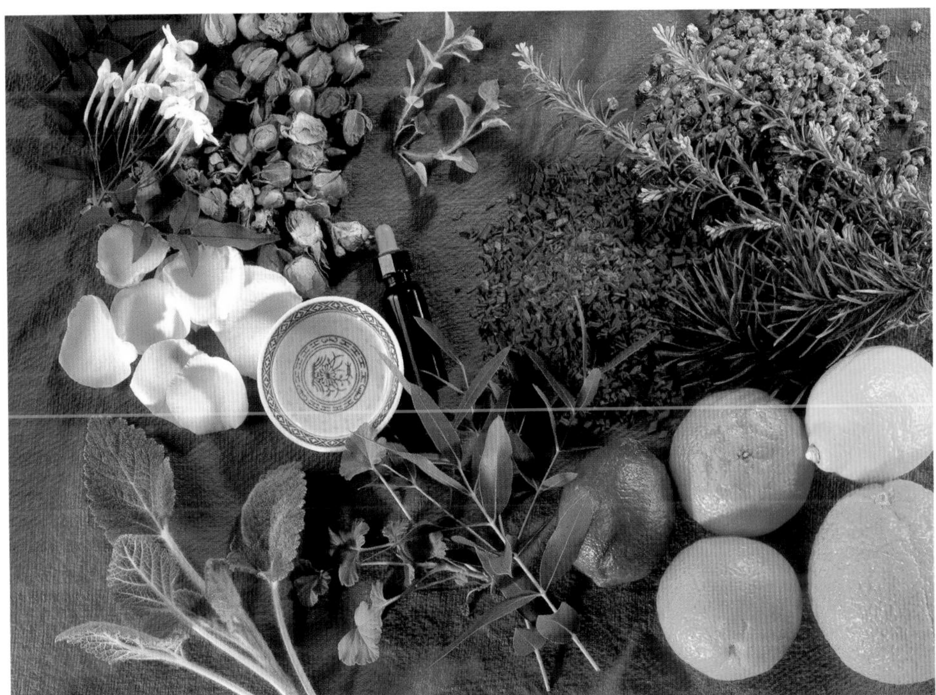

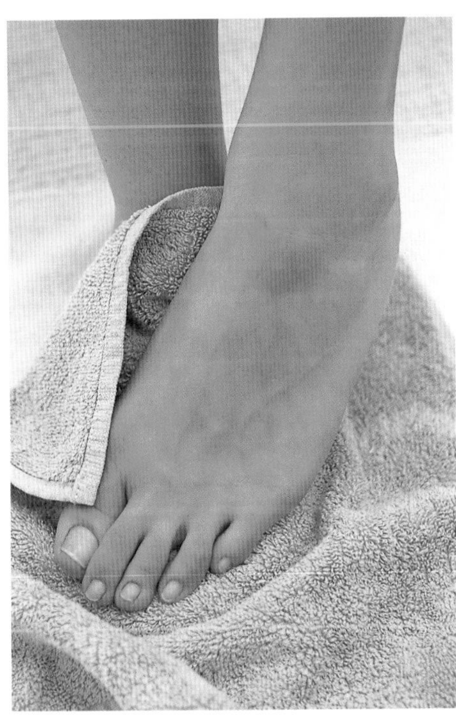

△ **Massage oil into the skin until it is well absorbed. Give the feet a quick wipe at the end of an oil-based treatment to ensure that there is no slippery residue left. You can use the sole of one foot to rub the towel over the top of the other, so that you do not have to bend down.**

adding essential oils

Essential oils are made from natural plant ingredients. They smell wonderful and also have healing qualities. Smell is the most evocative of all the senses, and aroma is a good way of creating instant relaxation. Some essential oils are soothing and calming, such as neroli or lavender; others are stimulating, such as rosemary.

Always smell an oil before you buy it, and choose only those oils with aromas that appeal to you. If you are massaging someone else, it is a good idea to have a small selection of oils so that you can offer them a choice. You may also select particular oils because of their medicinal qualities. However, be aware that not all oils are suitable for everyone.

There is a tendency to think that because essential oils are natural, they are completely safe, with no need for caution. However, this is not the case. Treat essential oil with respect, as you would any chemical or drug. Never use an oil unless you know it to be safe, and avoid using any oil with women who are pregnant, children, the very old and the sick unless you have specifically checked its suitability.

Aromatherapy for health

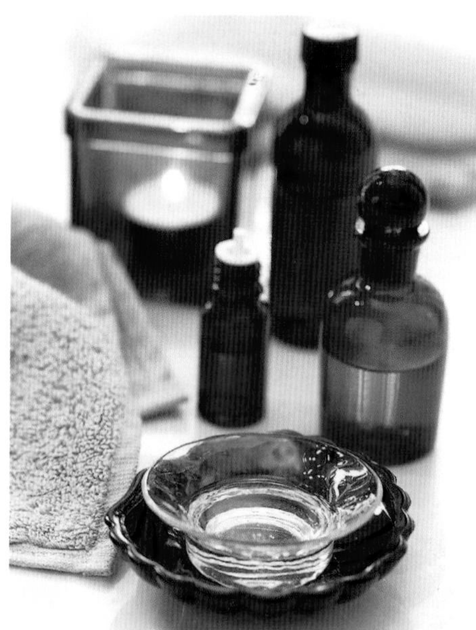

Essential oils bring an extra sense of pleasure and relaxation to any foot treatment. Smoothing a pleasant-smelling oil into the feet as you massage helps to create a deep sense of calm and can also have a beneficial effect on your general well-being. In aromatherapy, different oils are also used to create specific effects – such as relieving stress, increasing vitality or treating certain health problems.

Nobody knows exactly how the therapy works, but it is thought that the scents stimulate nerve endings in the nostrils. Messages are then sent to the areas of the brain that are concerned with moods and emotions, and may trigger a reaction here. Pleasant smells are also thought to have an effect on the hypothalamus, a mysterious organ deep within the brain which regulates our sleep, body temperature, metabolism and the libido.

The oils used in aromatherapy massage can also have a direct effect on the nerve endings in the the skin where they are applied. Lavender and tea tree, for example, have been known as healing plants for centuries. These and other oils with antifungal, antiseptic and anaesthetic ingredients have an instant first-aid effect at the point where they are rubbed in.

◁ It is easy to use essential oils. All you need are the oils of your choice, a good carrier such as almond oil, and a saucer to mix them together.

using essential oils

The most direct and effective method is to add a few drops of your chosen oil to a carrier oil, and then gently smooth it into the skin. Breathe deeply as you massage for maximum effect.

The routines in this book contain suggestions for good oils to incorporate, or you can experiment with your own favourites. If you do not like to use oil when you massage (or if you are giving a reflexology treatment), you could burn essential oils in a vaporizer instead. However, the effect will not be as strong.

Essential oils can be added to unscented powders, creams and potions, and used to for beauty and therapeutic treatments. Try the recipes in this book, or adapt them by substituting different essential oils (keeping to the quantities specified). To prevent the ingredients from spoiling, always transfer to a dark screwtop bottle or jar for storage.

baths and compresses

A warm bath or footbath allows you to absorb the oils through your skin as you lie back and relax. Soak for at least ten minutes, breathing deeply all the while. The oils do not disperse well in water so you will need to dilute them in a carrier oil or in full-fat milk. Add to the filled bath (not to running water) and swirl the water with your hand.

If you are having a footbath, keep a boiled kettle nearby (take care with hot kettles). You can then top up the water as it cools down. Footbaths can help to relieve aching or swollen feet; they are also a good way of softening feet before a pamper session.

For bruising, pain or arthritic joints, try an aromatherapy compress. Use a warm compress for general pain, aching or arthritic joints, and a cold compress if the area is inflamed, swollen or hot.

To make a compress, fill a bowl with hot or very cold water. Dilute your chosen essential oils in a carrier: a good blend is 4 drops geranium, 3 drops bergamot and 3 drops clary sage combined in 10ml/2 tsp grapeseed oil. Add to the water and swish around. Soak a clean cloth in the water, then wring it out and hold against the affected area. Replace the cloth often so that the temperature of the area remains constant.

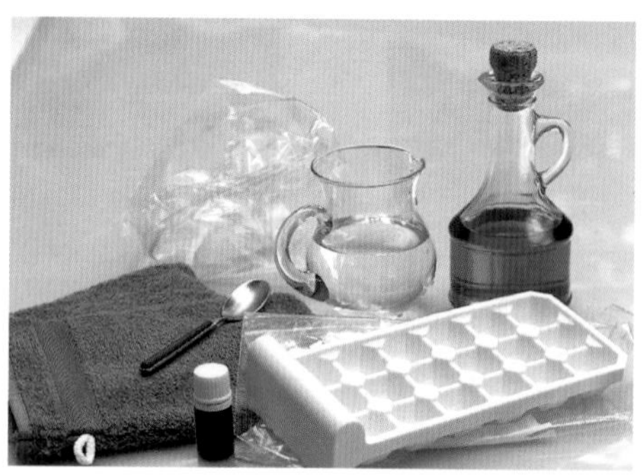

△ When making a cold compress, use chilled water or water with a few ice cubes added. You can place a sealed bag of crushed ice over the compress to help keep the area cold. You could also freeze the oil and water mix in an ice cube tray, and use it to produce your own aromatic ice-packs. Never apply ice directly to skin.

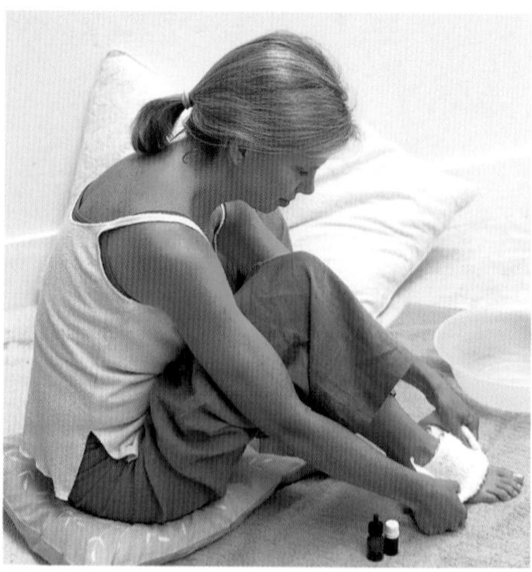

△ A warm aromatic compress effectively soothes an aching ankle. Secure in place with a bandage or a thin clean scarf, and rest with your feet above the level of your heart for 15 minutes.

healing oils for home treatments

Here are some of the therapeutic properties of popular essential oils. Not all these oils will be suitable for everyone. Always check the safety of an oil you use, particularly if the person suffers from a chronic condition, such as high blood pressure, or is pregnant. Men often do not like flowery scents, but these can be combined with a citrus or a woody oil to make them acceptable.

Oil	Description	Uses
Bergamot	A flowery aroma	Antiseptic and pain-relieving; uplifting antidepressant. A good insect repellent and helpful for skin problems. Do not sunbathe 12 hours after application.
Camomile	Blue oil with a gentle apple-like aroma	German camomile is ideal for treating blisters and inflammation; Roman camomile helps promote restful sleep and soothe aching, and it is good for skin conditions.
Frankincense	The aroma of camphor with a hint of lemon (good for men)	Calms anxiety and has an uplifting effect. May relieve heavy periods. Good for mature skin and also has antiseptic properties.
Ginger	Sweet, woody aroma	Helpful for aches, pains and sports injuries. Warming: helps arthritis, muscle spasm and poor circulation. Aids the digestion and helps with travel sickness.
Grapefruit	Tangy aroma that mixes well with flowery oils (good for men)	Uplifting and works as an antidepressant. A good cleansing oil. Can help boost the immune system.
Jasmine	Floral, slightly heady fragrance	Excellent for anxiety and menstrual problems. Considered an aphrodisiac. May be helpful in labour.
Lavender	Slightly mossy, woody scent	Suitable for stress-related or nervous conditions. It has anti-inflammatory, antiseptic properties, and can help with skin problems and healing.
Lemon	Sharp citrus scent that combines well with heavy floral oils	Helps aches, pains, depression, fluid retention, sluggish circulation and varicose veins. Astringent.
Mandarin	Faintly orange aroma	Both calming and uplifting; good for anxiety, stress, insomnia and PMS. Often recommended during pregnancy.
Neroli	Sweet floral scent with a seaweed-like note	Good for depression, shock, exhaustion and insomnia. May improve appearance of broken veins and scar tissue. Can cause drowsiness.
Peppermint	Strong fresh minty aroma (good for men)	Stimulates the circulation. Good for hot, aching feet. May cause skin reaction if overused; should not be used for people with epilepsy.
Rose	Rich floral fragrance	Good for the skin, and may help varicose and broken veins. Helps female complaints such as PMS, as well as grief, depression and fatigue.
Rosemary	Refreshing camphorous aroma	Soothes aches, pains and stiff muscles. Increases alertness, and good for stress and exhaustion. Do not use if you have high blood pressure or epilepsy.
Sandalwood	Warm, woody smell (good for men)	Relaxing oil, with antiseptic and anti-inflammatory qualities. Good for dry skin. Helps stress and exhaustion. Said to be an aphrodisiac.
Tangerine	Tangy, slightly sweet smell	Antispasmodic, helpful for pre-menstrual tension.
Tea Tree	Balsamic aroma (good for men)	Good first-aid oil for the skin: antifungal, antiviral, anti-inflammatory. Good as an insect repellent; soothes insect bites.
Thyme	Strong herbal scent (good for men)	Antiseptic, antispasmodic, antifungal, antiviral. Stimulating oil that boosts concentration. Do not use on sensitive skin.
Violet	A rich sweet floral	Encourages good circulation and feeds the skin. Pain-relieving and anti-inflammatory properties.
Ylang-Ylang	Powerful spicy scent	Eases tension, stress and fatigue. Over-use can cause headaches or irritation.

Simple self-massage

All that is needed for a simple self-massage treatment is an understanding of a few basic strokes. After that, it is a matter of practice so that you become comfortable with the different techniques involved.

Self-treatment is a great way of learning massage, because you have your own physical responses to guide you. It is important to get yourself into a relaxed position: you should not need to twist your back or the knee in order to reach the foot. If you are comfortable, you will find it much easier to detect the subtle differences between different strokes and types of pressure, and your reactions to them. You will instantly know when you have got the technique right, and when your touch is sufficiently sensitive and pleasing.

Once you have mastered the basic routine described here, you will be able to adapt the techniques to suit your particular needs and your different moods. You'll also find it much easier to learn the other treatments in this book.

easy self-treatment

This is a quick, simple and effective massage that helps to soothe the tired muscles. It can be used at any time as a treatment to relax and refresh the feet, as a quick pick-me-up or as a way to boost your vitality and energy. You can use a cream or massage oil if you like. This basic massage is best done while sitting on the floor, with the resting leg stretched out in front of you.

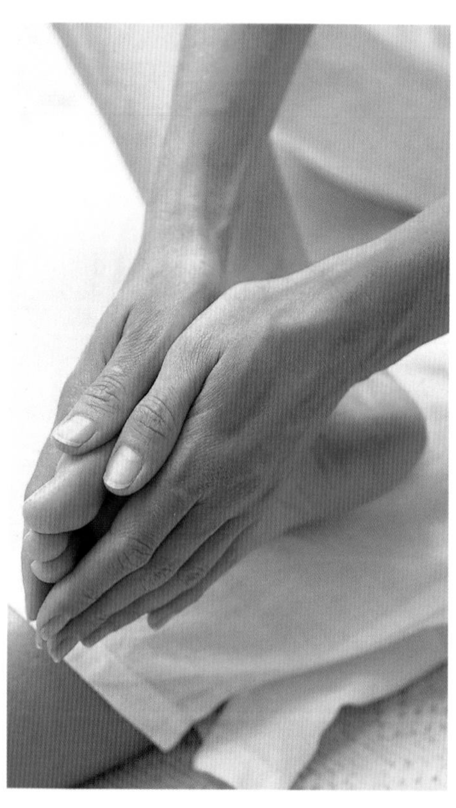

△ **1** Bring your right foot to rest on your left knee; make sure that you are sitting in a comfortable position. Start with gentle stroking. Grasp the foot between your hands, in a sandwich hold, then slide them up the foot, from your heel to the toes.

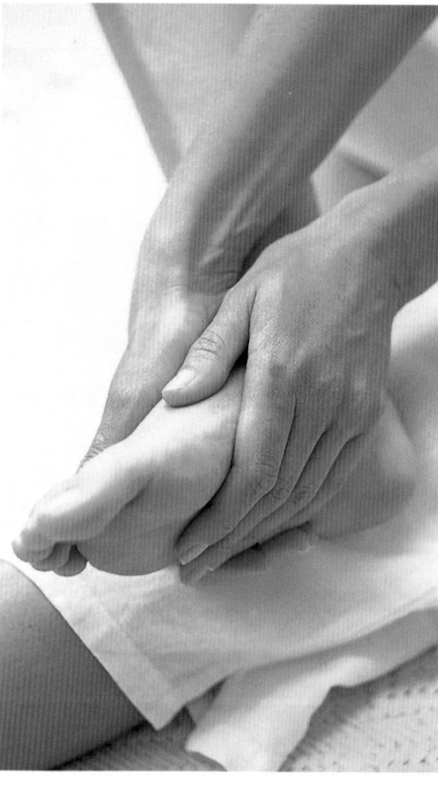

△ **2** Keeping the foot in the same position as before, slide your hands in the opposite direction – down the foot from the toes to your heel. Keep the pressure steady and firm. Now repeat these up-and-down sliding movements two more times.

△ **3** Place your foot on the floor, beside the knee. Hold the foot so that your fingers curl round the sole and your thumbs and heels are on top. Spread the top of the foot by sliding the thumbs apart, applying firm pressure and keeping your fingers in place.

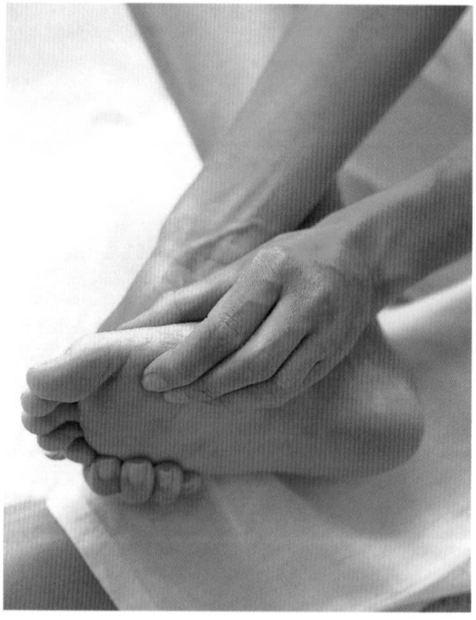

△ **4** Now lift up your foot and place it on your knee again. Place your hands in the same position as in step 3. Now, pull the fingers slowly outwards so that you stretch and spread the sole of the foot. Apply firm pressure as you do so.

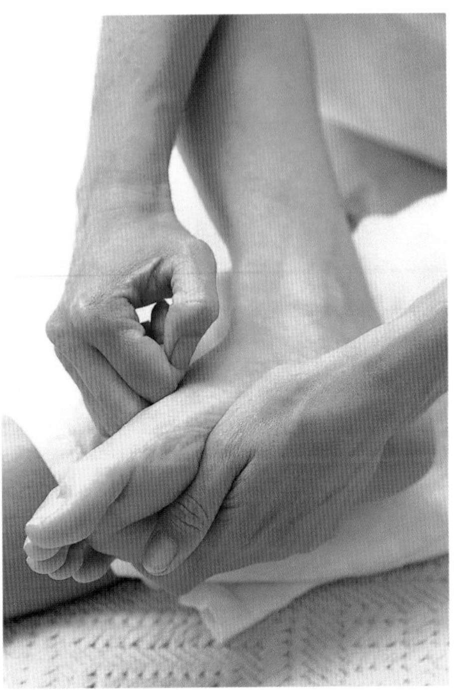

△ **5** Support the sole of the foot with your left hand. Make a fist with your right hand. Use your knuckles to apply light pressure to the top of the foot, making circular movements. Now support the top of the foot with your right hand. Use the knuckles of the left hand to work the sole, applying deeper pressure.

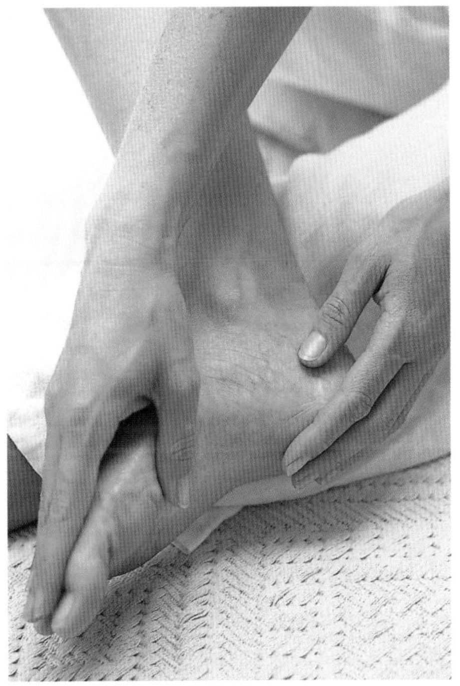

△ **7** Continue to support the heel of your foot with your left hand. Place the right hand over the top of the foot, placing your thumb on the sole. Now, gently stretch and push the foot downwards. Again, stretch only as far as feels comfortable. Do steps 6 and 7 once more.

different strokes

When giving yourself a foot massage, take the opportunity to experiment. Try out different strokes, levels of pressure and combinations of the two. People vary considerably in what strokes they like best, and in particular how much pressure they enjoy. What you like can also change depending on your mood and the part of the foot being worked. As a general rule:

Fast strokes are stimulating and energizing.

Slow rhythmic strokes have a hypnotic, relaxing effect.

Deep pressure can be used to release muscular tension, relieve stress or to enhance vitality.

Gentle pressure is soothing and has a calming effect on both the mind and the body.

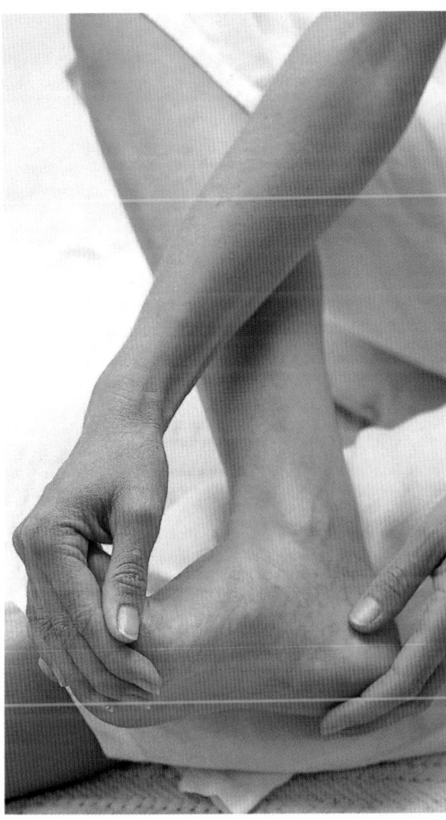

△ **6** Hold the heel of your foot with your left hand, then grasp the ball with your right. Pull the ball of your foot gently upwards so that you stretch the sole. Make sure that you stretch the foot only as far as feels comfortable.

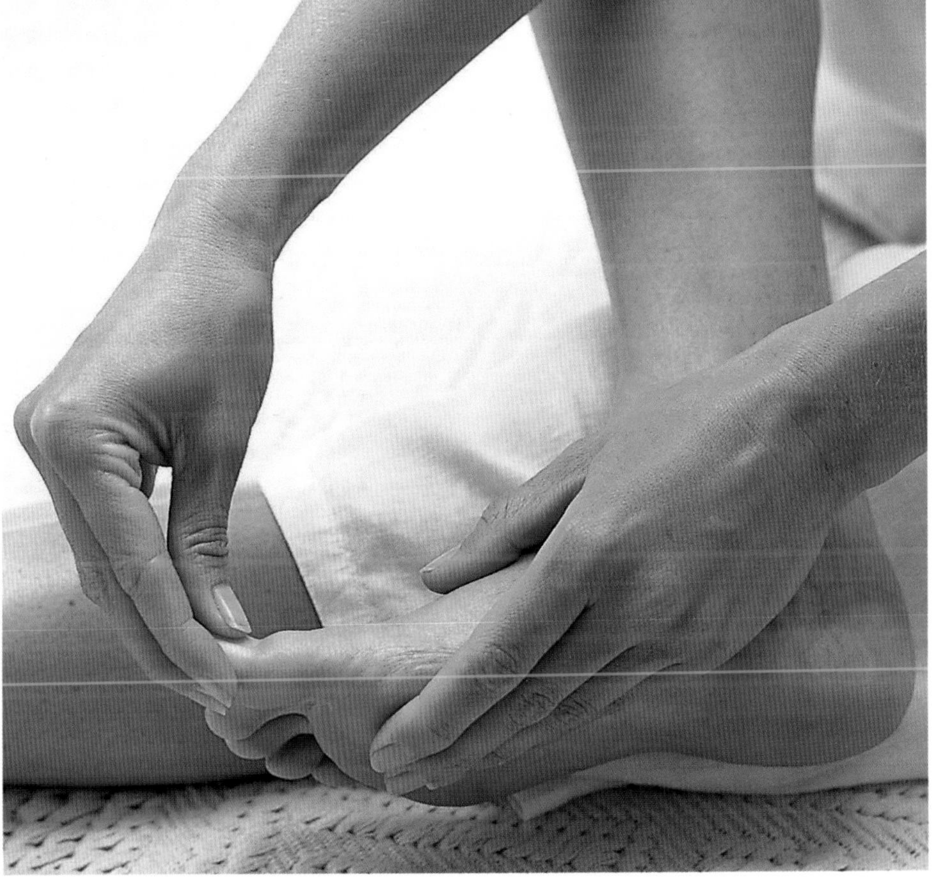

△ **8** Support the foot near the arch with your left hand. With your right hand, hold the big toe near the main joint. Gently rotate the toe first in a clockwise direction, then in an anticlockwise direction. Repeat the action on each toe, finishing on the little one. Now, repeat steps 1 to 8 on your left foot.

Soothing relaxer

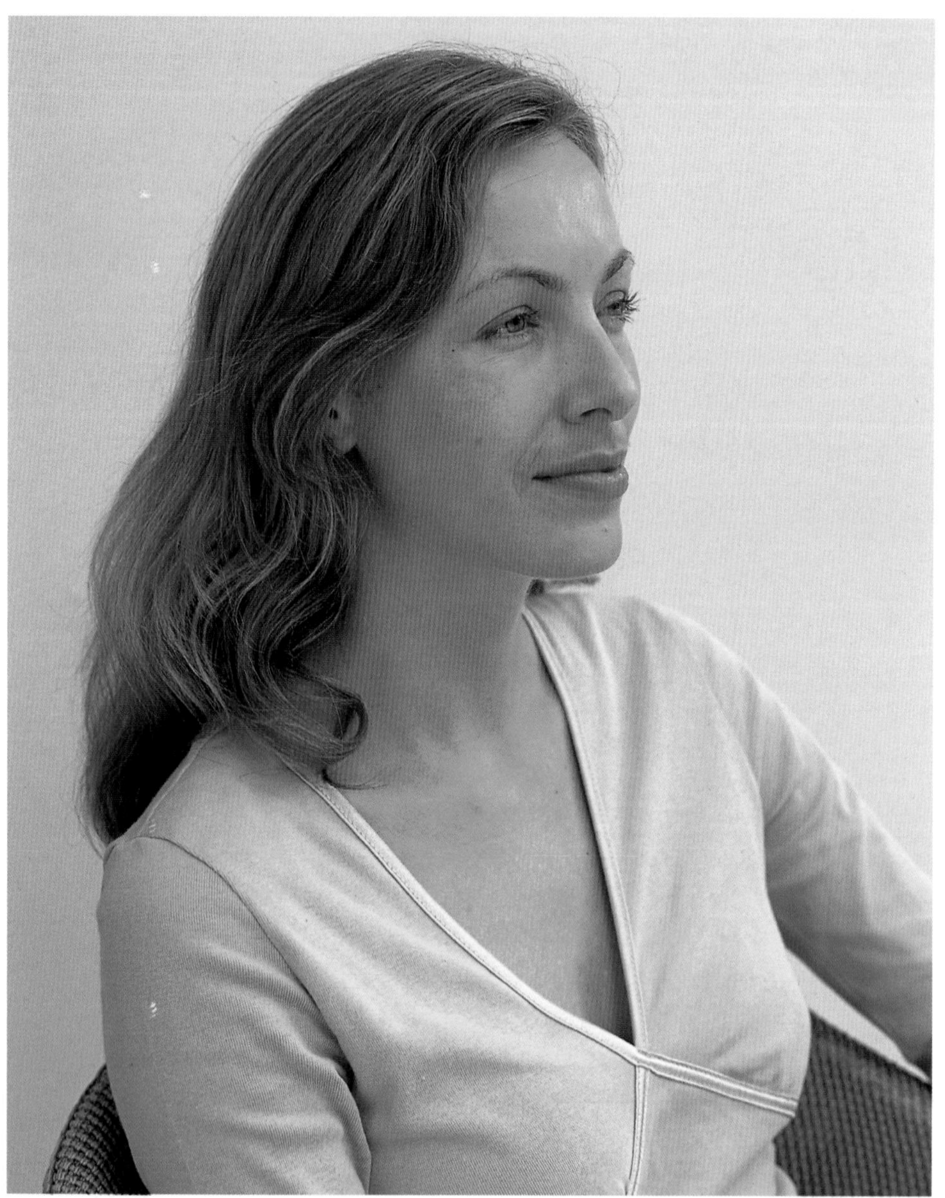

Self-treatment is wonderfully soothing. However, nothing you do to yourself can quite match the sensation of leaning back and letting someone else do the work, as in this routine. There is something utterly relaxing about having your feet massaged; tension seems to drain out of the whole body almost as though a tap had been opened. Perhaps because the feet are so far away from your head, it feels easy to let your mind release worries and anxieties, too.

teach a friend

A relaxing foot massage is a wonderful gift to be able to offer others. It's also worth persuading a friend to learn this short routine, so that you can benefit from it.

△ This treatment should leave you thoroughly relaxed. Take some time to sit quietly after the routine. If you are giving it to someone else, leave them alone for five or ten minutes so that they appreciate the full effects.

Anyone can do it even if they have never learned massage techniques before.

There is no need to make any special arrangements in order to do this massage. It can be done anywhere, and works well if the person is sitting on the sofa watching TV or if you are in the garden on a warm, sunny afternoon. You can use it to give a friend a pick-me-up after a late night, and it can also be done in the morning to set someone up for a long, stressful day.

calming massage routine

If you like, you can incorporate this massage into a longer pamper treatment for the feet. You may also like to use some favourite aromatherapy oils to heighten the effects. Neroli and sandalwood or rose and bergamot would be excellent soothing blends to use. Take some time to relax afterwards, too – perhaps with a cup of herbal tea.

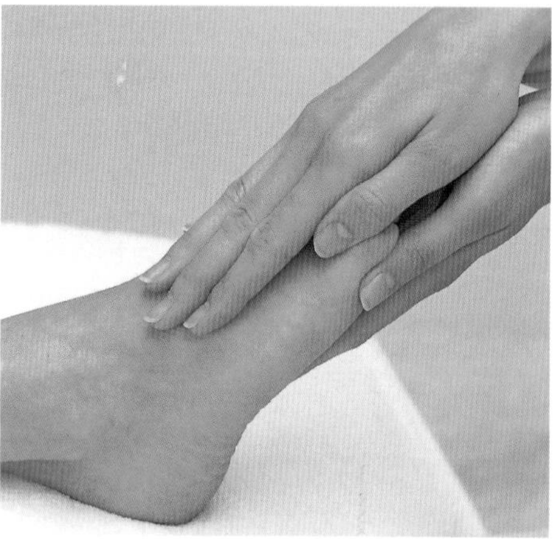

△ **1** Start with the right foot. Hold the foot between your hands – place one hand lengthways over the top of the foot, with the other underneath it. Slide the hands up the foot to the toes, then back down again. Repeat the action at least three times, increasing the pressure as you go.

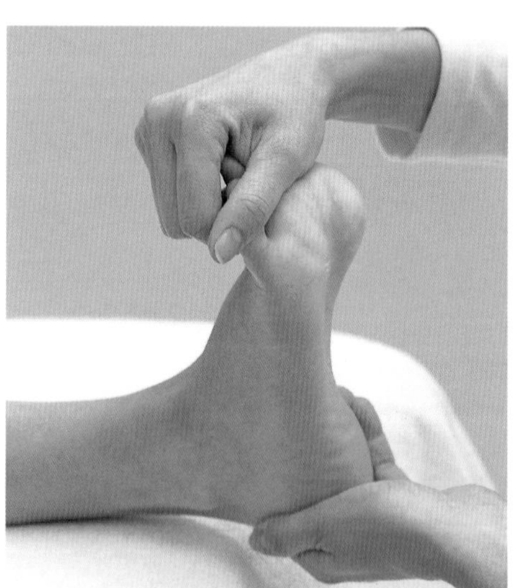

△ **2** Support the heel of the foot in your left hand. Gently grasp the toes with the other hand and then slowly push the top of the foot towards the leg. This gives the sole a good stretch, which helps to release tension. Do not push further than feels comfortable.

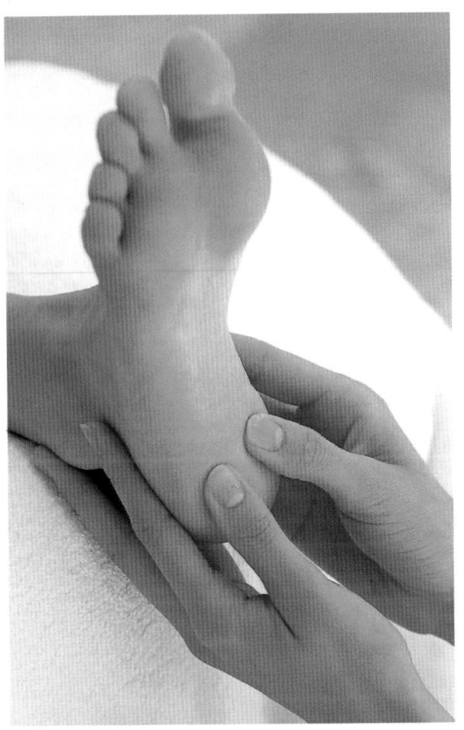

△ **3** Place both of your thumbs on the heel of the foot, with one thumb positioned slightly higher than the other. Now start to massage, by making tiny circles with the thumb, using alternate thumbs. Work your way right up the foot, to the top of the sole, and remember to use much lighter pressure on the arch than on the heel and ball.

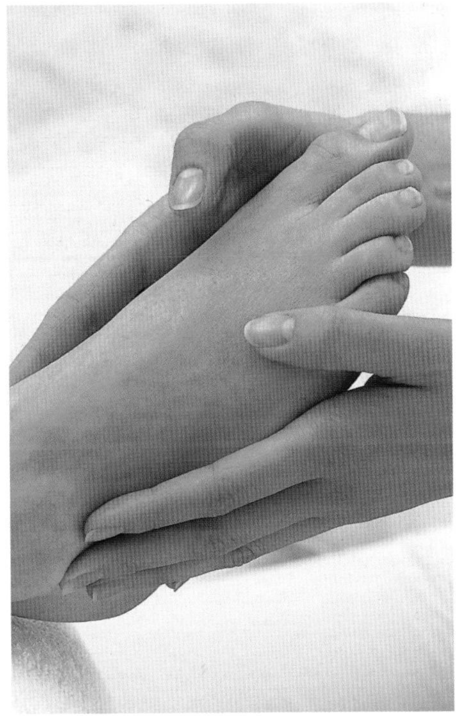

△ **5** Place both of your hands on either side of the foot, in such a way that your fingertips are positioned next to the ankle bones. Now, using firm (but pleasurable) pressure, massage in a clockwise direction around both ankle bones at the same time. Repeat the movement, but this time working in an anticlockwise direction.

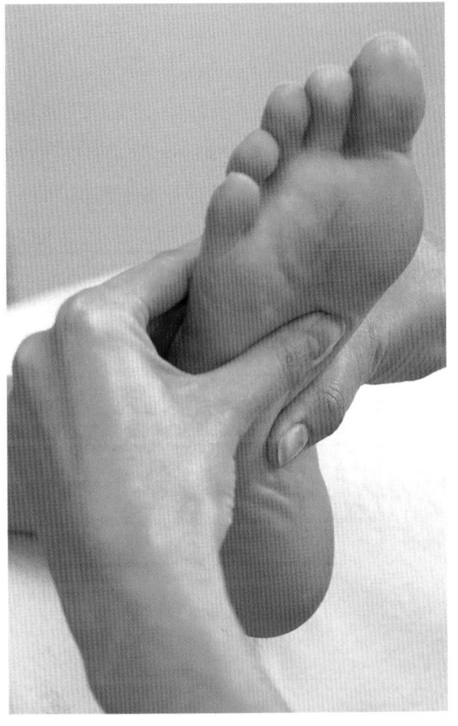

△ **7** Now place your thumbs on the sole so that they point in opposite directions. Wrap your fingers around the top of the foot to keep it steady. Slide the thumbs up the sole, making a criss-cross movement – so that first the left thumb slides above the right, then the right one slides above the left. Start at the toes and work down the foot; then work back up to the toes.

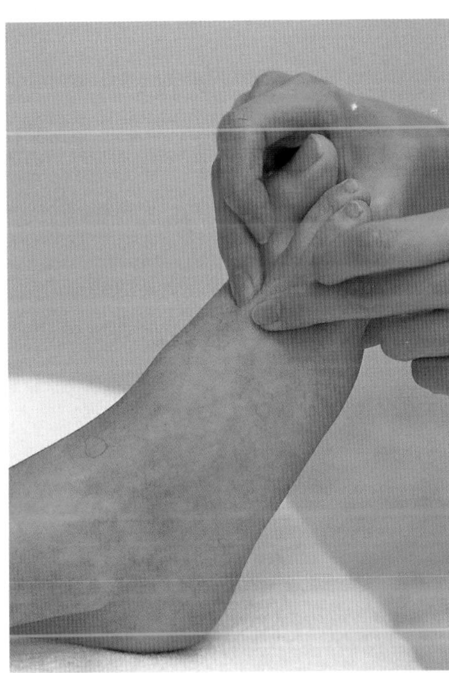

△ **4** Massage the top of the foot, using your two middle fingers to make tiny circular movements. Start in the groove between the big and second toe, and work down the entire foot to the ankle. Repeat the movement, this time starting in the groove between the second and third toes. Work across the foot in this way until you reach the little toe.

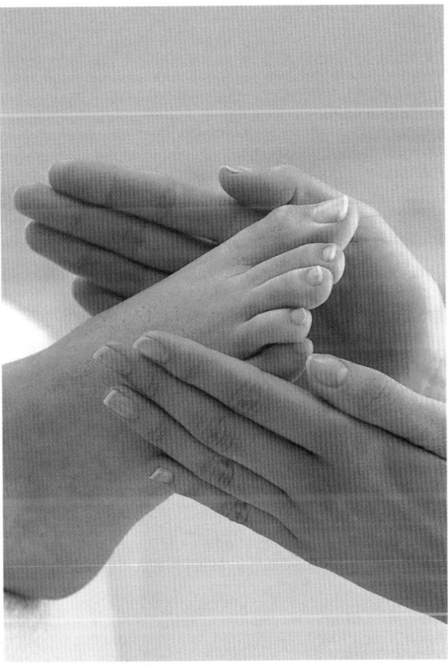

△ **6** Place your hands either side of the foot, so that it is wedged in-between them in a sandwich hold. Using a gentle push-pull action, pull one side of the foot towards you and push the other side away at the same time. Repeat, but this time reverse the action so that you push the first side away, and pull the other towards you. Do the movements twice more.

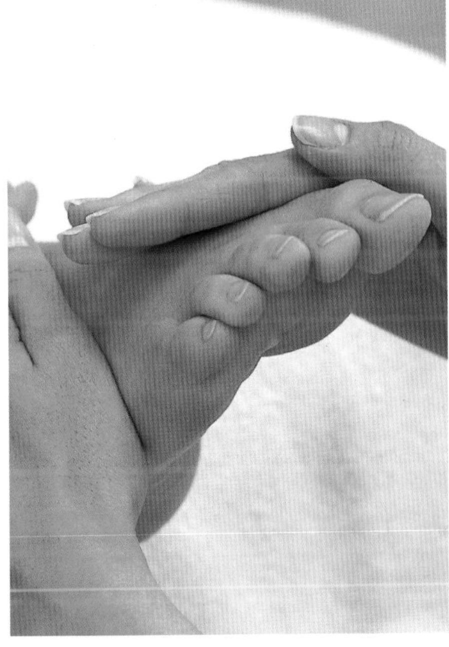

△ **8** Finish the massage by making feather-light strokes on the top and sole of the foot, using alternate hands. Cover the whole area two or three times, or longer if you feel that the person is really benefiting from this relaxing action. Now repeat the whole sequence on the left foot.

Reflexology and acupressure

The therapy of reflexology is based on the idea that health-giving energy flows around the body. When this energy flows freely, physical and mental well-being is maintained. If the energy flow is blocked or stagnant, we can become unwell or unhappy.

Reflexologists believe that gentle pressure applied to points on the feet – known as reflexes – can be used to stimulate energy flow and release any blockages. The feet contain a "map" of the entire body: every organ and body structure relates to a precise point on the top, side or sole of the foot. For example, the brain is connected to the top of the big toe, while the bladder point is at the base of the heel.

When an area of the body is out of balance, the related reflex will be tender to the touch. Sometimes small granules may be felt around the reflex. These granules are thought to be accumulated waste which has solidified in the form of calcium crystals or uric acid. A reflexologist will gently work a tender point, which helps to break down waste deposits and restore energy flow through the zone. The massage-like action also has the effect of stimulating the circulation of blood and lymph to the area, and it feels highly relaxing.

The hands also contain a map of the body. However, they are not as responsive as the feet so they are usually used only for self-help.

mapping the feet

Reflexology is a holistic therapy that aims to bring the whole body back to balance. For this reason, a full treatment always encompasses work on both feet. The majority of reflexes are on the sole of the foot, but some are on the top or along the side. In general the right foot relates to the right-hand side of the body, while the left relates to the left-hand side. Some organs are sited on only one side of the body, and therefore the related reflexes appear on only one foot.

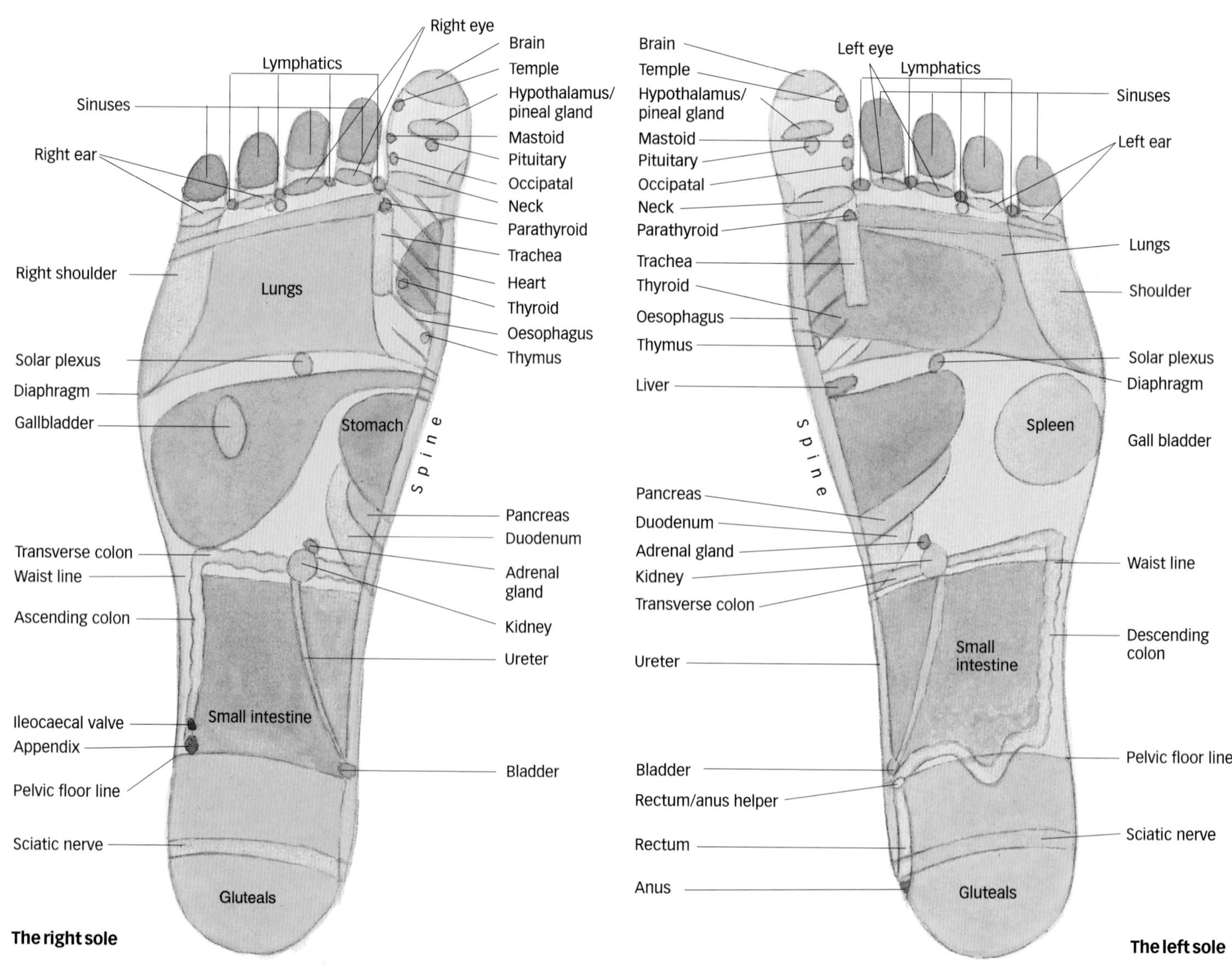

The right sole

The left sole

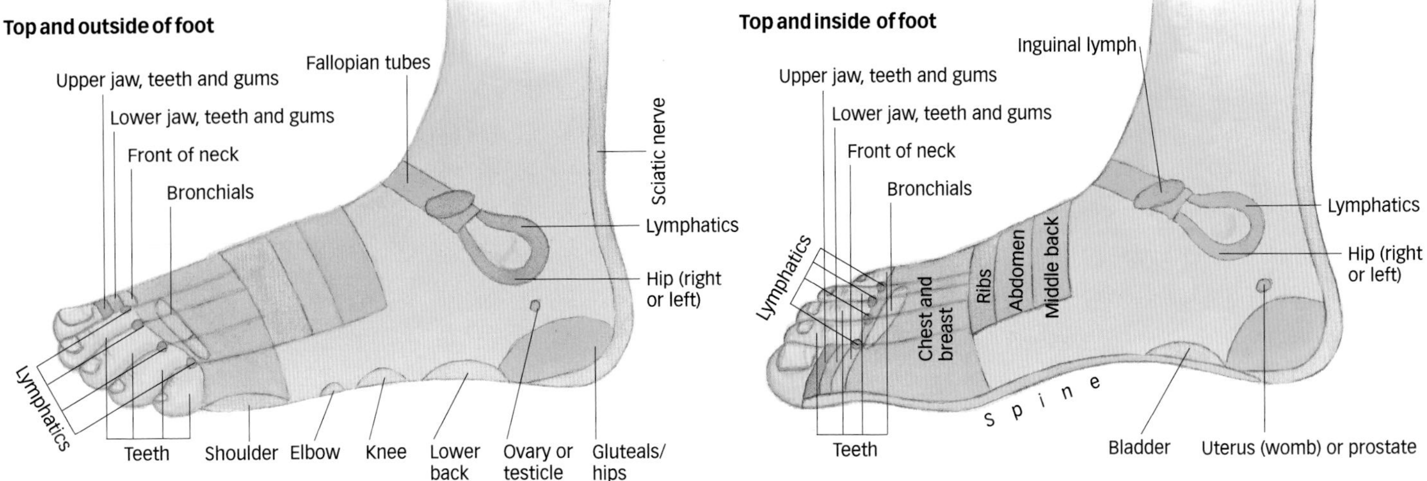

acupressure

Like reflexology, acupressure aims to restore our natural ability for self-healing by encouraging energy flow around the body.

In acupressure, energy is said to flow through invisible channels, called meridians. Most of these are named after the organs of the body – Liver, Heart and Kidney are all important meridians. In Chinese medicine, our organs represent aspects of our emotional well-being as well as physical health: the kidneys are associated with grief, while the heart is connected to joy.

As in reflexology, gentle pressure is used to stimulate the energy points, and points in one area of the body are used to promote healing elsewhere. However, while reflexology concentrates on the feet, acupressure involves points all over the body.

Stomach 45 is on the outside of the base of the nail of the second toe. Press if you have indigestion, or are recovering from a late night.

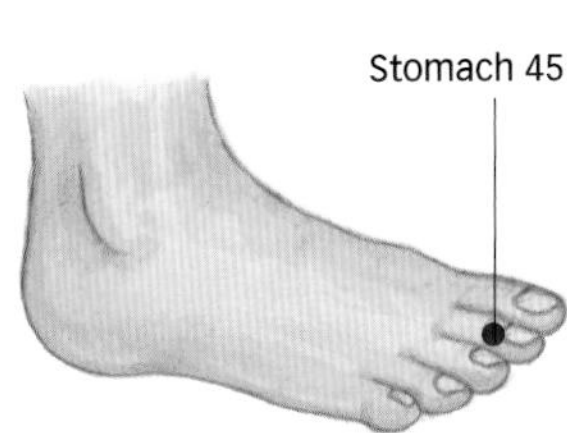

Liver 3 – known as Bigger Rushing – is a useful point to press if you are feeling stressed. It is in the groove between the big toe and second toe, where the bones meet.

Liver 2 is in the webbing between the big toe and the second toe. It is another good stress-relieving point, and it can help to ease constipation.

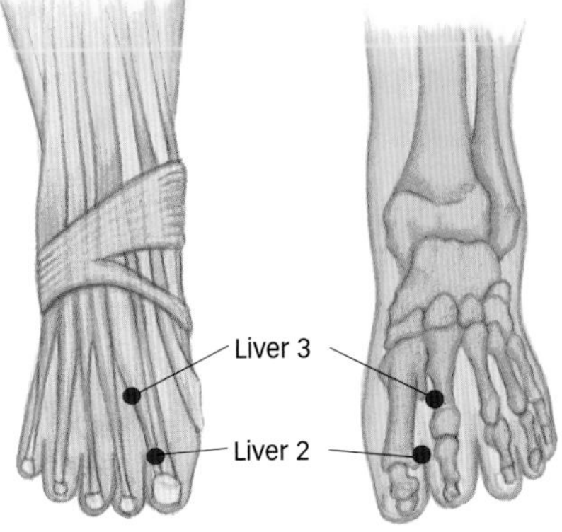

useful acupressure points for self-help

To stimulate an acupressure point, place the tip of your thumb over it. Press gently for a minute or two, making a small rotational movement as you do so. You may notice some tenderness or tingling in the area; ease the pressure if you feel any discomfort. Do not use these points if you are pregnant or seriously ill, unless otherwise recommended by a professional acupuncturist.

Bladder 62 is known as Calm Sleep. It is a very soothing point, and can help to ease insomnia. It is in the first indentation directly below the outer anklebone – about one-third of the distance from the outer anklebone to the bottom of the heel.

Gallbladder 41, which is called Above Tears, is on top of the foot. It is 2.5cm (1in) above the webbing of the fourth and fifth toes, in the groove between the bones. It is good for migraines and headaches that affect one side only.

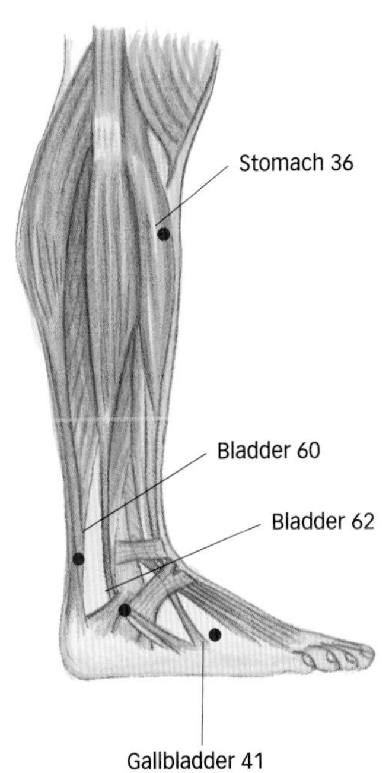

Try pressing **Stomach 36** if you need a quick energy boost. It is called the Three Mile Point – supposedly because it was used by the Chinese army when they needed to push themselves a few miles further. You will find it four finger-widths below the kneecap, and one finger-width from the outer edge of the shinbone. To check you are on the right spot, move your foot up and down – you should feel the muscle flexing beneath your fingertip.

Bladder 60, also known as High Mountains, is midway between the back edge of the outer ankle bone and the achilles tendon. This is a good general relaxation point.

Spleen 6 is a good first-aid point to press if you are feeling faint. It can also help relieve period pain and aids the digestion. The point is four finger-widths above the inner anklebone, close to the back of the shinbone. **Spleen 4** is found in the upper arch of the foot, one thumb-width from the ball – a helpful point if you are fighting off a cold.

Kidney 6 is also known as the Illuminated Sea. It is good for insomnia and can also ease the symptoms of menopause. The point **Kidney 3**, or the Bigger Stream, is helpful if you are feeling depleted and drained.

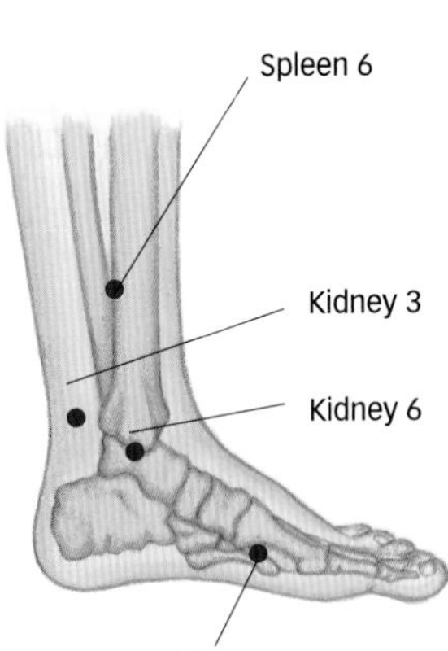

Reflexology techniques

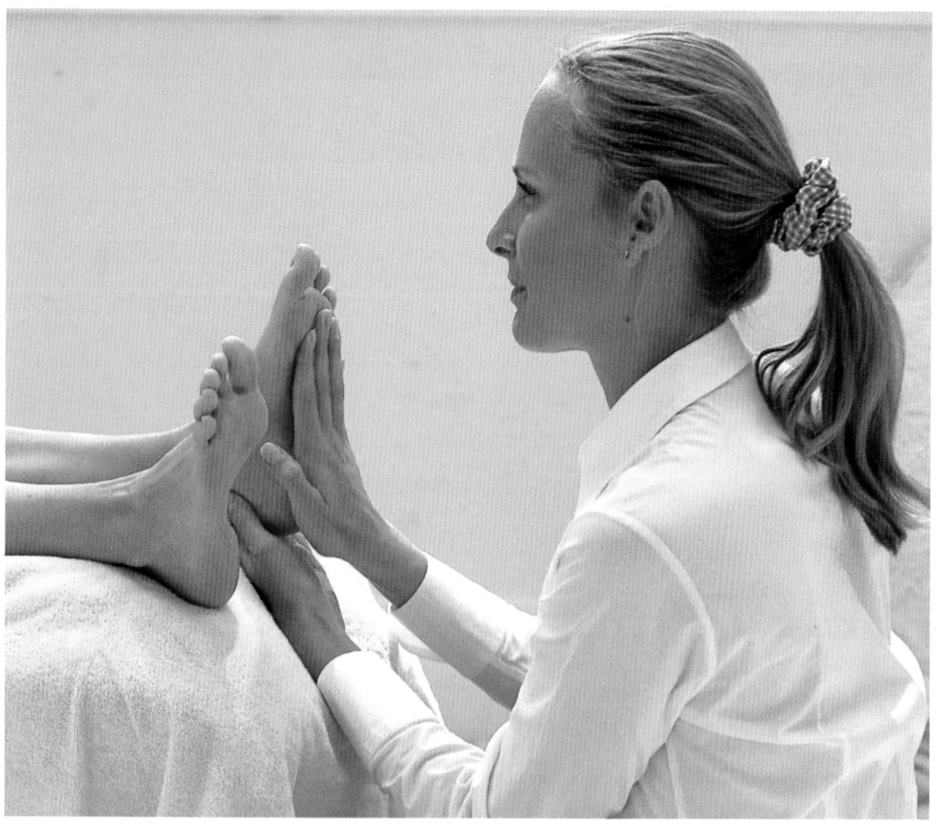

◁ **Establish a connection with the person you are treating before starting a reflexology treatment, and always ask the recipient how he or she is feeling. Placing your hands on the soles of the feet before you begin is a reassuring and centring experience for both giver and receiver.**

Reflexology is a method of self-healing that can easily be done at home. The basic movements are simple to learn. Once you have become familiar with them, you can use reflexology to treat minor ailments as well as to boost the general well-being of yourself and your family and friends.

When doing reflexology, wear comfortable clothing that does not restrict your movements: in particular, do not wear a tight top. Maintain good posture throughout; try to keep your back straight and your shoulders relaxed. Remember to breathe naturally and deeply – many people tend to hold their breath when they are concentrating.

What every reflexologist needs is a good touch. To a certain extent, this comes with practice. However, it is always very important to check the responses of the recipient, and to ask him or her for feedback. Practise the hand exercises given in this book regularly: this will help you to develop suppleness in your wrist and fingers.

Have a glass of water after giving a treatment. If you are treating another person, offer him or her a drink as well.

giving a treatment

Always start a reflexology treatment by giving the feet a gentle massage. This helps you to connect with the person you are treating, and it will help you to connect with your own body when self-treating. Massaging also gets the fingers mobile, and it encourages both you and the recipient to relax. The simple self-massage and relaxing massage treatments on the previous pages are good routines to do at this point. A short massage should also be given after the reflexology treatment.

You can either give the full reflexology routine – described on the following pages – or you can focus on a particular area of the body, or on a symptom. If doing a full treatment, remember to work gently, and do not repeat the routine more than once a week. If you are working on specific points rather than doing the full routine, then two or three treatments a week should be sufficient. Do not treat anyone with a major illness or severe problem, or a woman in the first three months of pregnancy.

getting the pressure right

Reflexology should neither hurt nor tickle – aim for firm, pleasurable pressure. The pressure will need to be varied depending on the size of the person's foot, his or her general health and individual tolerance level. In general, the pressure applied to bony areas such as the top of the foot should always be lighter than that applied to fleshy areas, such as the heel or ball. The pressure used when treating a child or an elderly person should always be significantly lighter.

Start off using a light pressure, then gradually increase to tolerance level. Do not overtreat particular points – keep to the number of times suggested.

hand preserver

This great lotion can be used every day to keep your hands soft.

ingredients

- 15ml/1 tbsp avocado oil
- 15ml/1 tbsp almond oil
- 15ml/1 tbsp petroleum jelly or glycerine
- 1ml/⅕ tsp vitamin E oil
- 10 drops essential oil. Use any one or a combination of these: rose, sandalwood, geranium, lavender, neroli.

Combine the ingredients in a small bowl. Transfer to a 50ml (2fl oz) screwtop jar.

basic techniques

Anyone giving a reflexology treatment needs soft skin, so moisturize daily. Always check that your nails are clean and short before treating. This is even more important for reflexology than for massage since you press into the skin.

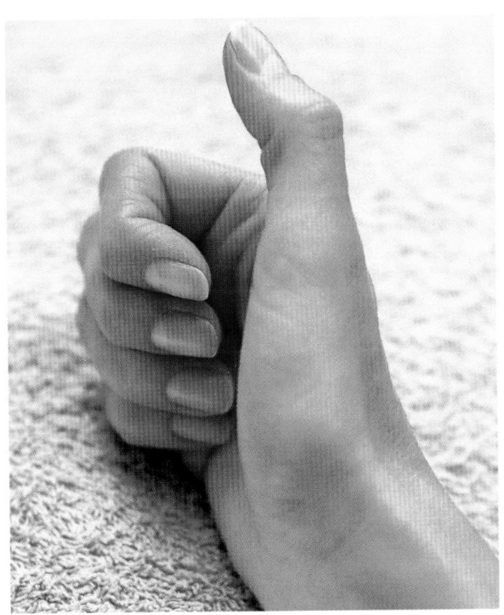

△ **Thumb walking or crawling**
Hold your thumb straight up in front of you, then bend it from the first joint and straighten it again – this is the basic technique used in thumb walking. Place the thumb on the skin, and use alternate bending and straightening movements to "walk" across the area. This has been likened to the crawling movement of a caterpillar.

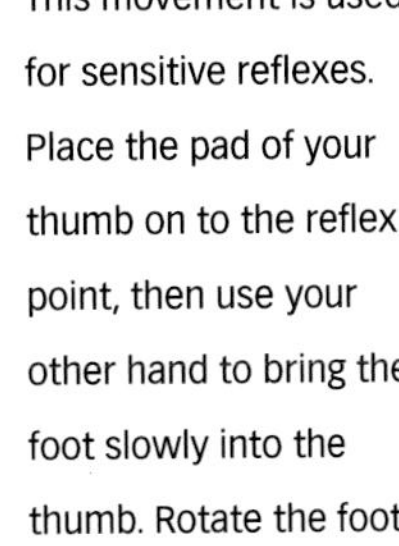

▷ **Rotation on a point**
This movement is used for sensitive reflexes. Place the pad of your thumb on to the reflex point, then use your other hand to bring the foot slowly into the thumb. Rotate the foot in a circular movement around the thumb.

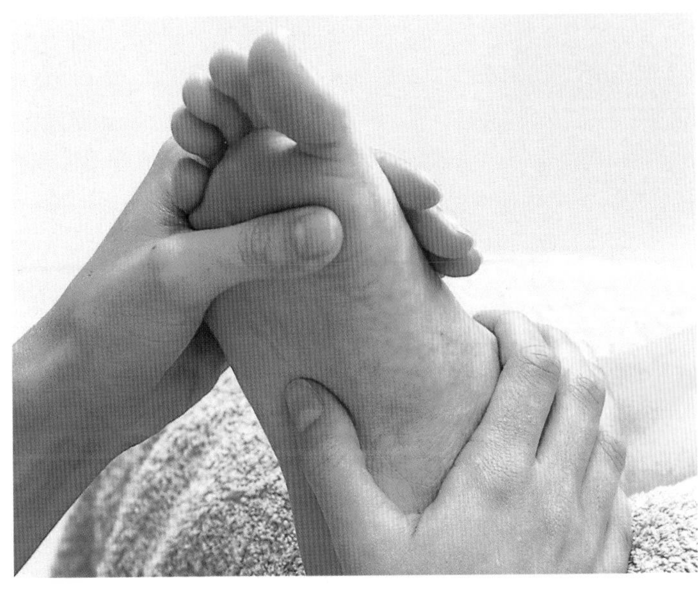

▷ **Pinpoint, or hooking**
This is used for small reflexes or those that are difficult to locate. Place your thumb on the point, and apply pressure. Now, keeping the pressure steady, move the thumb on to the uppermost tip in a "hooking" action. Move the thumb back to the original position.

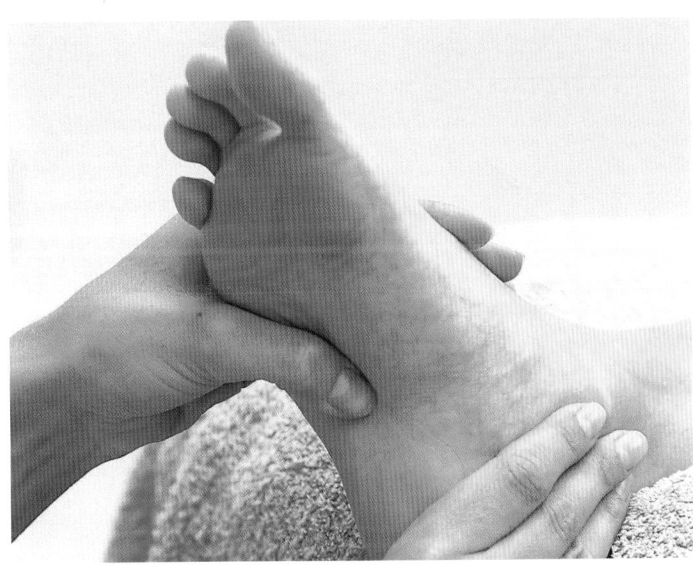

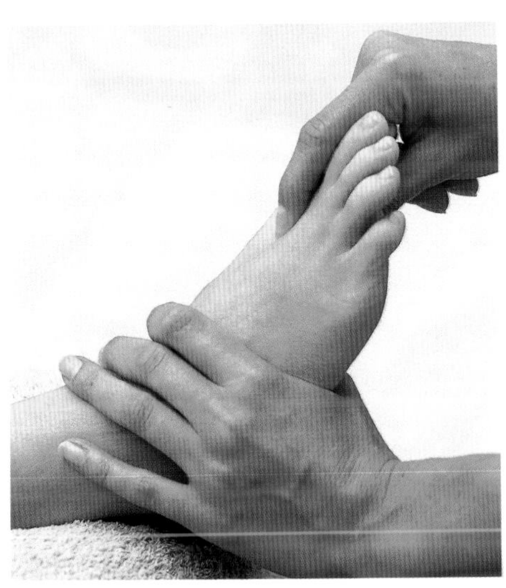

△ **Finger walking or crawling**
This technique is the same as the thumb-walking technique described above, but you use the index (first) finger instead. The action is used on the top of the foot and other areas where the flesh is thinner and less pressure is required. You can use another finger if you find that easier.

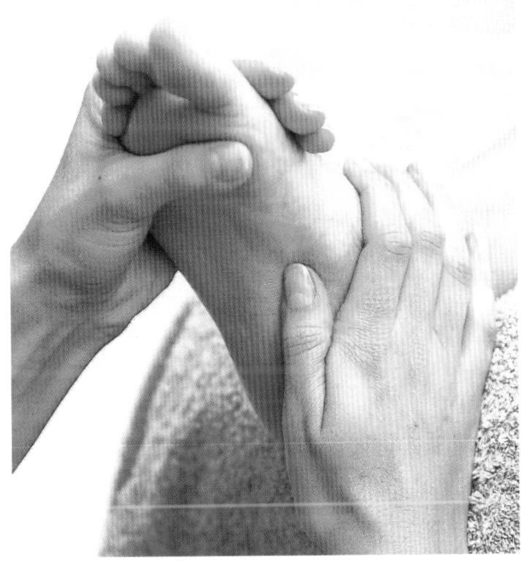

△ **Holding and supporting**
One hand is used to support while the other works the reflex. Always support the foot while you are working. Position your working hand close to the holding hand: this allows you to support and control the movement of the foot. It also gives the recipient a feeling of security.

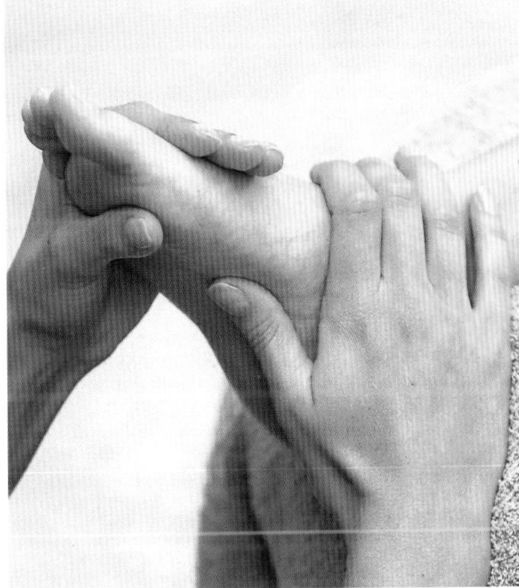

△ **Pressure circles on a point**
Hold the foot comfortably with one hand and place the flat pad of the working thumb on the reflex. Press into the area and then slowly circle your thumb gently on the point. This movement is usually used for very sensitive areas.

A complete reflexology treatment

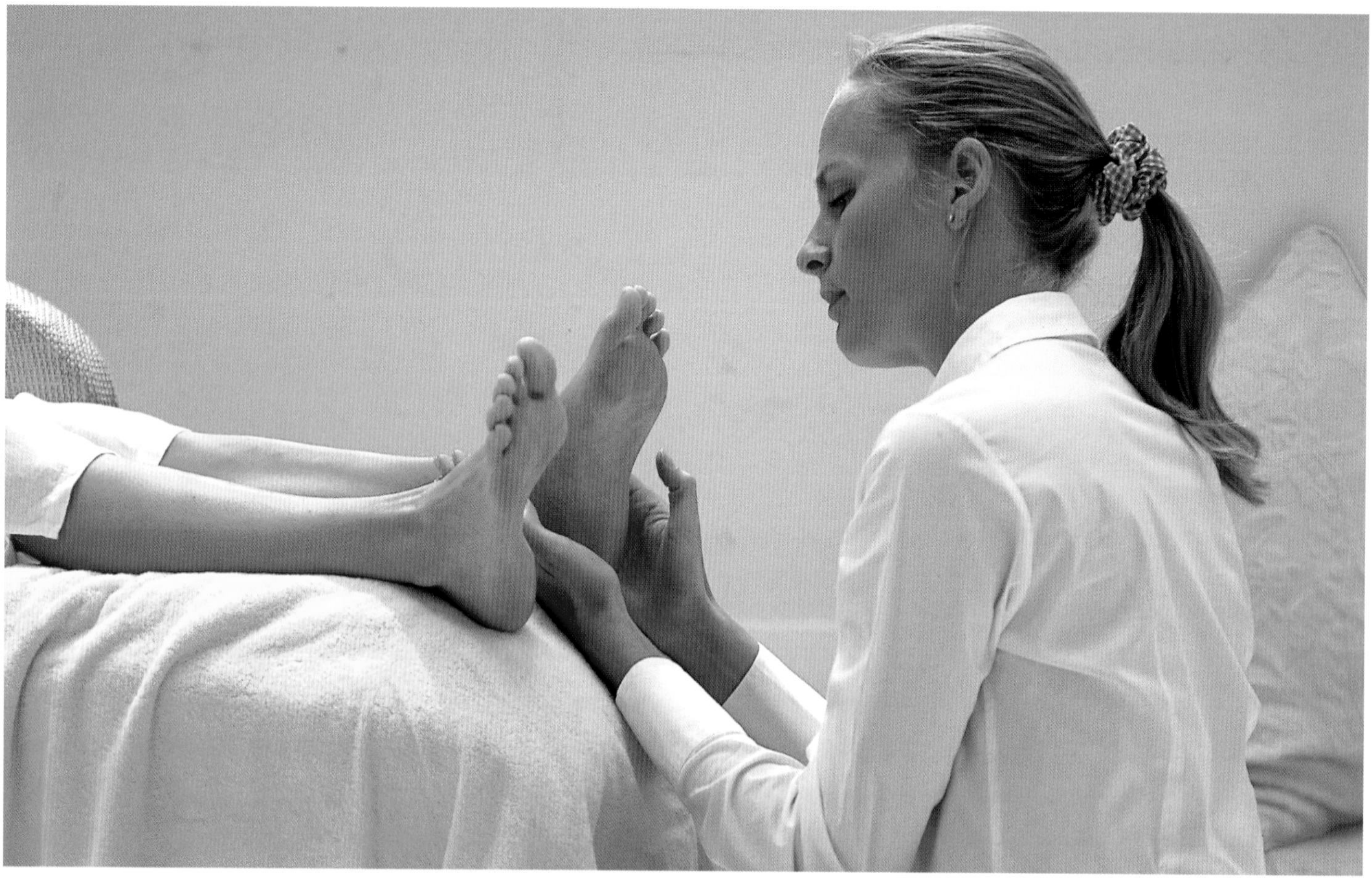

A full reflexology routine treats the whole body, and can be a great way to enhance general well-being, and boost energy. Reflexology treatments work best if the recipient is mentally and physically relaxed, and if he or she is breathing well. For this reason, the first movements in the routine work on the diaphragm and solar plexus reflexes. These points are powerful relaxants which encourage natural, deep breathing. The third movement in the routine treats the head and brain. Stimulating this reflex helps to clear the mind, and also prepares the brain to receive and send messages to and from the rest of the body.

Although each reflex point relates to a specific organ or part of the body, it will also have an effect on other areas. For this reason, it is important that you work round the foot in the exact order given. Be sure to treat all the reflex points on both feet. Ideally, you should perform reflexology on the right foot first (unlike massage, where it is not so important which foot is attended to first).

Reflexology can be very powerful, so it is important that you do not repeat a movement more than the amount of times specified here. You should also not give more than one treatment to the same person – or to yourself – in a week.

△ This is a long routine so make sure that both you and the person you are treating are comfortable. In particular, it is important that the feet are at the right height so that you do not have to bend to reach them. The recipient can lie on a couch, or sit in a chair with the feet propped up on a footstool, with you sitting or kneeling directly in front.

in the hands

The hands, as well as the feet, contain a stylized "map" of the body. Reflexologists tend to treat the feet because they are more sensitive, but the hands can be easier to use for self-treatment. A person's hands may also be used for treatment if they are very frail or have a foot problem.

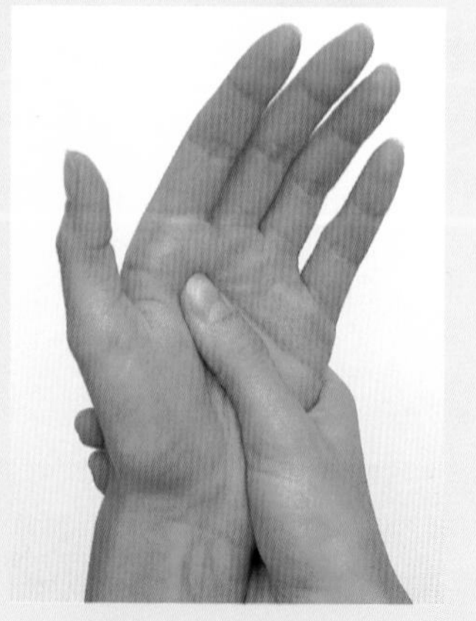

▷ The point being pressed here is connected to the solar plexus. It is an excellent reflex to stimulate if you are feeling anxious or stressed. Breathe deeply as you work it.

holistic reflexology routine

Before starting the treatment, give the person a short foot massage. This helps to release tension in the foot, and allows the person to get used to your touch. You may use a massage oil or cream, but you should blot this off with a towel to prevent your hands from slipping when you are working on the reflexes. At the end of the treatment, massage the feet again. This time, you can leave the oil or cream to sink in. Here the right foot is treated first, then the left.

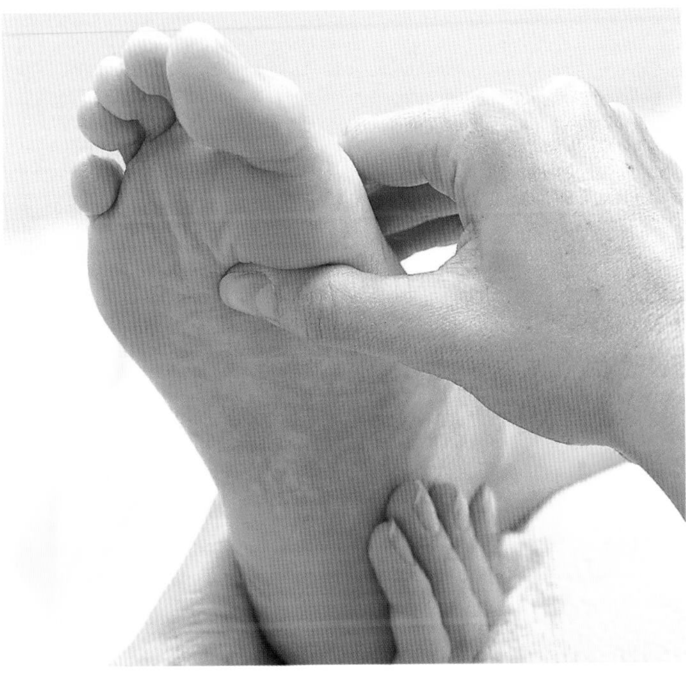

△ 1 **Diaphragm (sole)**
Cup the right heel in your left hand. Place your right thumb on the edge of the foot, so that it is on the big toe side just below the ball. It should be pointing across the foot, towards the inside edge. Now walk the thumb across the sole in a crawling motion, remaining just below the ball. Repeat the movement once more.

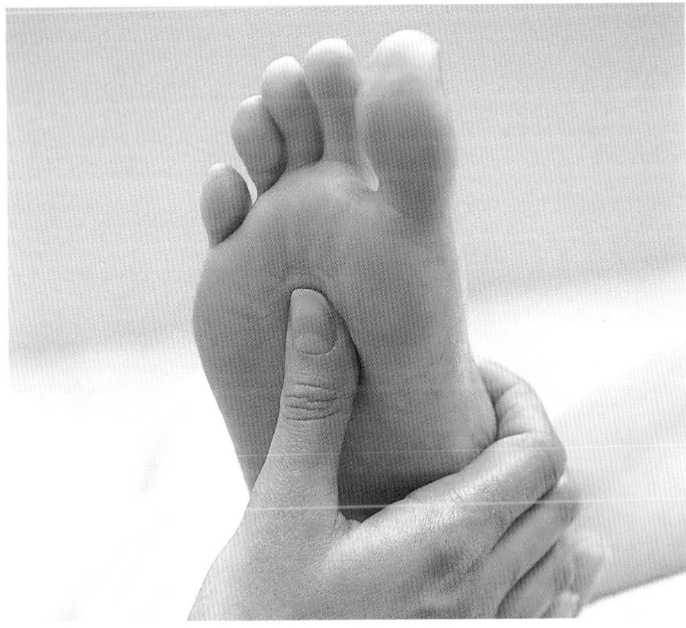

△ 2 **Solar plexus (sole)**
Repeat the action described in step 1, but this time stop when you reach the point directly below toes two and three. Turn the tip of your thumb so that it points towards the toes and press three times on the solar plexus reflex. Then continue the crawl to the outer edge of the foot. Do this movement twice.

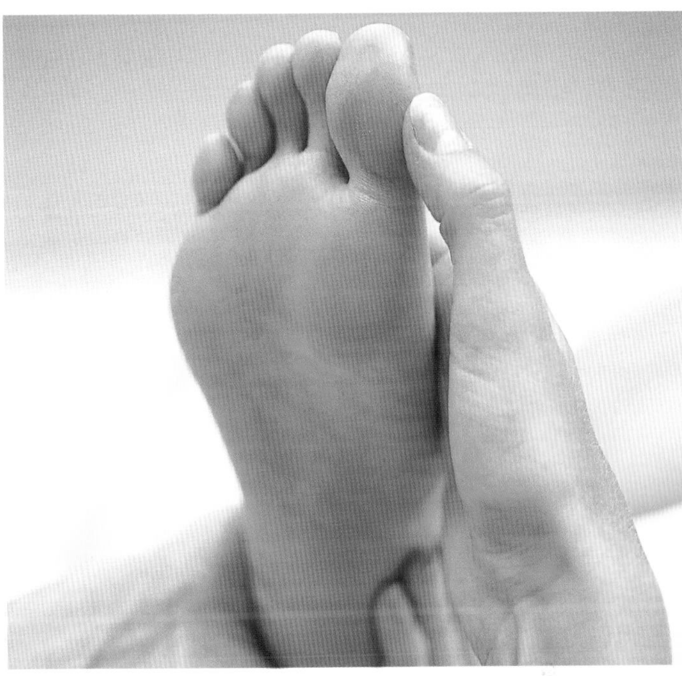

△ 3 **Head and brain (big toe)**
Continue cupping the heel. Use the right thumb to crawl up the outside of the big toe, going over the top and down the inner edge, in a large horseshoe shape. Then crawl up the back of the big toe from the base to the top. Do as many crawls as necessary to cover the entire surface area.

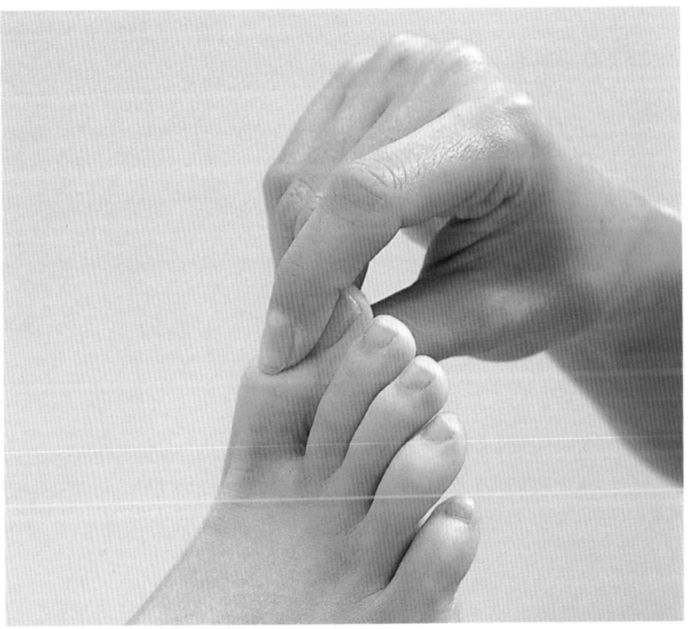

△ 4 **Face (front of big toe)**
Continuing to cup the heel, use the right index finger to crawl down the front of the big toe (finger walking). Use your thumb to keep the toe steady as you do this. Crawl from the top of the toe to the base, and do as many crawls as necessary to cover the entire surface area.

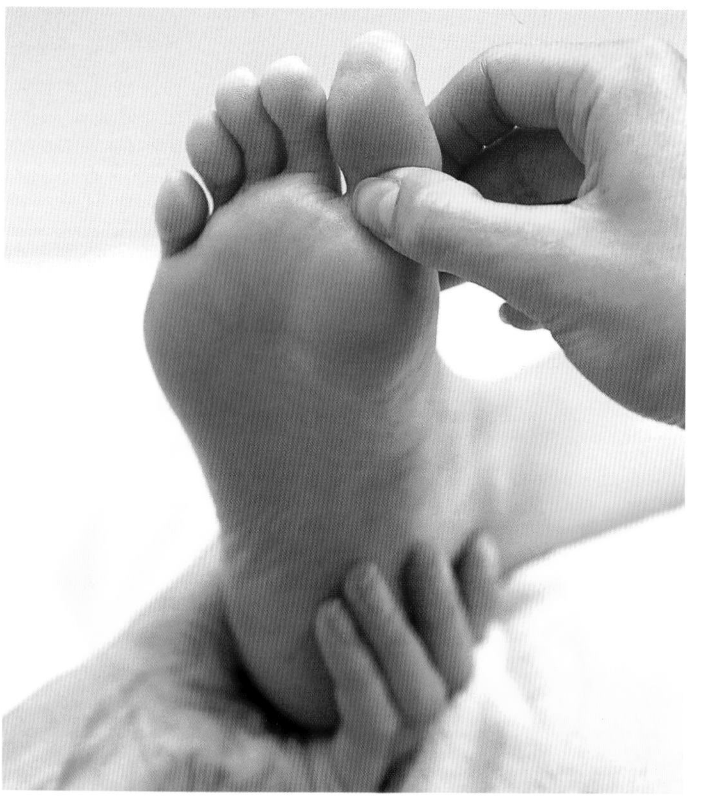

△ 5 **Front and back of neck (base of big toe)**

Place your index finger on the base of the big toe, at the edge of the foot. Finger-walk around the front of the big toe, until you reach the join between the big and second toes. Now use your thumb to crawl around the back of the toe, again starting from the edge of the foot and stopping at the join between the toes.

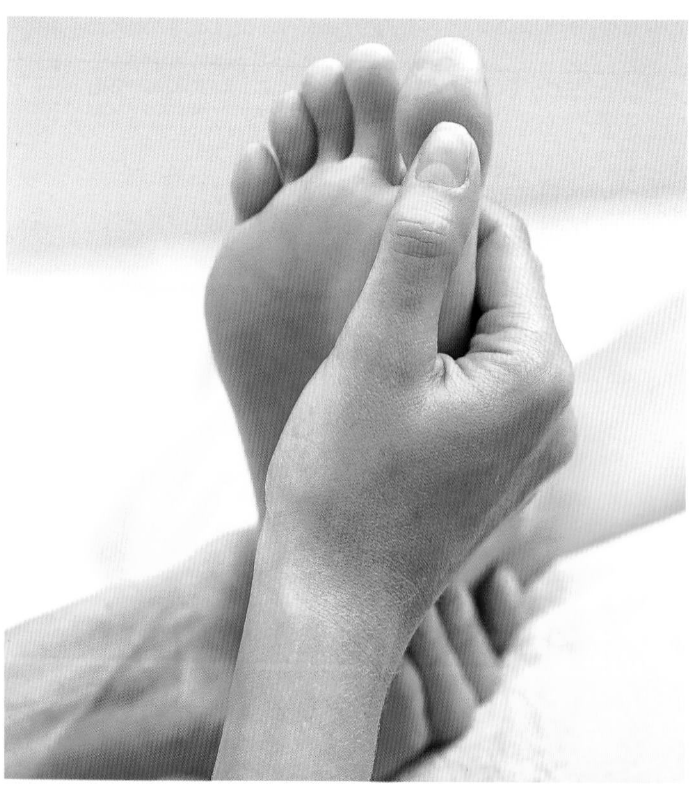

△ 6 **Pituitary (back of big toe)**

Continue cupping the heel. Place your right thumb in the centre of the widest point on the big toe and press deeply on the reflex here three times. **Do not work this point on a woman who is pregnant.**

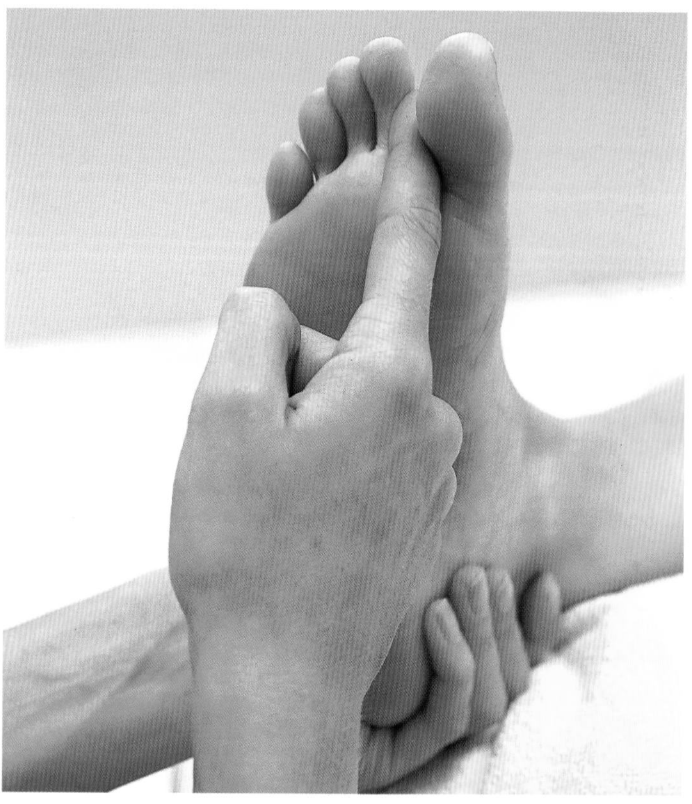

△ 7 **Cranial nerves (four small toes)**

Place your right index finger in-between the big and second toes, angling it towards the second toe. Finger-walk up the second toe and down the other side, making a horseshoe shape. Finger-walk over the next three toes in the same way. Now repeat the whole movement.

treating between meals

You should not give reflexology to someone who has eaten a heavy meal within the last two or three hours. On the other hand, a person should not have reflexology treatment on an empty stomach, as their energy levels will be depleted and they will not respond to the treatment as well as they should. If the person that you are treating has not eaten for several hours, or if he or she is hungry, offer a small snack such as juice and biscuits before starting the routine.

▽ **A glass of orange juice and a couple of biscuits will help to boost the person's energy before a reflexology treatment.**

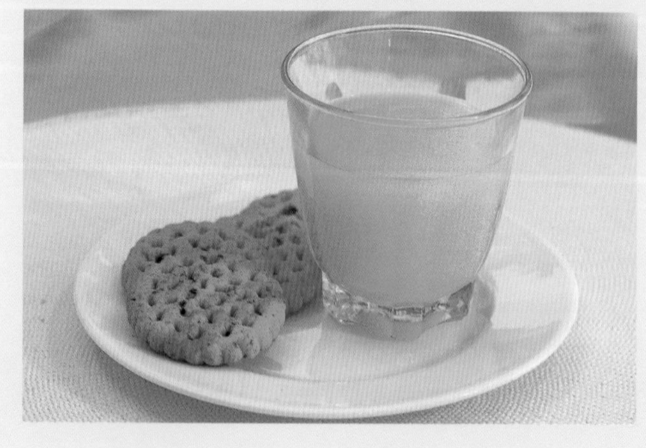

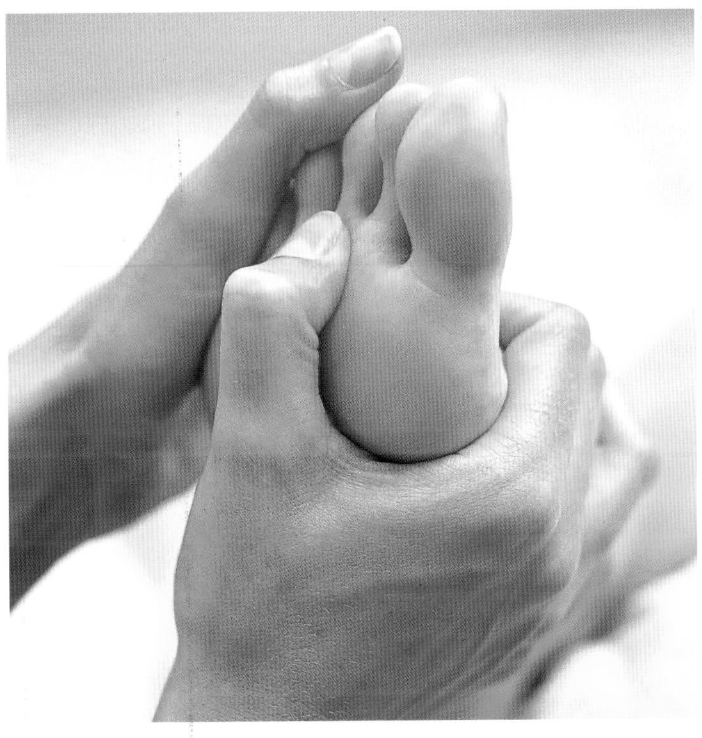

△ **8 Sinuses, teeth and gums (back and front of four small toes)**
Support the toes with your left hand. Thumb-walk up the back of each toe: start at the base and crawl up the centre-line to the top. Repeat the movement, but pause when you reach the fleshy bulb of each toe, press in and slide the thumb up to the top. Now, use your index finger to walk down the front of each toe – start at the top and support the base of the toe. Do as many crawls as needed to cover the area.

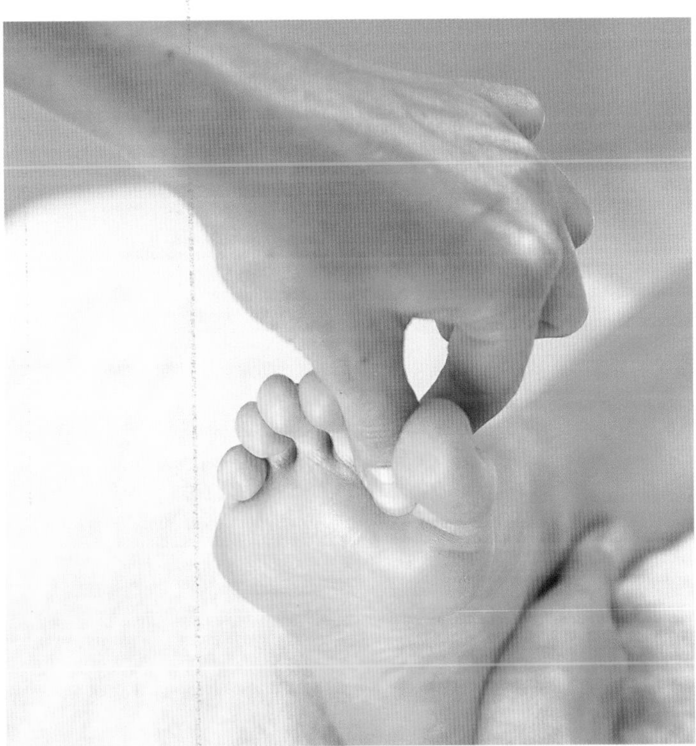

△ **9 Lymphatic glands (webbing between toes)**
Support the foot by cupping the heel. Use your index finger and thumb to pinch and release the webbing between the big and second toes. Repeat on the webbing of the other toes in turn, working gently. Now place your index finger between the big toe and second toe. Slide the finger down the groove on the top of the foot, by a distance of about half its length. Draw back along the same groove.

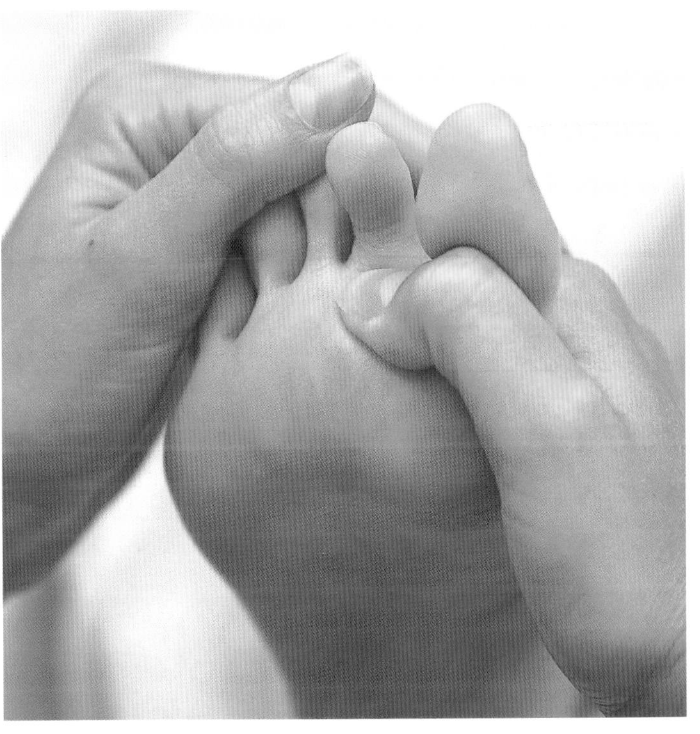

△ **10 Eyes and ears (under the toes on the sole)**
Use your left hand to hold the tops of the toes and bend them back slightly; this exposes the ridge on the sole underneath the toes. Starting on the inner edge of the foot, use the right thumb to crawl along the ridge to the outer edge. Exert a good downward pressure as you thumb-walk. The eye reflex is located under toes two and three, while the ear reflex is under toes four and five.

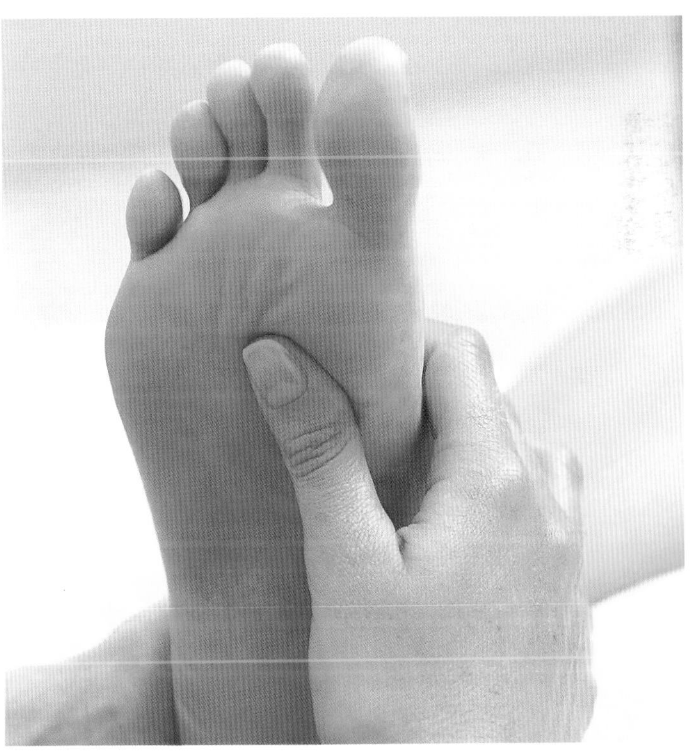

△ **11 Thyroid, parathyroid, thymus (sole)**
Cup the heel in your left hand again. Use the thumb of the right hand to crawl along the diaphragm line, which runs across the foot at the base of the ball: start at the inner edge of the foot and thumb-walk until you are directly in line with the point between the big and second toe. Turn the thumb to point upwards, and thumb-walk up until you reach the base of the toes.

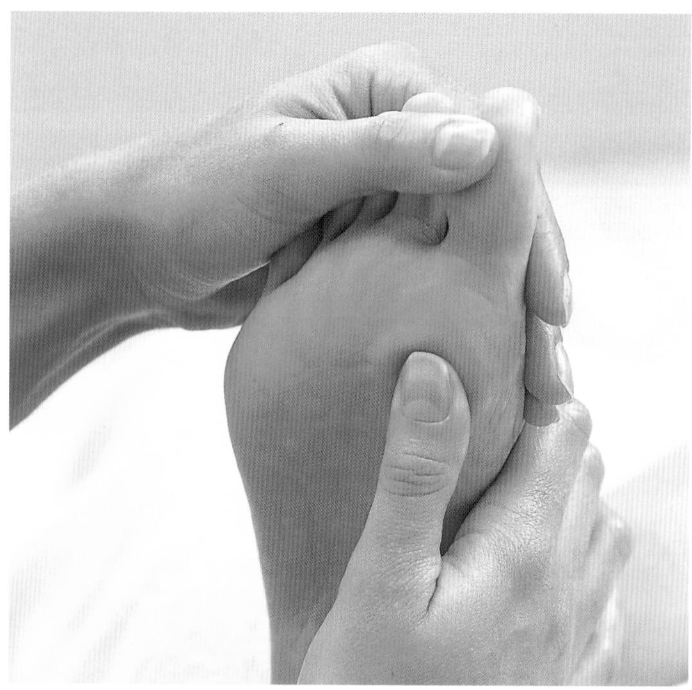

△ **12 Oesophagus, chest, lungs, heart, shoulder (sole)**
Now gently grasp the top of the toes. Place your right thumb on the diaphragm line at the edge of the foot; this thumb should be pointing up, towards the big toe. Using your thumb, make crawling movements up the ball of the foot to the base of the big toe. Do as many crawls as necessary to cover the area. Now, work in the same way to cover the area of the ball of the foot from toe two to toe four. Finally, cover the area under the little toe.

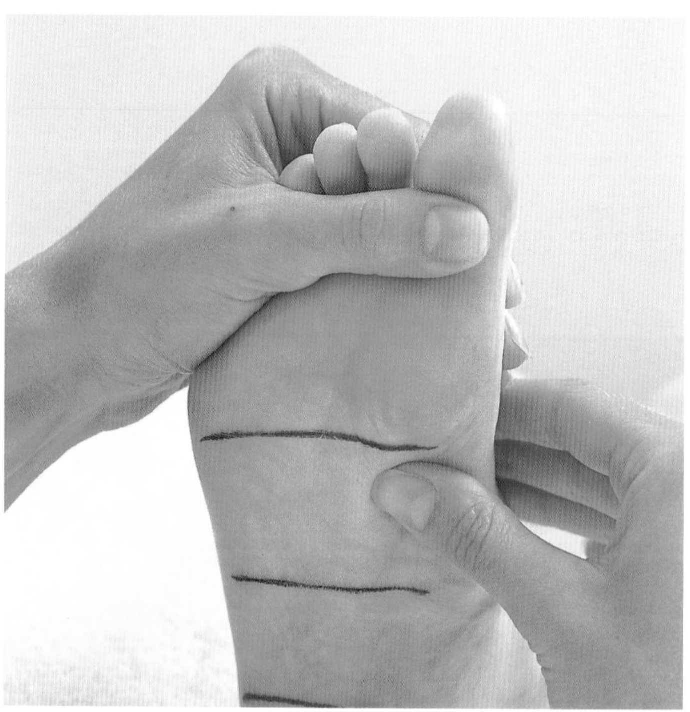

△ **13 Upper abdominal area (sole)**
The upper abdomen reflex is located between the diaphragm line and the waist line, which is in the arch of the foot (marked above). Use the right thumb to crawl across the foot from the inner edge to the outer edge. Repeat the movement as many times as you need to in order to cover the entire area twice. The reflexes for the liver, gall bladder and duodenum reflex are in this area on the right foot; the stomach, pancreas and spleen reflexes are on the left foot.

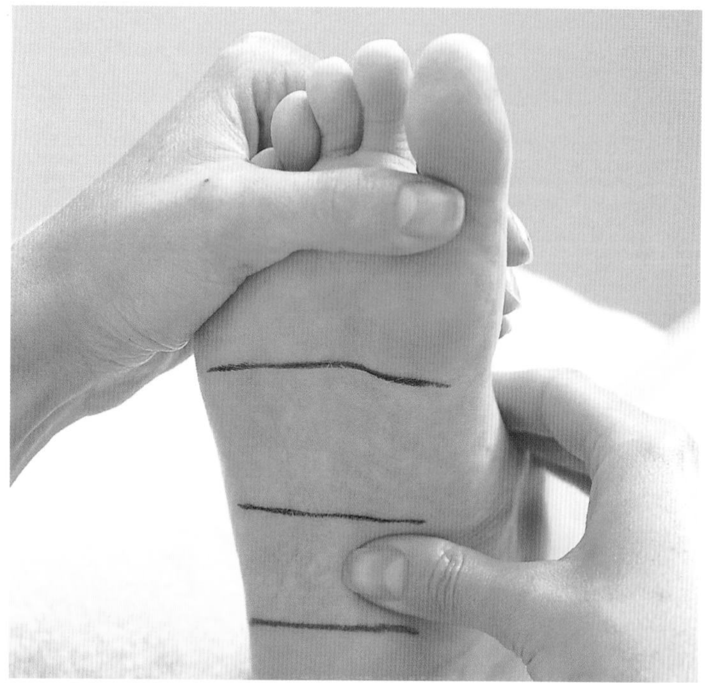

△ **14 Lower abdominal area (sole)**
Here you work in the same way as for Step 13, but you cover the area between the arch (waist line) and the edge of the heel pad (the pelvic floor line.) Again, crawl with the right thumb across the foot as many times as necessary to treat the area. Do the movement twice. The reflex for the small intestine is in this area.

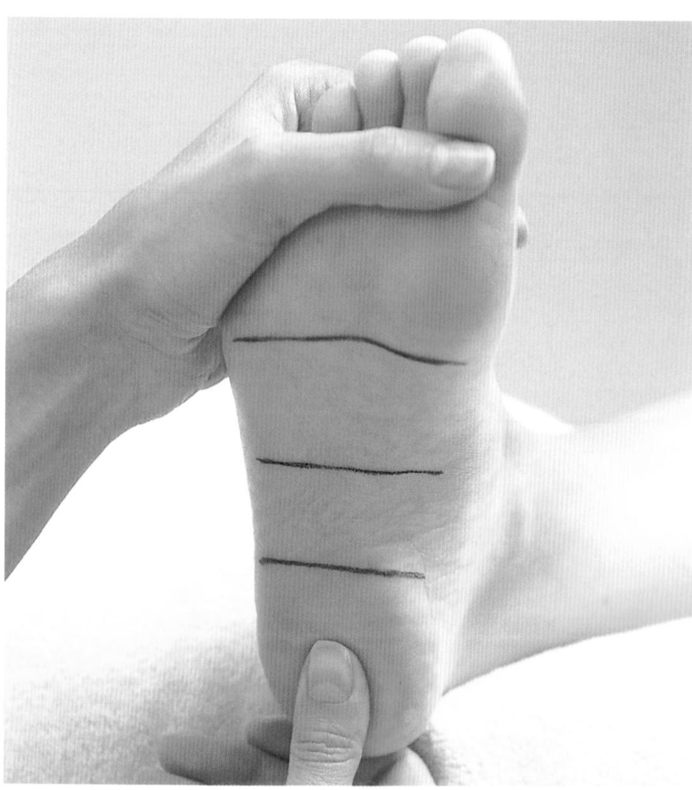

△ **15 Lower back pelvic and sciatic (sole)**
Continue to support the foot at the toes. Start at the back of the foot, and use the right thumb to crawl up through the heel pad, stopping when you reach the soft flesh. Use as many crawls as needed to cover the entire pad, always working in the same direction. Now, place the thumb on the inner edge of the heel, so that it points across to the outer edge. Crawl across the heel as many times as necessary to cover the entire area.

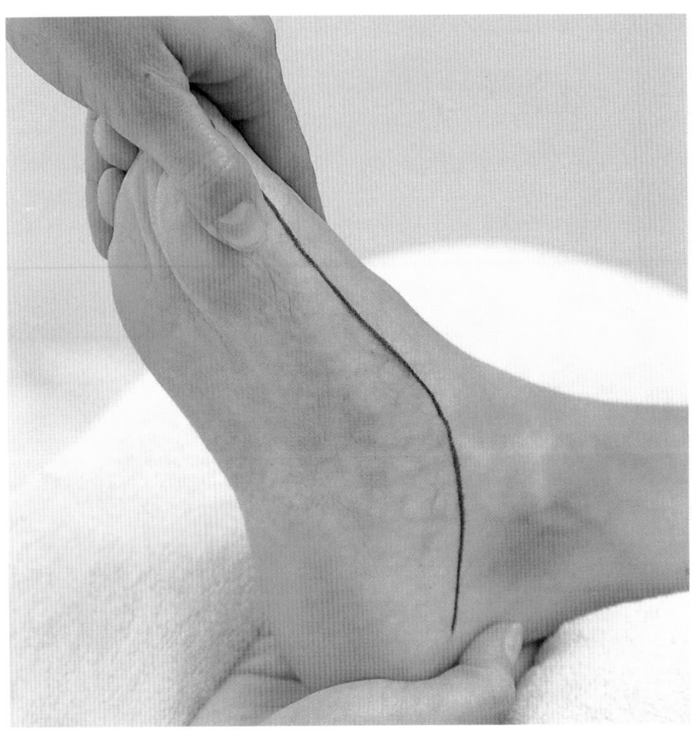

△ **16 Spine (inner edge of the foot)**
Cup the heel with your right hand. Crawl the left thumb down the inner edge of the foot. Start from the first joint of the big toe and work to the heel, following the bone (as marked above). Change hands and crawl back upwards, this time pressing upwards into the bone as you crawl. Do the movement twice in both directions. Most conditions benefit from work to the spine, because nerves run from here to all areas of the body.

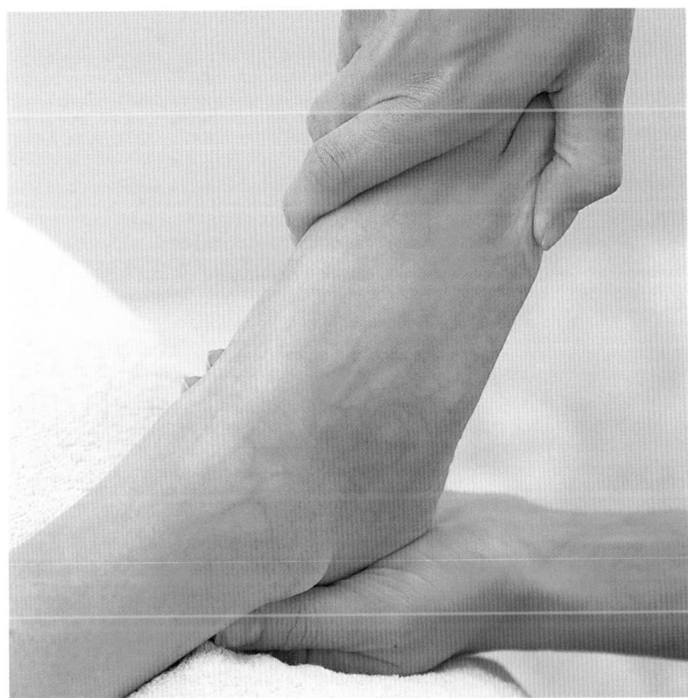

△ **17 Shoulder, hip and knee (outside edge of the foot)**
Now cup the heel firmly but gently in your left hand. Thumb-walk right down the length of the outside edge of the foot, from the base of the little toe to the heel. Then work back up to the toe along the same line. Do this movement twice in both directions. It is important to work this area of the foot thoroughly as you are treating three very different parts of the body.

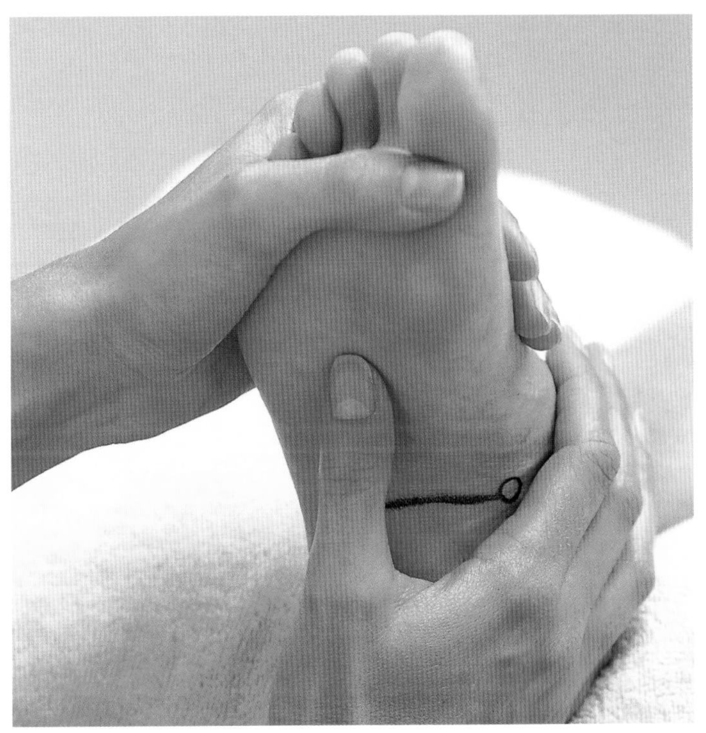

△ **18 Kidney (sole)**
Support the foot by gently holding the base of the toes. Put your right thumb on the waist area, which crosses the centre of the arch; the tip should be pointing towards the join between toes two and three. Make one tiny crawl up the foot; this is the kidney reflex. Press twice, rotating the thumb as you do so (pressure circling). Release the pressure for a second, then make two further pressure circles on the same point.

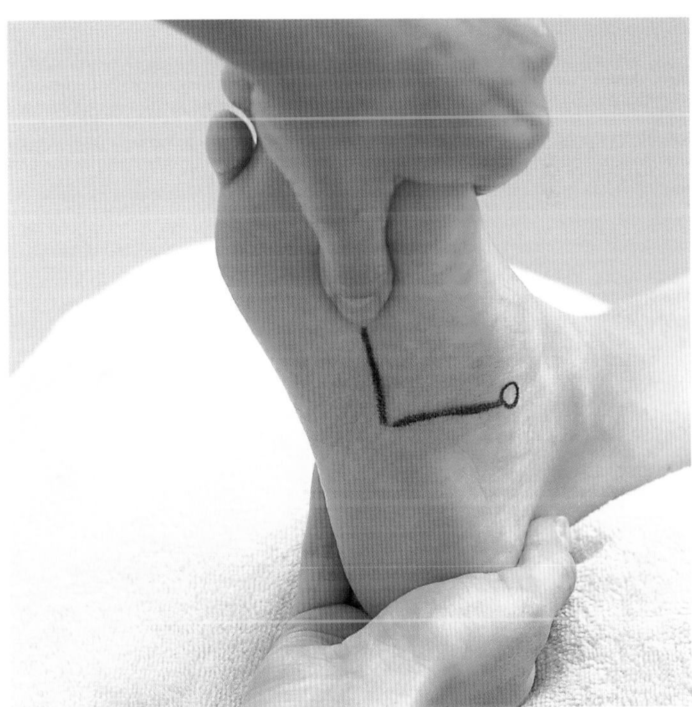

△ **19 Ureter and bladder (sole)**
Now use the right hand to cup the heel. Turn the left thumb to point towards the heel and crawl down the ureter reflex to the line where the heel pad and the soft flesh of the foot meet (as marked). Now, turn the thumb again and crawl up on to the inner side of the foot. You will reach a soft, fleshy mound, which is the bladder reflex (circled). Press on this point three times.

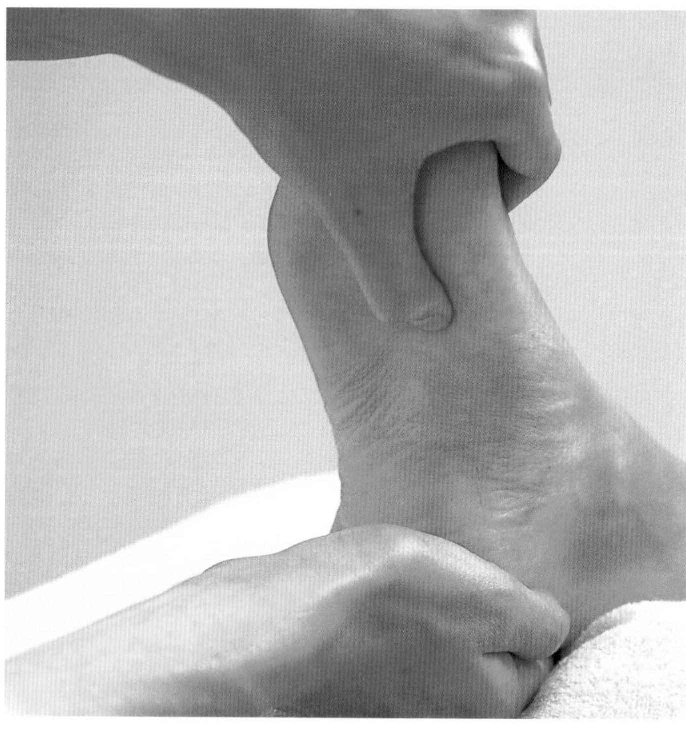

△ **20 Adrenal gland (sole)**

Continuing to cup the heel with the right hand, place your left thumb on the kidney reflex again. Move the thumb across the foot so that it is directly below the second toe. Turn the thumb around so that it is pointing towards the heel, then hook into the flesh and pull back towards the toes. Do three distinct hook-in and back movements on this point.

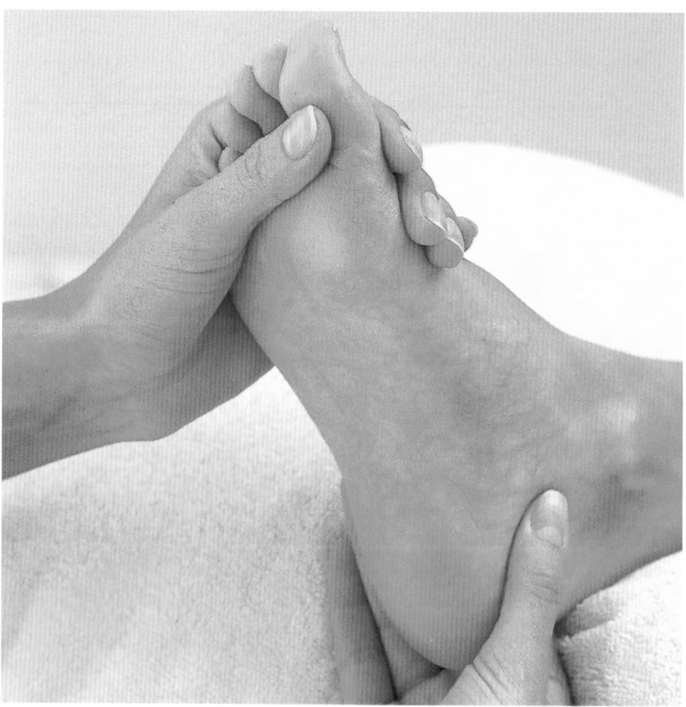

△ **21 Uterus (female) or prostate (male) (inner side)**

Hold the toes with your one hand (whichever feels easiest to you). With the other hand, place the thumb midway along an imaginary line running between the ankle bone on the inside of the foot and the back corner of the heel. Press this point three times. As you press, rotate the thumb slightly (pressure circling) so that you are covering an area the size of a large coin. **Gently stroke rather than press the area if you are treating a woman who is pregnant or has an IUD fitted.**

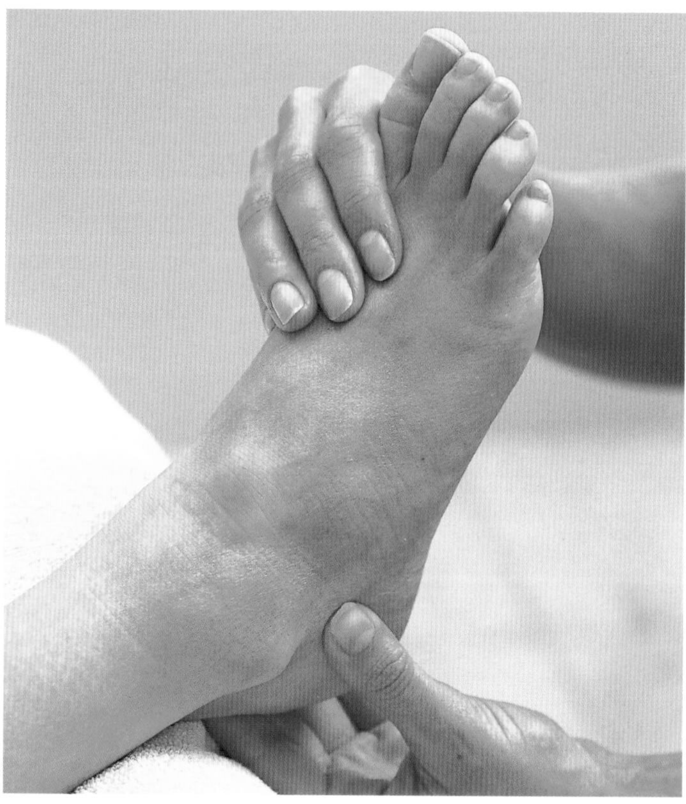

△ **22 Ovaries (female) or testes (male) (outer edge of foot)**

Find the same midpoint on the outer side of the foot. Press in the same way. (You may find it easier to swap your hands over.) **Stroke rather than press this area if you are treating a woman who is pregnant.**

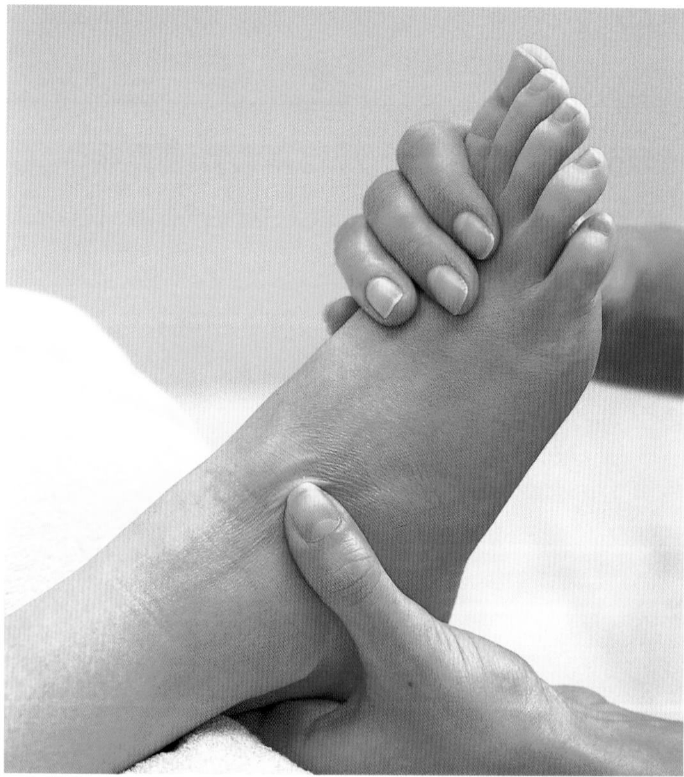

△ **23 Fallopian tube (female), vas deferens (male) (top of foot)**

Continuing to hold the toes with one hand, use the thumb of the other hand to crawl across the top of the foot on the crease line between the leg and foot. Work from the outside ankle area to the inner ankle area. Repeat.

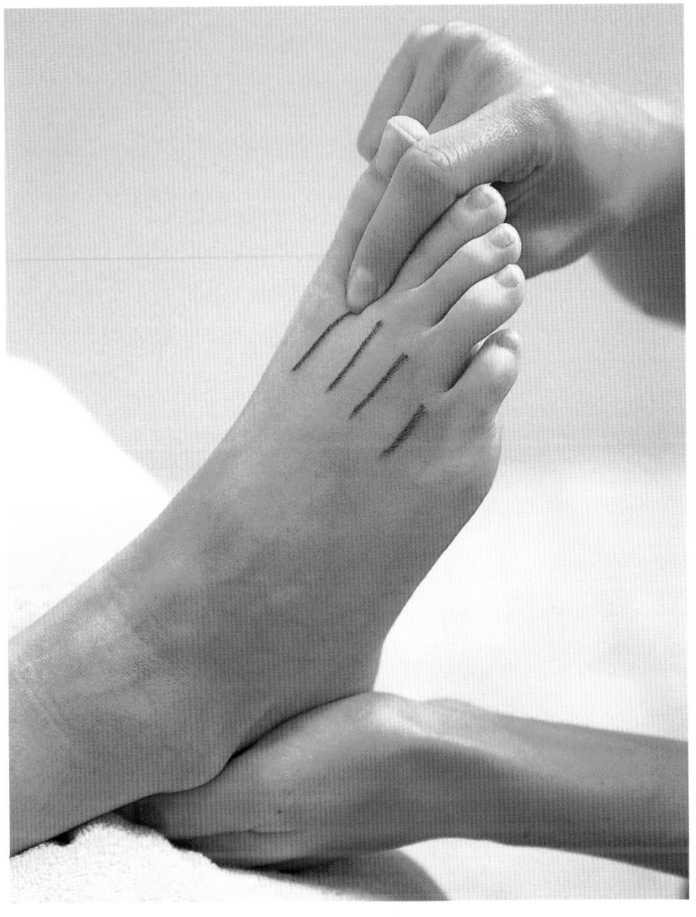

△ **24 Breast area (top of foot, at base of toes)**
Cupping the heel in your left hand, use the index finger of the right hand to crawl down the top of the foot from the base of the toes to a point corresponding with the diaphragm line (the base of the ball). Now, crawl backwards over the same area. Do as many crawls as needed to cover the breast reflex, which starts between the big and second toes and ends between the fourth and little toes. Repeat steps 1-24 on the left foot, then bring both feet together to finish.

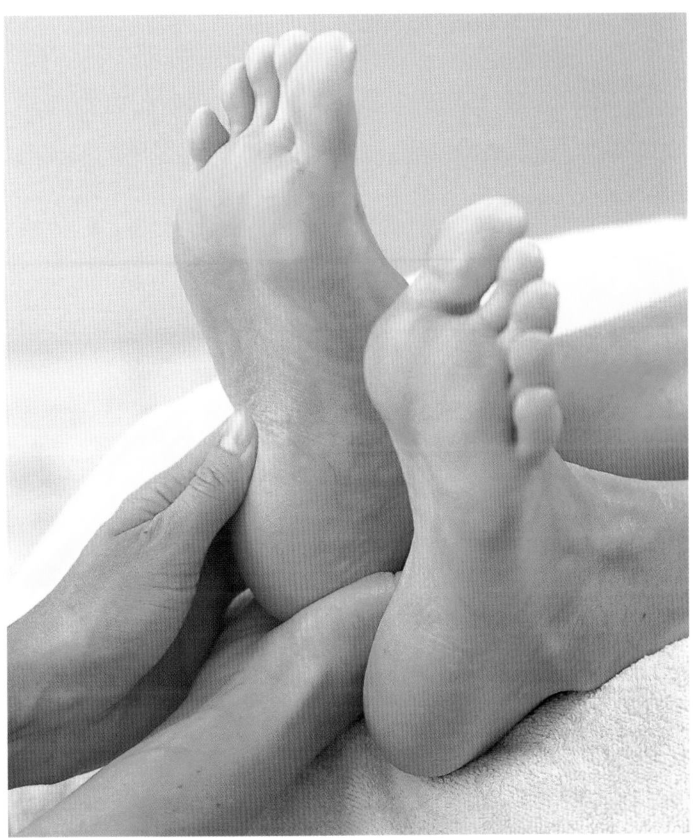

△ **25 Colon/large intestine (soles of both feet)**
Start at the edge of the right heel, in line with the join between toes four and five. Thumb walk up the right sole to the middle of the foot. Now thumb-walk across both feet until you are in line with toes four and five on the left foot. Crawl down to the left heel pad, then a little way across the foot until the thumb is in line with toes three and four. Turn the thumb to point towards the heel and make three deep pressure circles here. Crawl to the inside of the left foot, make two pressure circles, then crawl down about two-thirds of the heel – to the anus reflex. Make three deep pressure circles. Repeat the movement three times.

treating with care

Being able to offer friends and family a reflexology treatment is very satisfying. However, it is important to be sure that you are treating people safely and responsibly. Always ask if someone has any major illnesses. If so, it is probably wisest to offer a gentle massage rather than reflexology. Similarly, if the person is experiencing any severe or unusual symptoms, advise him or her to get a diagnosis and treatment from a doctor before giving reflexology. People with conditions such as arthritis can benefit from reflexology, but they should ideally check with their doctor before receiving treatment, and you should always work very gently.

If treating a woman, check whether there is any chance that she is pregnant. Do not treat a pregnant woman in the first three months, or if she has experienced any problems. Some points must not be pressed at all during pregnancy.

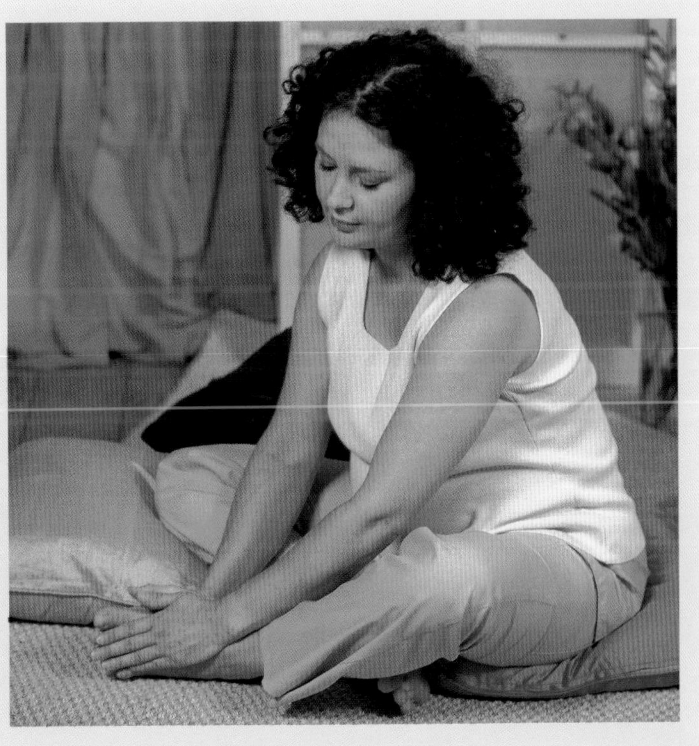

▷ **Reflexology can help to alleviate some of the common symptoms of pregnancy. However, you should not treat if the pregnancy is unstable.**

For Pleasure and Relaxation

Your feet can transport you into realms of pleasure. They are one of the most sensual and sensitive parts of your body, and a loving touch applied here can be wonderfully relaxing, energizing or stimulating. Here are some fabulous foot treatments that will soothe your spirits, and restore your soul.

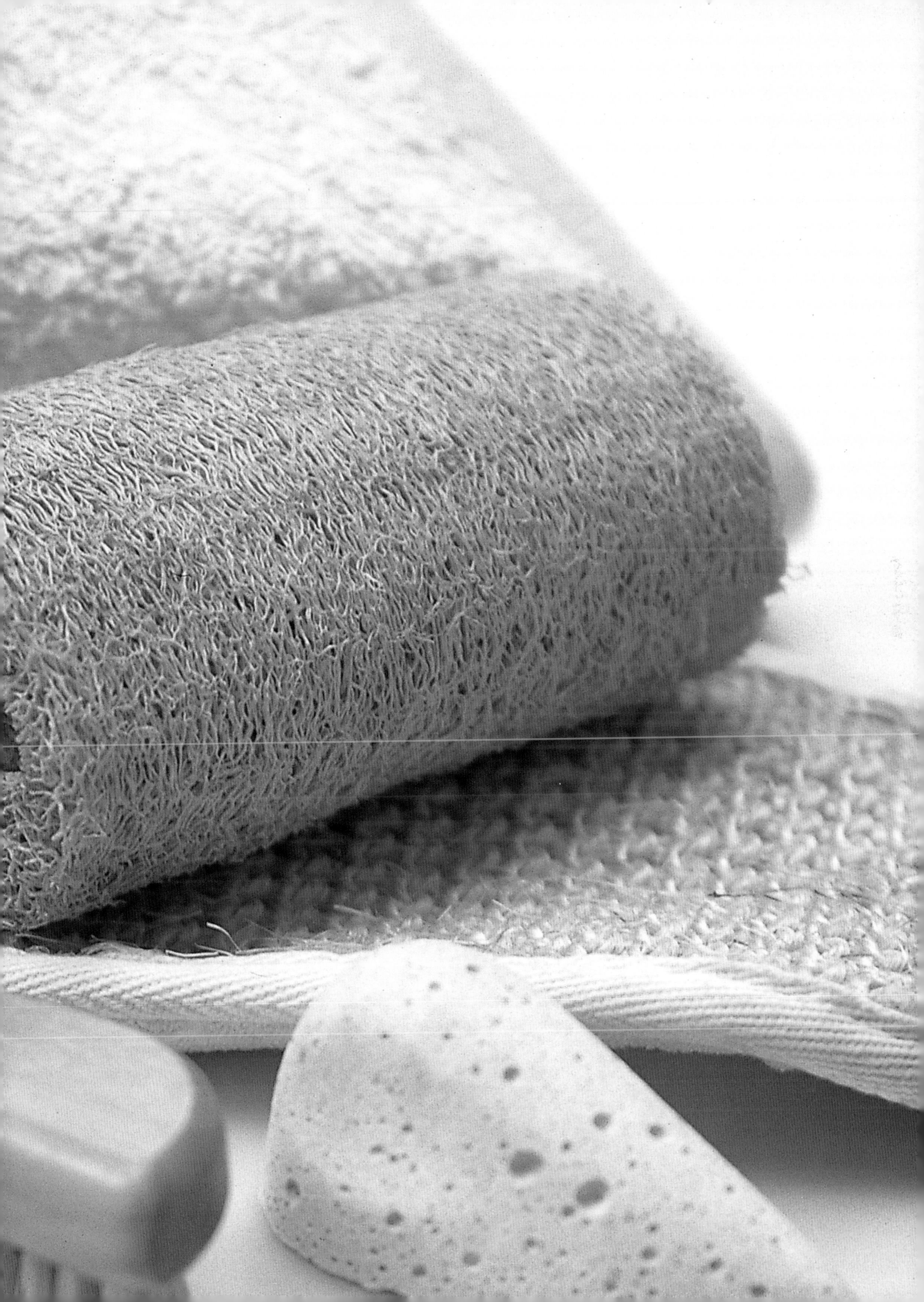

Start the day massage

The ancient Greeks believed that a daily massage was one of the best ways of keeping the body healthy. Few of us have time for a full treatment, but a quick self-massage for the feet is a great way to start the day. This routine is designed to be relaxing yet invigorating – a real wake-up call.

▽ It's worth getting up 15 minutes early so that you can enjoy a relaxing start to the day. A foot massage doesn't take long, but it can make all the difference to the way you feel.

wake-up routine

Ideally you will be relaxed before starting this sequence. However, don't worry if you wake up feeling anxious; you will find it almost impossible to remain so once the massage is underway. Start with the right foot, then repeat on the left.

▷ **1** To start, get into a comfortable position in a peaceful spot. Have a glass of juice and some fruit on hand to enjoy after the massage. Choose a favourite cream or essential oil blend to apply to the feet – they should have reasonable slip but should not be dripping.

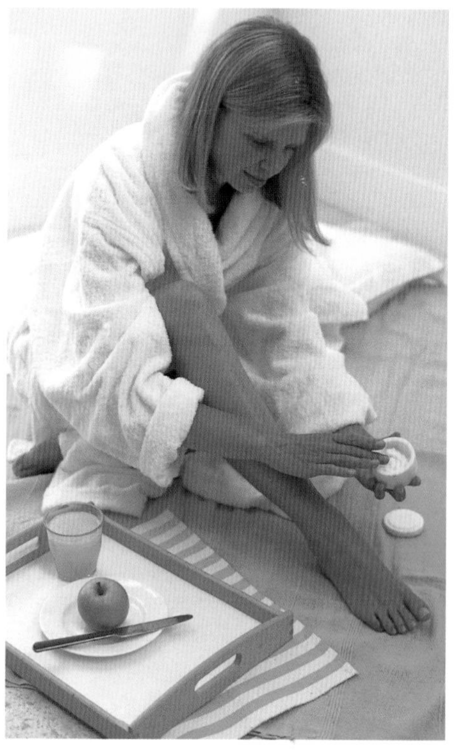

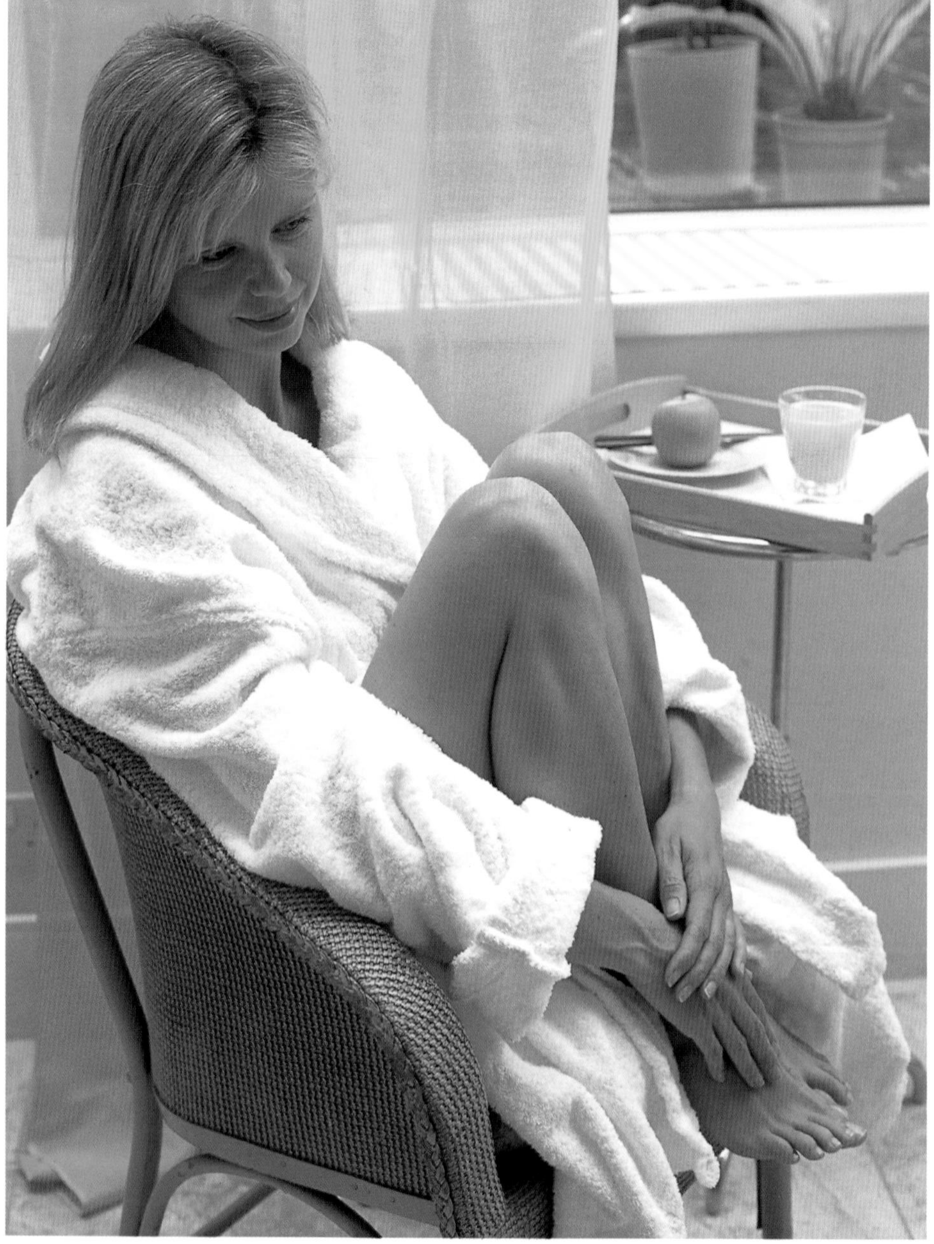

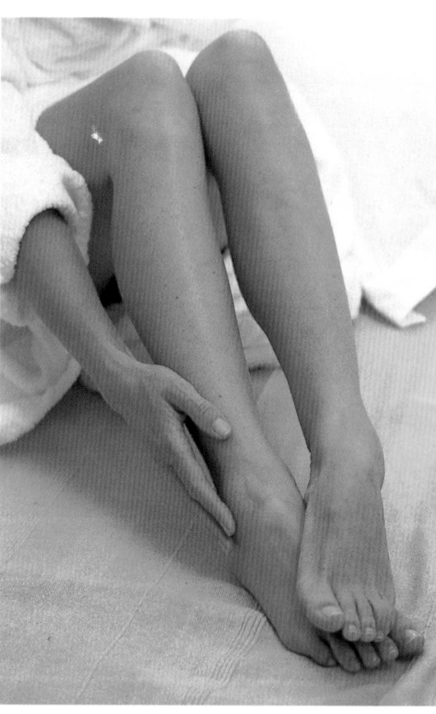

△ **2** Use your fingers to rub the cream or oil liberally over the top of the right foot. Then place your left foot on top, and use the sole to massage from the toes to ankle. Apply heavier pressure on the toes than to the top of the foot, which is more delicate. Take particular care around the ankle area.

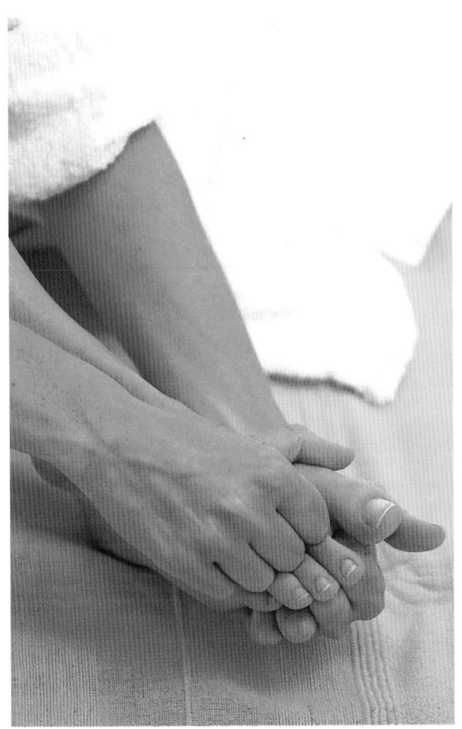

△ **3** Now smooth the cream or massage oil all over your toes. Make loose fists with both of your hands, and place the left one underneath your toes, with the right one on top. Slowly but decisively slide your knuckles across each toe in turn – from the big toe to the little one. You should keep the pressure firm, but it should not be painful.

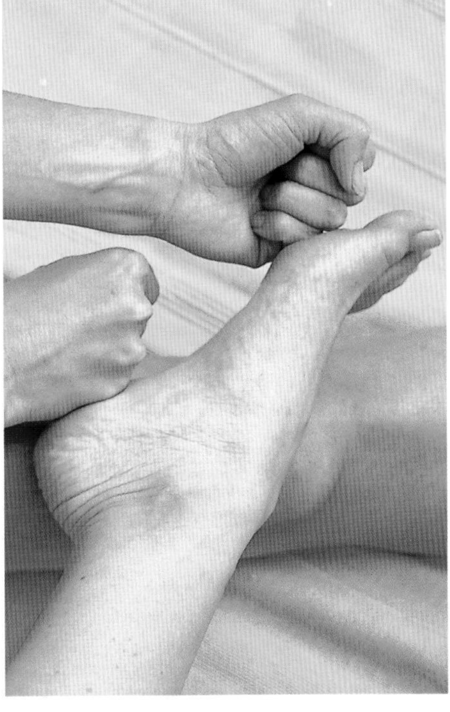

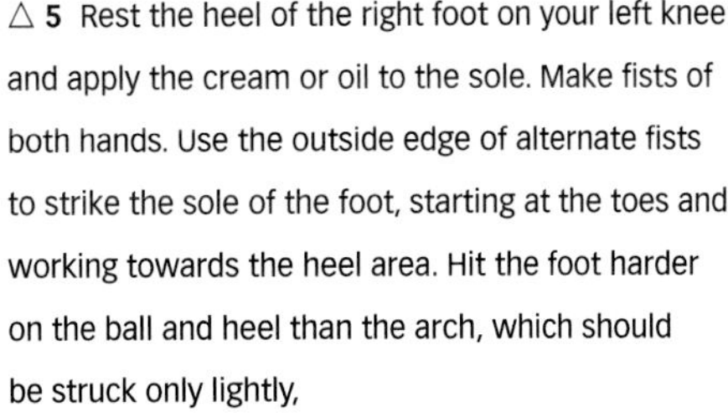

△ **5** Rest the heel of the right foot on your left knee and apply the cream or oil to the sole. Make fists of both hands. Use the outside edge of alternate fists to strike the sole of the foot, starting at the toes and working towards the heel area. Hit the foot harder on the ball and heel than the arch, which should be struck only lightly,

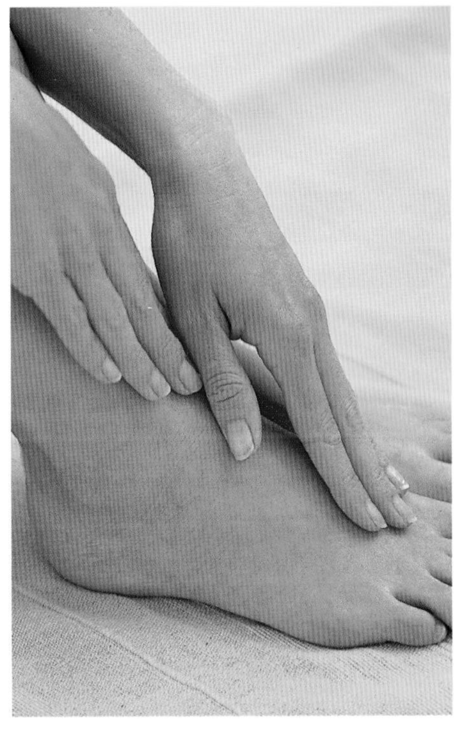

△ **6** Add more oil or cream to your hands, then rub the palms together to spread it evenly. Use alternate hands to stroke the top of the foot, starting from the toes and working down to the ankle. Begin with a feather-light touch to encourage relaxation, and then increase the pressure to a strong energizing level. Keep it pleasurable at all times.

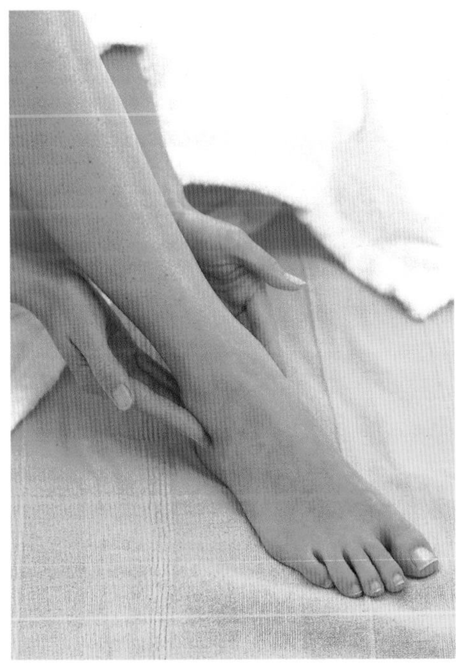

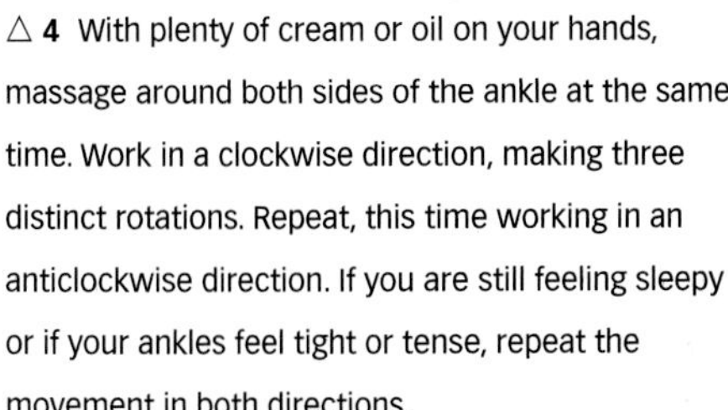

△ **4** With plenty of cream or oil on your hands, massage around both sides of the ankle at the same time. Work in a clockwise direction, making three distinct rotations. Repeat, this time working in an anticlockwise direction. If you are still feeling sleepy or if your ankles feel tight or tense, repeat the movement in both directions.

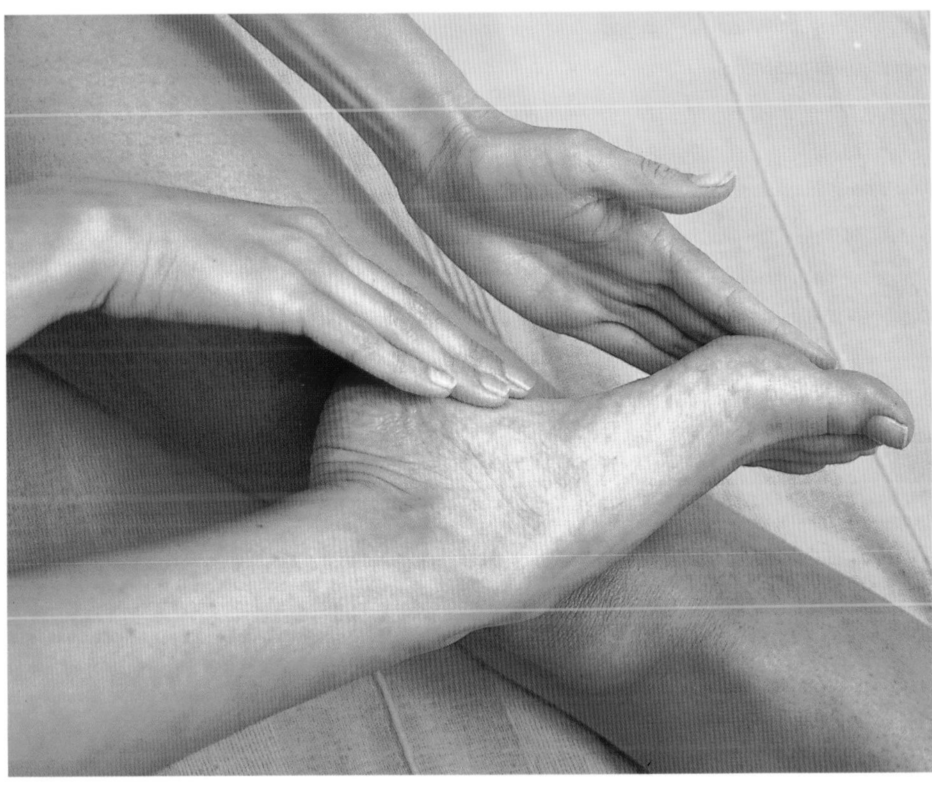

△ **7** Now rest the heel on your left knee, exposing the sole. Add a little more oil or cream to your hands and rub the palms together to spread it evenly through them. Use alternate hands to make long sweeping strokes down your foot from the toes to the heel. Again, start with light touch to aid relaxation, then gradually increase the pressure. Now repeat the sequence on the left foot.

Recharge your batteries

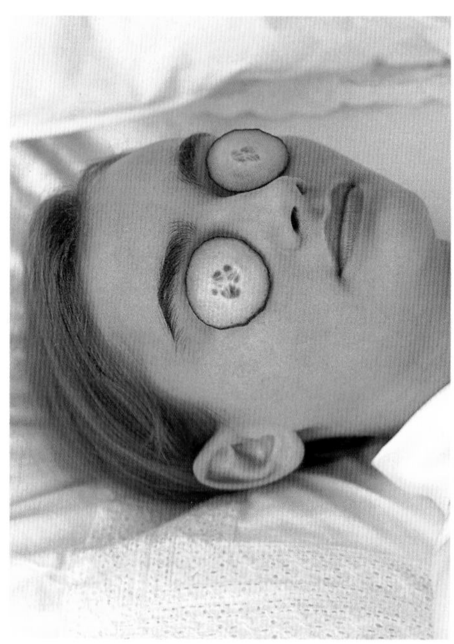

◁ Slices of cucumber or potato placed over the eyes while your feet are being massaged will enhance the general revitalizing effect.

Most of us don't have enough time in our lives to relax and recharge. Ideally, we should stop and rest whenever we feel tired or low in energy, but we often need to keep going because of work, home or social commitments.

This treatment is designed to soothe and revitalize at the same time, so it should leave the recipient feeling refreshed and energized. It is an excellent treatment to do if someone is going out in the evening after a hard day at work, or in the middle of a busy or stressful week.

The routine can easily be adapted for self-treatment – and used as an instant pick-me-up wherever you happen to be. It is great for days when you can't stop – but feel you can't go on.

the power of silence

Try to work in silence except when you need to ask for and receive feedback – a few minutes of calm can help to increase the restorative effect of this massage. The person you are treating may like to cover his or her eyes with slices of cucumber or raw potato; these will have a restorative effect, and closing the eyes will also reduce any temptation to chat.

Give the recipient a glass of water to sip before and after the massage – dehydration can increase feelings of fatigue. It is also good to eat a small snack – a piece of fresh fruit would be ideal – to boost energy levels. If possible, he or she should take a short walk in the fresh air after doing the routine.

revitalizing routine

Make sure the recipient is sitting comfortably. Suggest that he or she takes a few moments to relax the shoulders and face muscles, and to take a few deep breaths before you start.

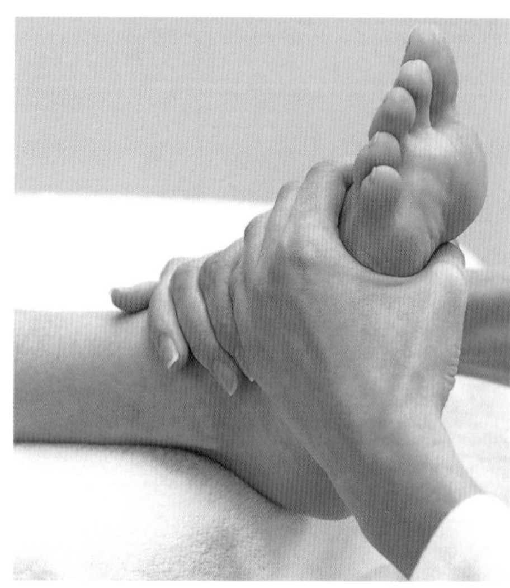

△ **1** Stroke the sole and top of the right foot, using alternate hands. Cover the foot three times or more. Now place your thumbs on the sole and the fingers on the top, one hand slightly above the other. Move the hands in opposite directions, in a gentle twisting action – as if wringing out a wet cloth. Start near the ankle and work up to the toes, then work back down the foot. Repeat the action once more.

tonic massage cream

This thick cream works well with the revitalizing routine, and it is suitable for any skin type. Made in the following quantity, it will last for about 12 treatments. You can substitute other essential oils for the peppermint and petitgrain if you like. Try cypress and lemon to aid detoxing, rose and mandarin for total indulgence, or rosemary and geranium for an uplifting effect.

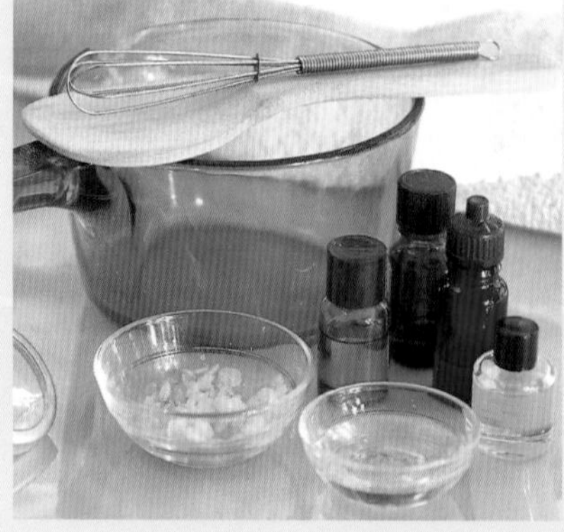

△ **You can make a superb massage cream using just a few natural ingredients.**

ingredients

- 20ml/4 tsp almond oil
- 40ml/8 tsp avocado oil
- 20ml/4 tsp rosewater
- 5ml/1 tsp lecithin granules
- 10g/¼fl oz beeswax
- 8 drops each petitgrain and peppermint essential oils

Put the almond oil, avocado oil and beeswax into a ceramic or stainless steel jug. Stand in a saucepan that is half-filled with water. Heat on a low temperature, stirring occasionally until the wax melts. Remove the jug from the water. Add the lecithin and beat the mixture vigorously, then stir in the rosewater. Allow the mixture to cool (but not to become completely cold). Now mix in the essential oils. Scrape the cream into a clean, screwtop jar.

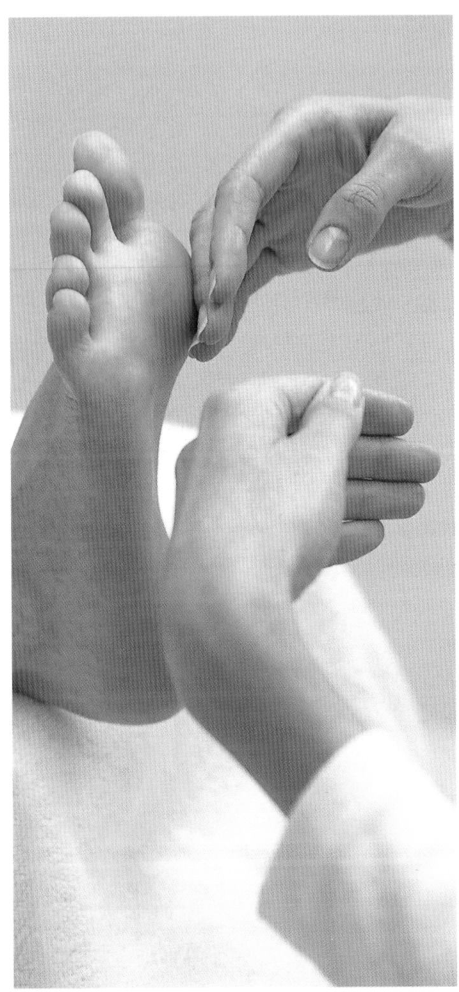

△ **2** Briskly but lightly, use your palms to slap all over the top of the foot, working from the ankle to the toes. Then use the back of your hands to slap all over the sole – the pressure can be heavier here. Do this a few times. It helps to increase the circulation, removing toxins and bringing nutrients and oxygen to the area.

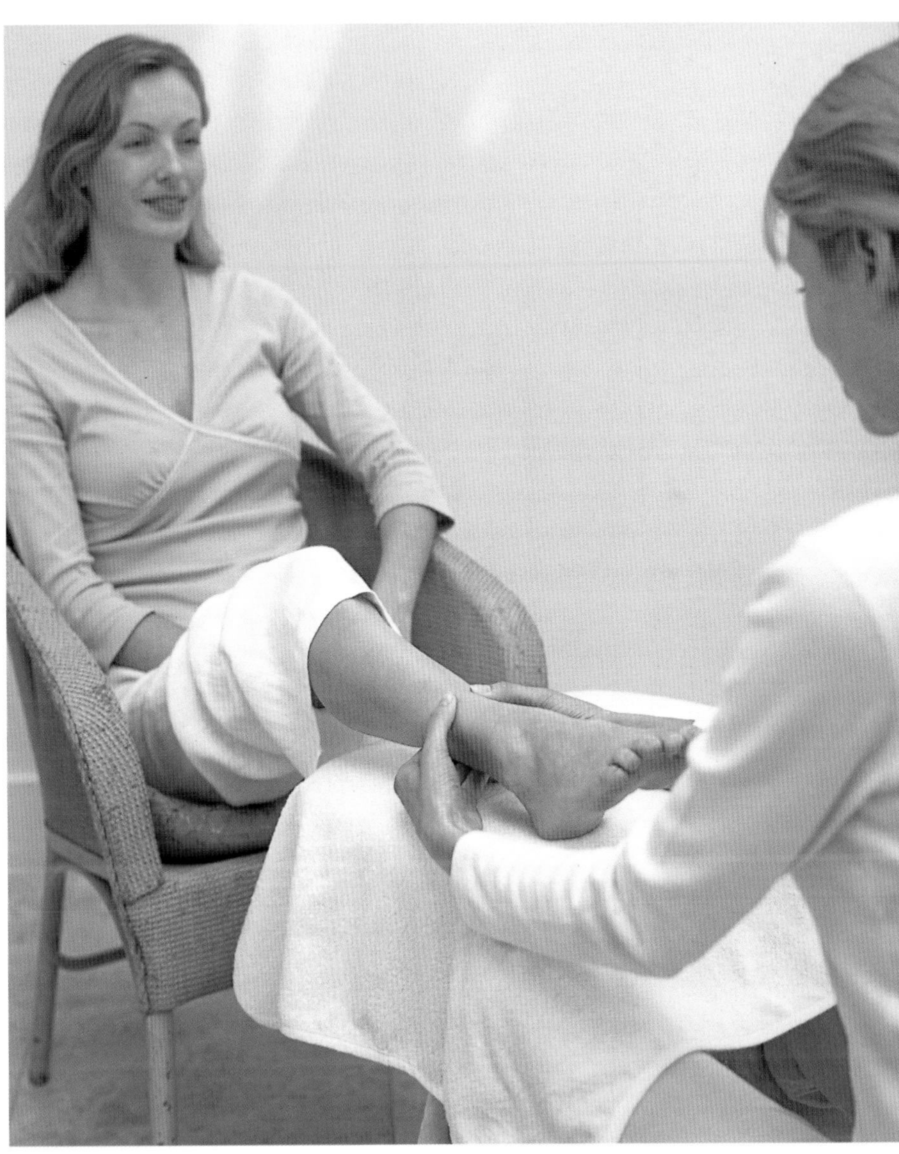

△ **4** Place your thumbs either side of the shinbone. Use the tips to massage, making little circles. Work up the leg from the ankle to the knee. Slide the hands back down to the ankle, without applying any pressure. Repeat.

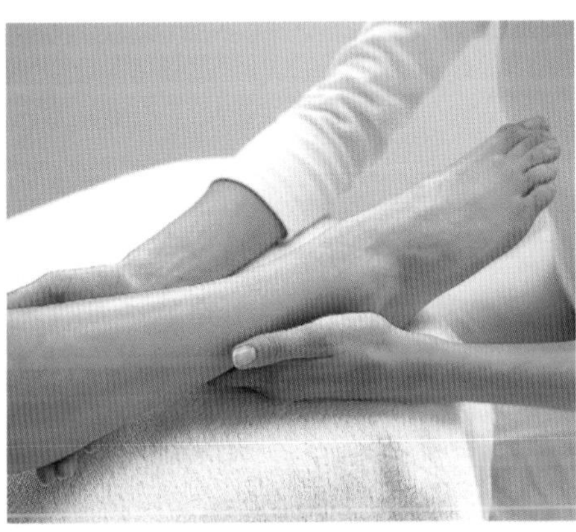

△ **3** Hold the foot behind the ankle to keep it steady. Cup the other hand around the calf muscle, then squeeze and release. Start from just above the ankle and work up the leg to just below the knee, squeezing every part of the muscle. Now slide your hand back to the ankle and work up the leg in the same way twice more. Tension often collects in the calves, and this is a good way to release it.

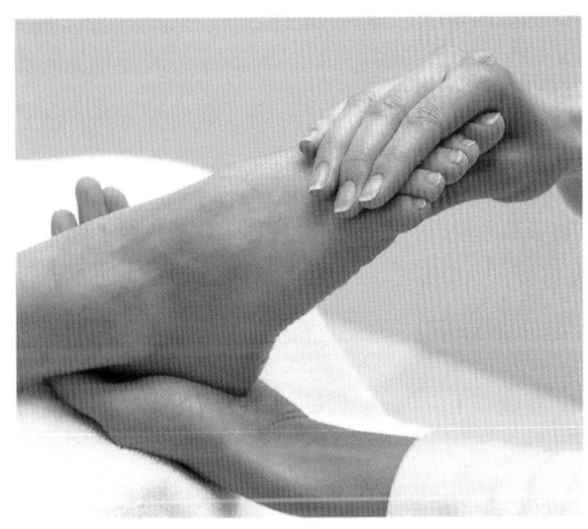

△ **5** Cup a hand around the heel to support the foot, while resting your other hand against the base of the toes. Gently push the foot away from you three times – remember that you should never push it further than it will go naturally. Now do a forward stretch (shown): place the hand on top of the foot near the toes and pull them gently towards you. Do this pulling movement three times.

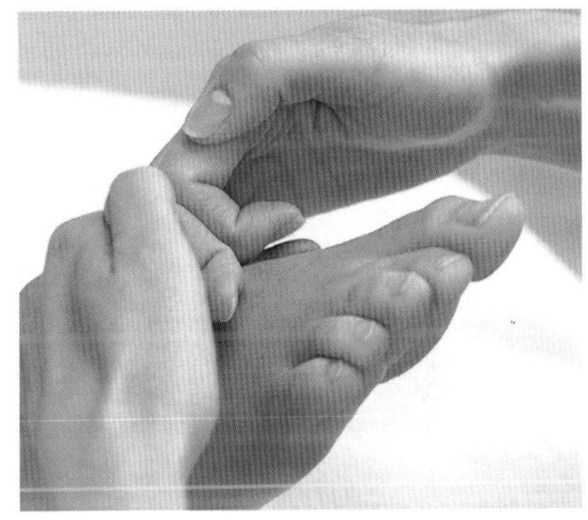

△ **6** Curl your fingers to make very loose fists with your hands. Rest the flat area between the top two joints of each fist on top of the foot, and use to massage, making small circular movements. Start near the toes and work down the foot to the ankle, then work back up again. Repeat. End the routine by stroking the sole and top of the foot, as in Step 1. Repeat the whole sequence on the left foot.

And so to sleep

When you sleep well, you wake up feeling refreshed and ready for the activities of the day. Sleep is also essential for good health: while we rest, the cells in our body repair and regenerate, our detoxifying organs do their work unimpeded, and our blood pressure drops. All this helps to combat stress and improves our ability to fight off illness.

Regular sleep is a key element of a healthy lifestyle, along with exercise, a good diet, and drinking plenty of water. Exercising helps tire you out, so it can aid sleep, as can certain foods such as starchy carbohydrates.

getting into a routine

Your sleep is likely to be better if you have a regular routine before bedtime. Having a warm bath and a warm, milky drink each night will help you to relax. If you do these things each evening, you will start to associate them with bedtime, and this will get you in the right frame of mind for sleep.

A foot massage is another great way of relaxing. It is particularly good if your mind is buzzing with thought, because it redirects your attention from the head to the feet – the grounded part of your body.

sleep enhancer

This is a very simple self-treatment routine that you can do before bedtime. You use the feet to massage each other, so that there is no need for you to bend down. An oil-based spray is used, so that you can massage without pulling the skin. You can do the routine sitting on your bed, but put a towel down to protect the cover.

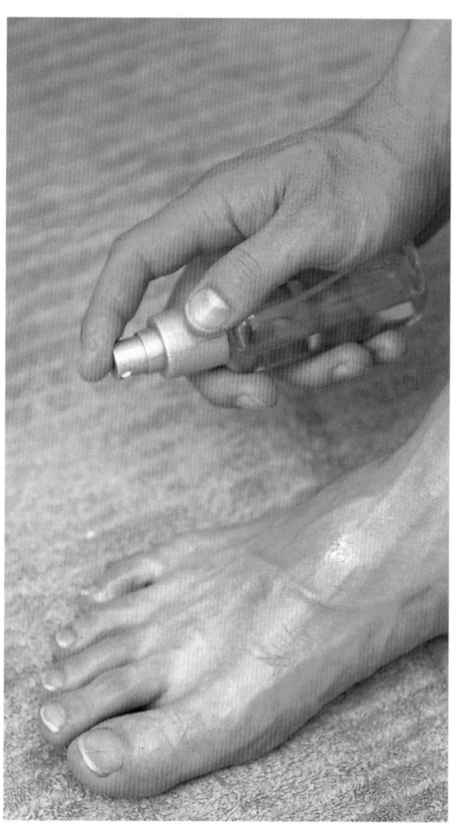

△ **1** Place a large towel underneath your feet. Spray a large, clean tissue with the sleep-time oil spray (see box, right), then spray the top of your right foot. Drop the tissue on top of the foot, and use the sole of the left foot to wipe it all over the top of the right one. Discard the tissue. Repeat on the left foot, so that the top and sole of both feet are lightly perfumed.

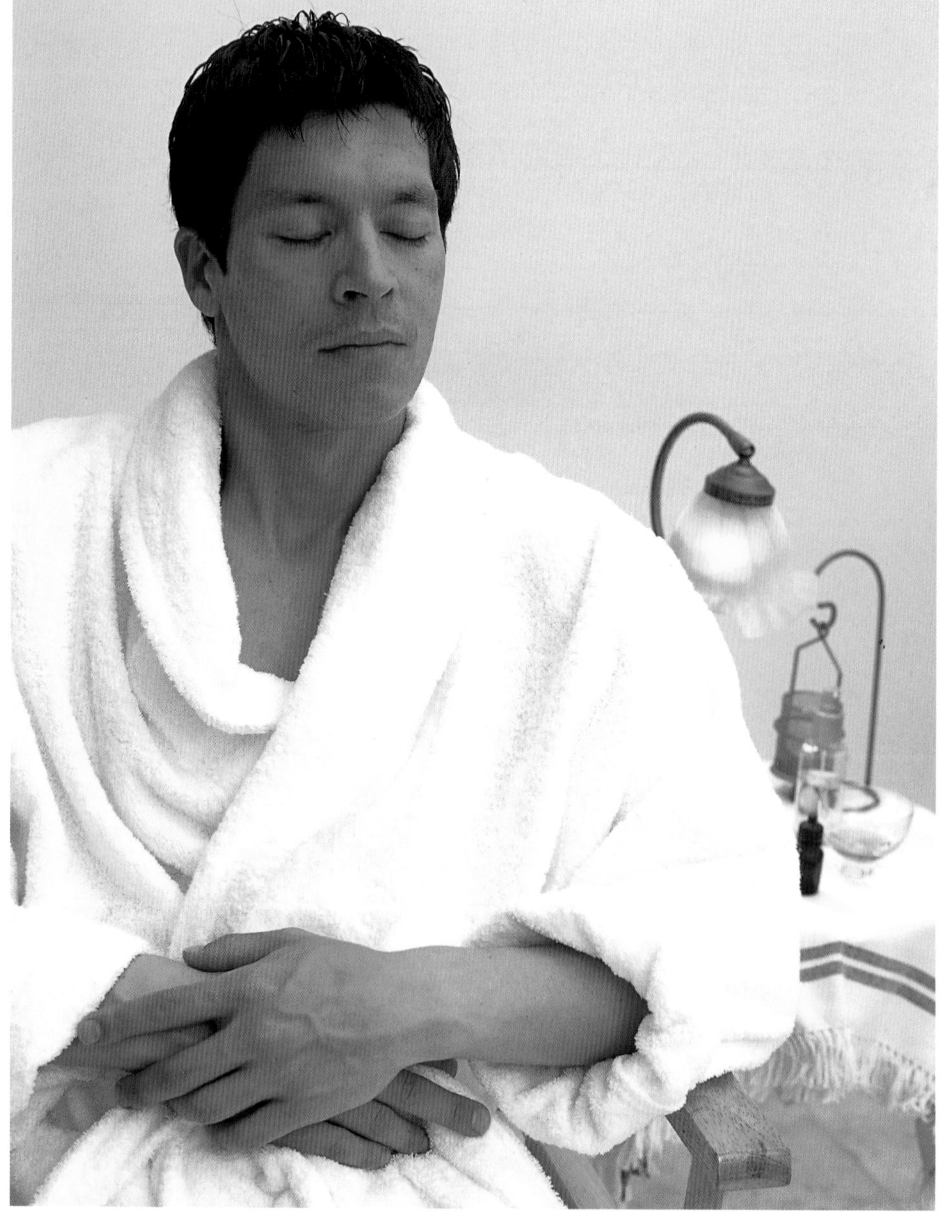

◁ **It is good to get ready for bed before doing this treatment. Ideally you should do it in the bedroom, either sitting in a comfortable chair or lying down in bed, in which case you can go straight to sleep afterwards. If you find yourself getting sleepy, do not feel you have to finish the routine but simply let yourself drift off.**

sleep-time oil spray

This oil spray uses camomile and lavender oils, which are prized for their relaxing and sedative properties. Neroli and marjoram can also be used, if you prefer their aromas. You can adapt the spray for other occasions by changing the oils: a combination of bergamot, clary sage, geranium and lemon, for example, will make a cleansing spray that is great after a workout and shower.

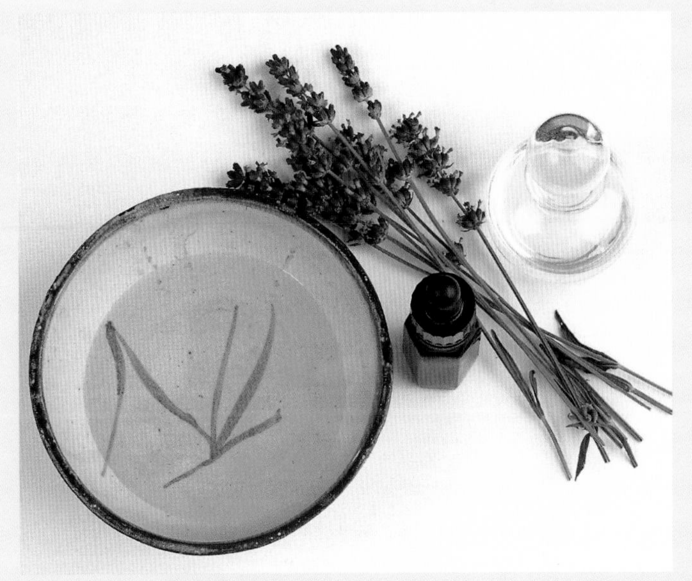

ingredients

- 25ml/5 tsp grapeseed oil
- 25ml/5 tsp almond oil
- 20ml/4 tsp jojoba oil
- 10ml/2 tsp rosewater
- 10ml/2 tsp glycerine
- 20 drops each lavender and camomile essential oils.

Mix the first five ingredients together, then stir in the essential oils, mixing well. Transfer to a clean 100 ml/3 ½ fl oz spray bottle. Shake before use.

△ **Essential oil distilled from lavender is well known for having a calming effect and for promoting deep, peaceful sleep**

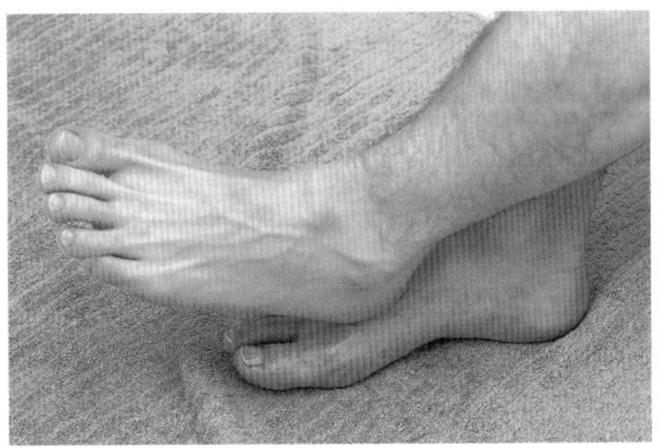

△ **2** Bend your right knee so that the right foot lies flat on the floor or bed. Use the heel pad of the left foot to massage the right toes. Work up and down each toe in turn.

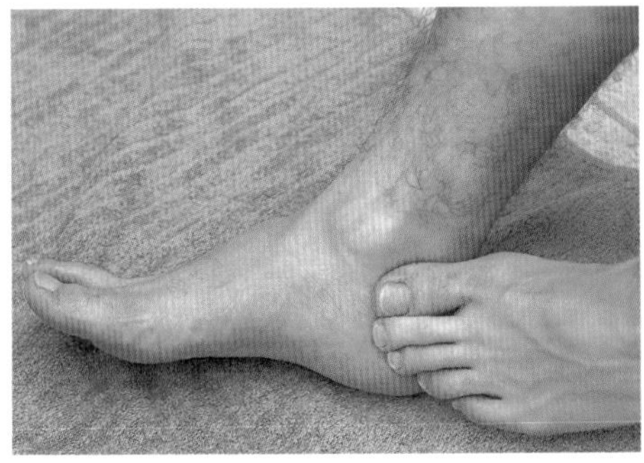

△ **3** Slide the left heel up to the right inner ankle. Use the left heel to massage all around and on top of the ankle bone. Then massage all over the same area with the toes of the left foot. Try to establish a soothing rhythm to the movements. The beauty of these kinds of self-massage techniques is that they can be done anywhere and at any time. So, you can easily try this kind of movement as you sit and watch television or sit on an aeroplane, for example.

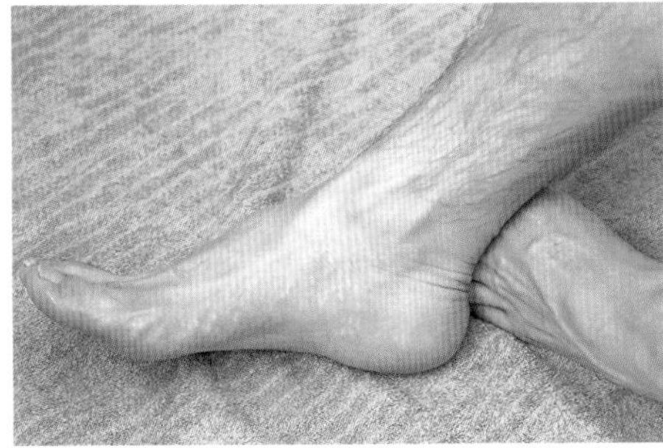

△ **4** Push the left foot around to the back of the right heel, as shown. Now use the toes and the top of the left foot to massage all round the right outer ankle – a quick and easy self-massage technique.

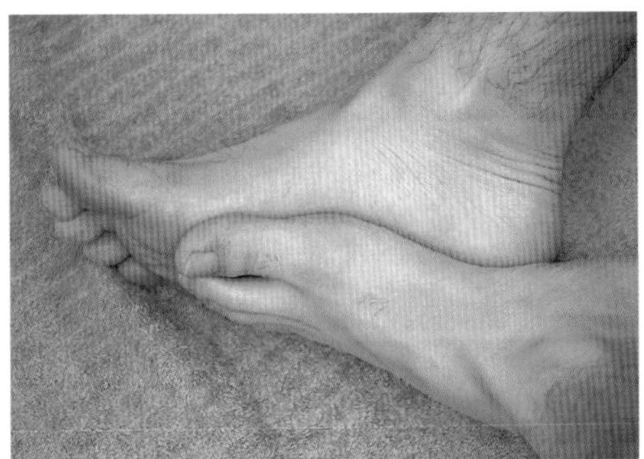

△ **5** Turn the right foot so that it is resting on its outer edge. Use the sole of the left foot to massage up and down the sole of the right. Now repeat steps 2-5 on the left foot. To end, rub the soles of the feet on a towel to ensure they are free from any residue of oil. If you are sitting up, close your eyes, lean back into the chair and relax for ten minutes. If you are in bed, then simply switch off the light and get into your normal sleeping position.

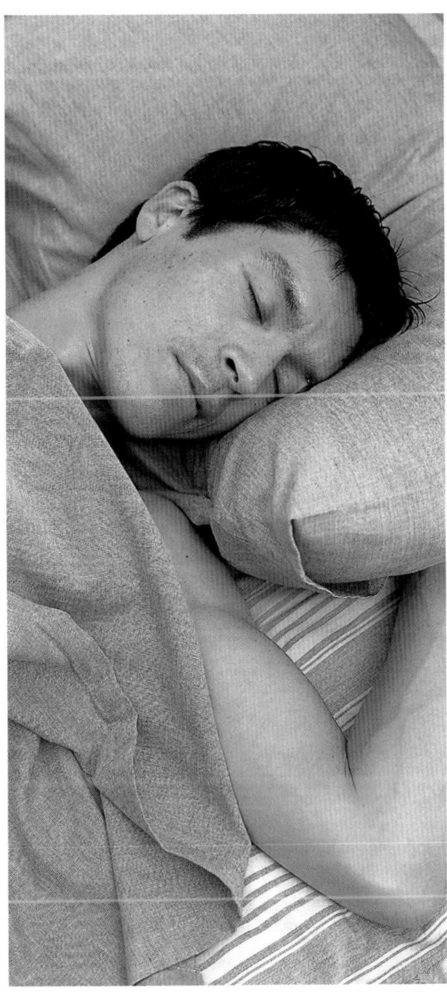

△ **How much sleep you need depends on how old you are and also on your individual constitution. Babies sleep up to 16 hours a day, while older people may need only six hours a night. Most adults need between seven and ten hours a night.**

Foot pamper session

Most of us neglect our feet – particularly in the winter months when they are not on show. Setting aside time for a regular treatment will help you to care for your feet and keep them healthy all year round.

This is a great routine to do at the weekend, or whenever you have some time to yourself. You'll need at least an hour to do it properly – or you can really indulge yourself and take two hours over it.

Think of a pamper session as a time to relax; working on the feet is a great way of taking your mind off day-to-day worries and allowing yourself to focus on feeling good. It is also great to share a pamper session with a friend – set aside an afternoon so that you can really indulge yourselves. You may like to give each other a foot massage at the same time, using one of the relaxing treatments in this book.

Doing a full pamper session once a month will greatly improve your feet's appearance, and will also soften the skin and help the circulation. It is also an excellent way of pepping up your feet at the start of the summer or before going on holiday. You can also shorten the routine and use it as a basis for a mini-pamper session. You may like to do this each week, to keep your feet looking and feeling good in-between full pamper sessions.

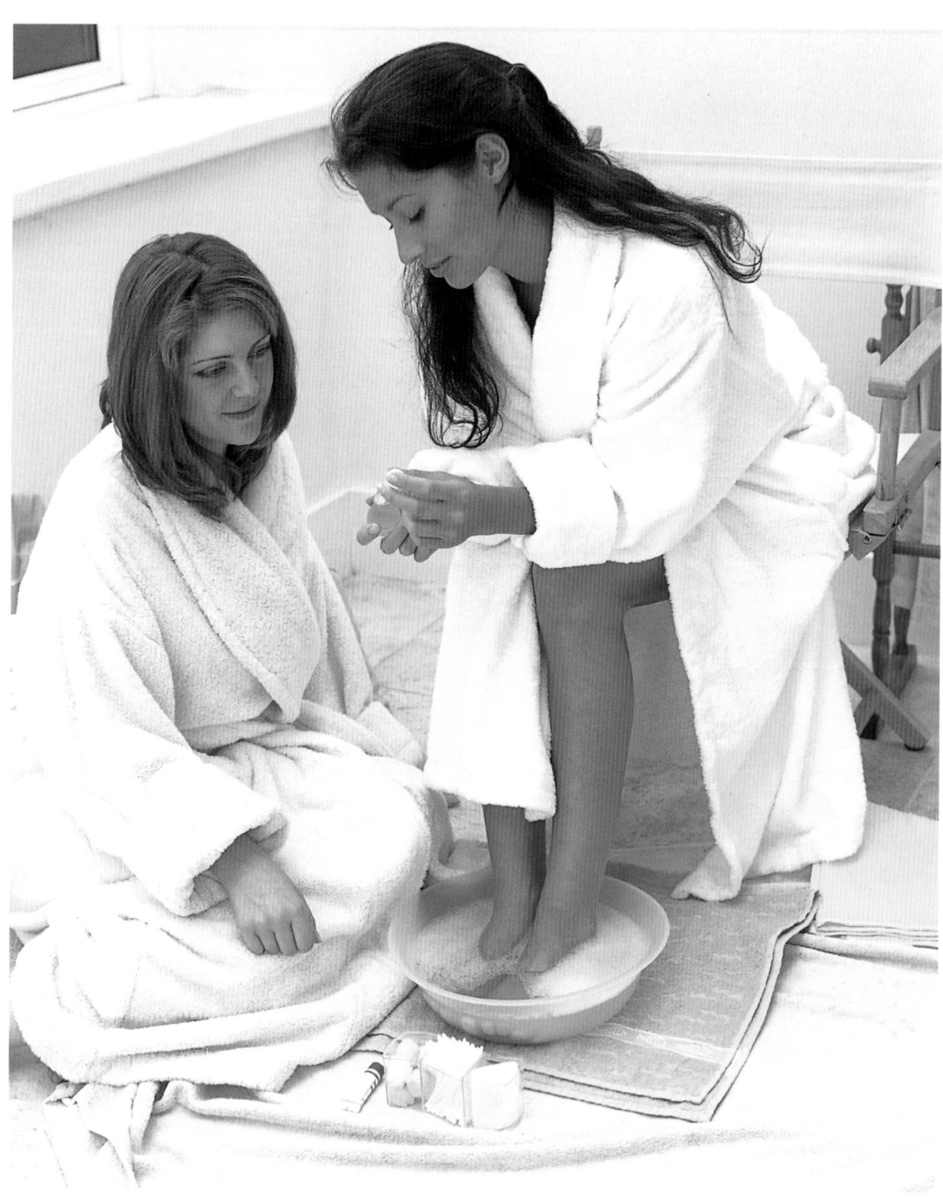

△ Instead of meeting a friend in a bar or restaurant, suggest that you spend an afternoon or evening enjoying a pamper session. It is a good way of spending some relaxed time together, and you could give each other a foot massage at the same time.

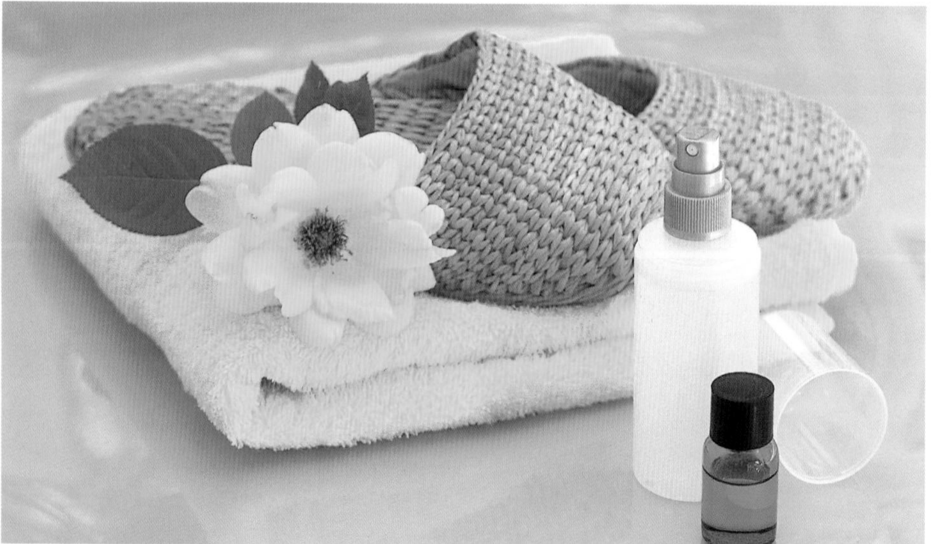

◁ Once you start the foot treatment, you won't want to stop, so get everything ready beforehand: lotions, oils, sprays and thick, fluffy towels. Make sure you have a pair of comfortable slippers to slip your feet into after the treatment.

foot care routine

This routine uses the luxury foot scrub described overleaf. If you don't have time to make it, buy one that includes essential oils so that you can benefit from their soothing properties. You'll also need foaming bath or foot gel, a large foot bowl, one large towel and two smaller ones, two plastic bags to slip your feet into, a pumice stone and other items for the pedicure.

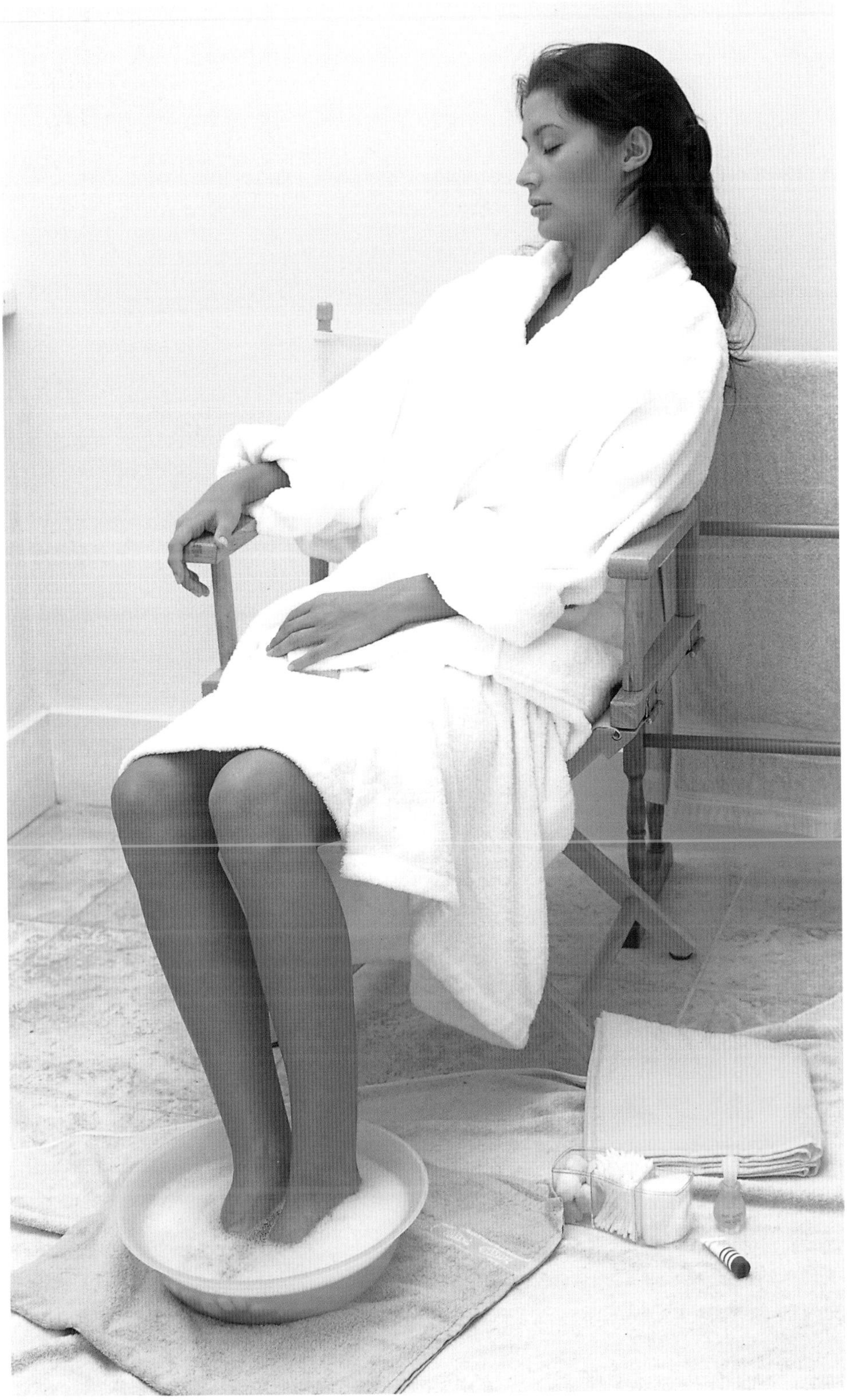

△ **1** Half fill a large bowl with warm water. Place the bowl on a large towel on the floor. Add a little foaming gel, and perhaps a couple of drops of essential oil which have been diluted in a carrier oil or in full-fat milk. Swish the water around with your hand to create plenty of bubbles and to release the aroma of the essential oil. Put both feet into the water, then sit back and relax as you soak them for a good five minutes. Remove your feet from the bowl and rub on the floor towel to remove most of the water.

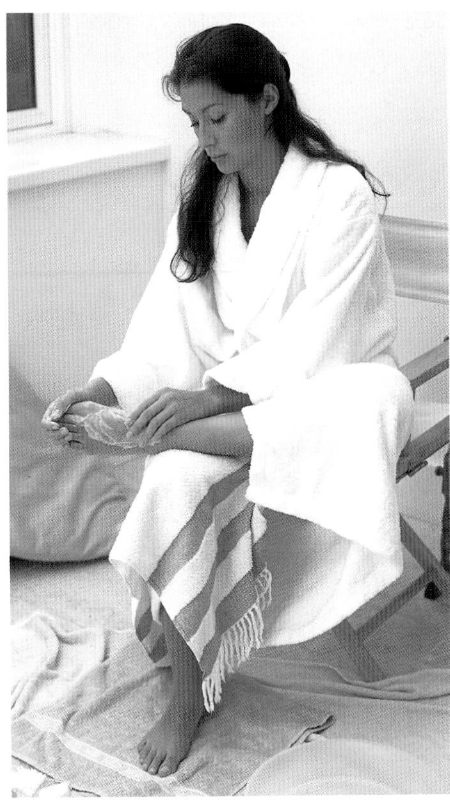

△ **2** Put a towel on one knee and rest the foot of your other leg on top. Massage the foot scrub all over the sole and toes: pay extra attention to any rough skin. Place the foot in a plastic bag and secure.

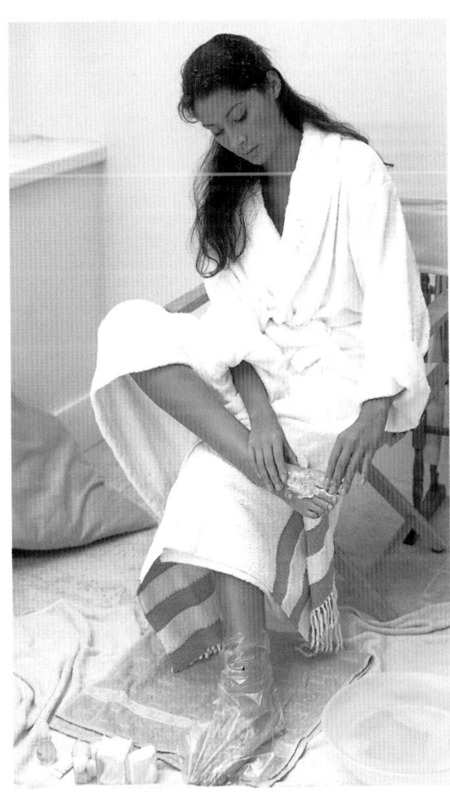

△ **3** Repeat on the other foot. Relax for ten minutes, then remove the bags from your feet, sliding the bags down so that they remove most of the scrub. Dip your feet back into the water. This will now be cool, and will stimulate the circulation.

grooming the feet

A pedicure will keep your feet looking great, and will also help to keep them healthy. You need a few special items in order to give yourself a pedicure. Once bought, they will last for ages, so it is worth the investment. Leave out the polish if you prefer to keep your nails natural.

what you need

- Nail polish remover – choose one with a conditioner.
- Cotton wool – to separate the toes while applying polish.
- Nail brush or orange stick (with the tip covered with cotton wool) – for cleaning under the nail.
- Hoof stick or cotton wool buds – to push back cuticles.
- Toe nail clippers – these are easier to use than scissors.
- Emery board – toe nails are harder than finger nails, so you'll need a strong one.
- Cuticle remover – to soften and loosen the cuticle.
- A base coat – to create an even surface.
- Polish colour of your choice.
- Clear top coat – to help seal the polish and prevent chipping.

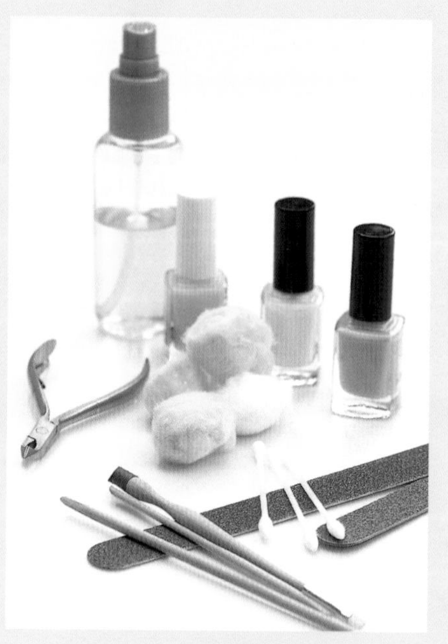

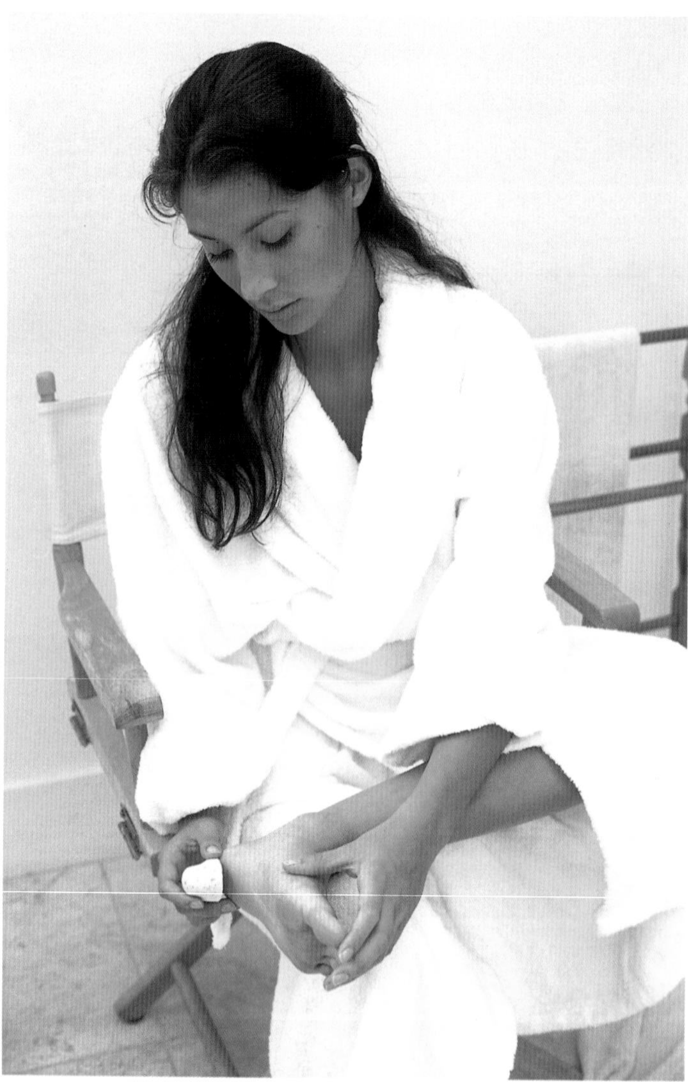

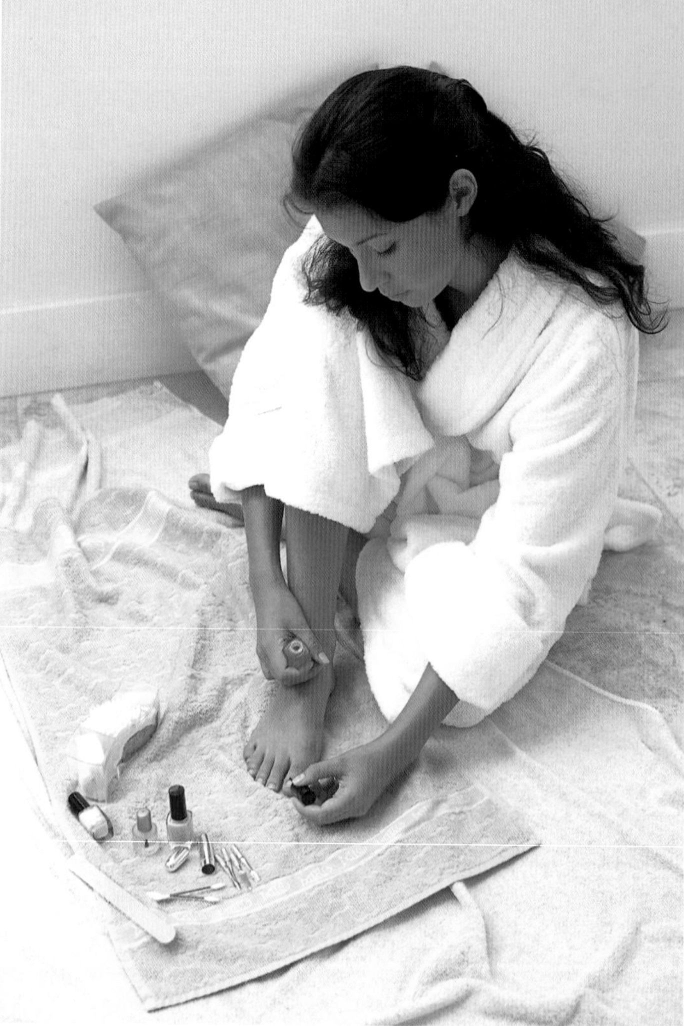

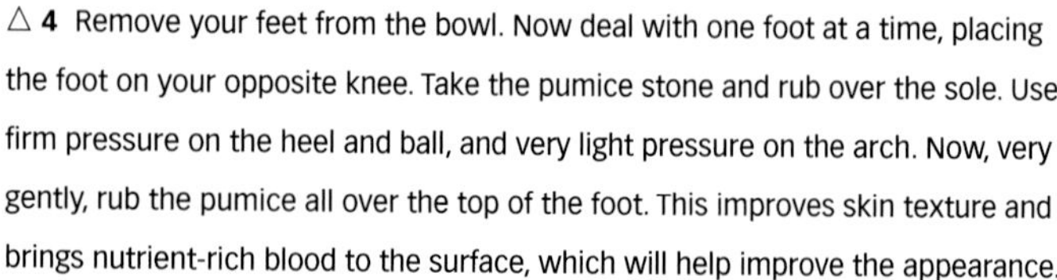

△ **4** Remove your feet from the bowl. Now deal with one foot at a time, placing the foot on your opposite knee. Take the pumice stone and rub over the sole. Use firm pressure on the heel and ball, and very light pressure on the arch. Now, very gently, rub the pumice all over the top of the foot. This improves skin texture and brings nutrient-rich blood to the surface, which will help improve the appearance.

△ **5** Trim the nails straight across, then smooth the edges with an emery board. Use a cotton-wool bud to apply cuticle remover, wait a few minutes, then gently push the cuticle back with a hoof stick. Soak the feet again, then carefully clean under the nail. Dry the feet, then apply base coat, polish and top coat; use cotton wool to separate the toes and allow each layer to dry before applying the next.

luxury foot scrub

This grainy scrub is an excellent cleanser and exfoliator for the feet.The oils and glycerine have a nourishing, moisturizing effect, while the Fullers earth and salt help to soften and deep-cleanse. The essential oils are added for an aromatic, feel-good factor. Choose whichever oils you like best, or use the blends suggested.

This scrub can be used whenever you feel that your feet need a bit of a boost. It should be applied after a warm bath or shower when the feet are damp but not sopping wet. For the best results, though, use it as part of the full pamper session, as described on these pages.

ingredients

- 5ml/1 tsp almond oil
- 5ml/1 tsp jojoba oil
- 5ml/1 tsp glycerine
- 5g/1 tsp each Fullers earth and rock salt
- 10ml/2 tsp foaming foot or bath wash
- 2 drops mandarin and 1 drop geranium essential oils – you could also use lavender and lemon here.

In a small, clean bottle, mix together the foaming wash, essential oil and glycerine. Shake and set aside while you prepare the other ingredients. Put the Fullers earth and rock salt into a medium-sized dish and mix together well. Add the almond and jojoba oils, and mix well. Add the glycerine mixture to the bowl, and mix all the ingredients together with a metal spoon. You should now have a paste with a runny consistency, which can easily be applied to the feet.

▽ Always soak your feet before applying the foot scrub. You can use a foot spa if you have one. This will give a strong massage at the same time as you soak. However, be aware that foot spas are not advised if you have high blood pressure.

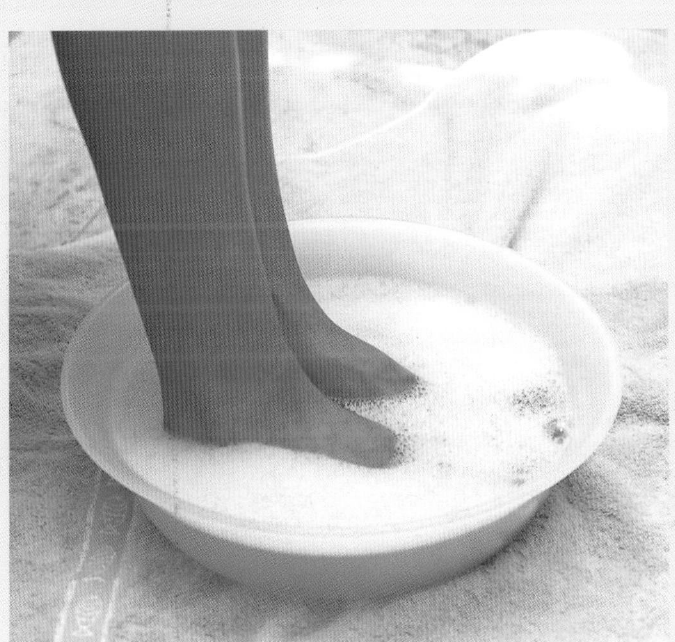

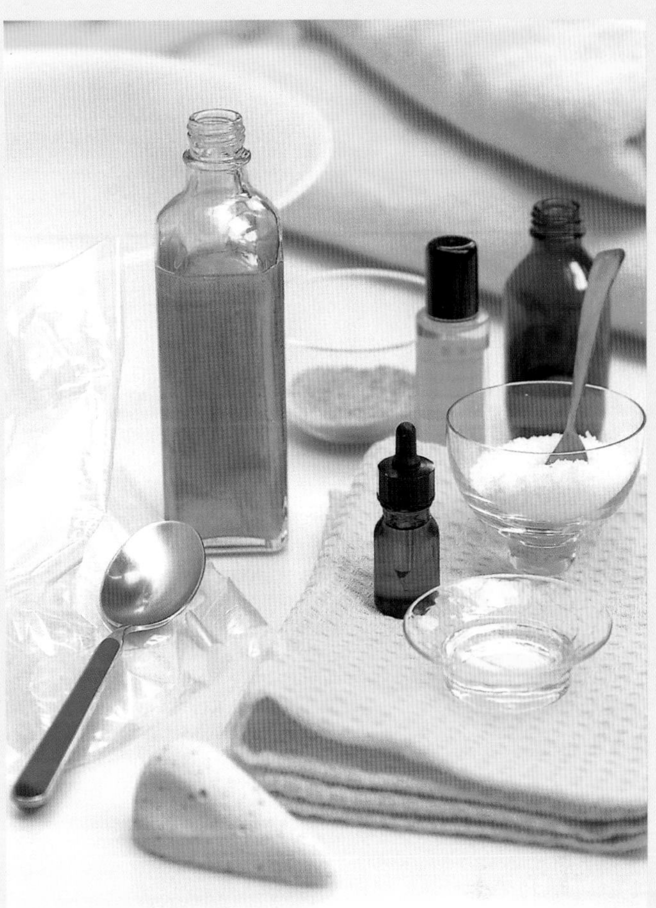

△ To make the luxury foot scrub, you'll need a mixing bowl that is large enough to hold all the ingredients, a metal spoon and a small clean bottle. Other equipment used in the pamper routine includes a pumice stone, a couple of freezer-type bags to put on your feet and three towels, one large one to protect the floor and two smaller ones for resting and rubbing the feet.

▽ A mini pamper session can be achieved by soaking the feet in warm suds for ten minutes. Use a loofah or nail brush to scrub and deep cleanse, then pumice all over the soles of the feet. Pat them dry, then give a quick massage using a blend of neroli and lemon essential oils well diluted in almond oil.

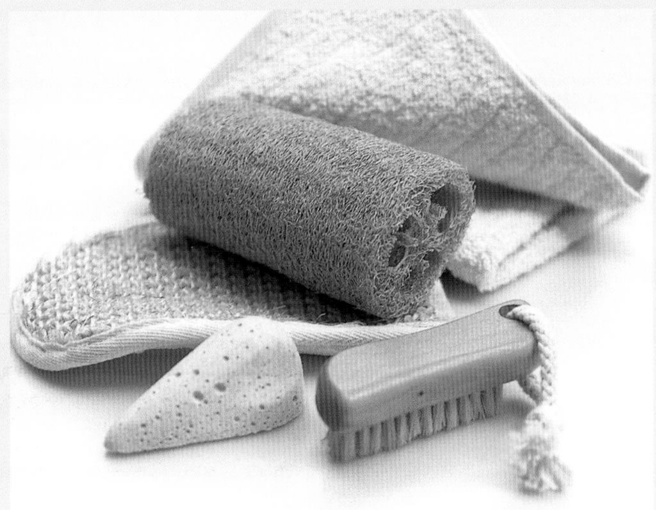

Getting closer

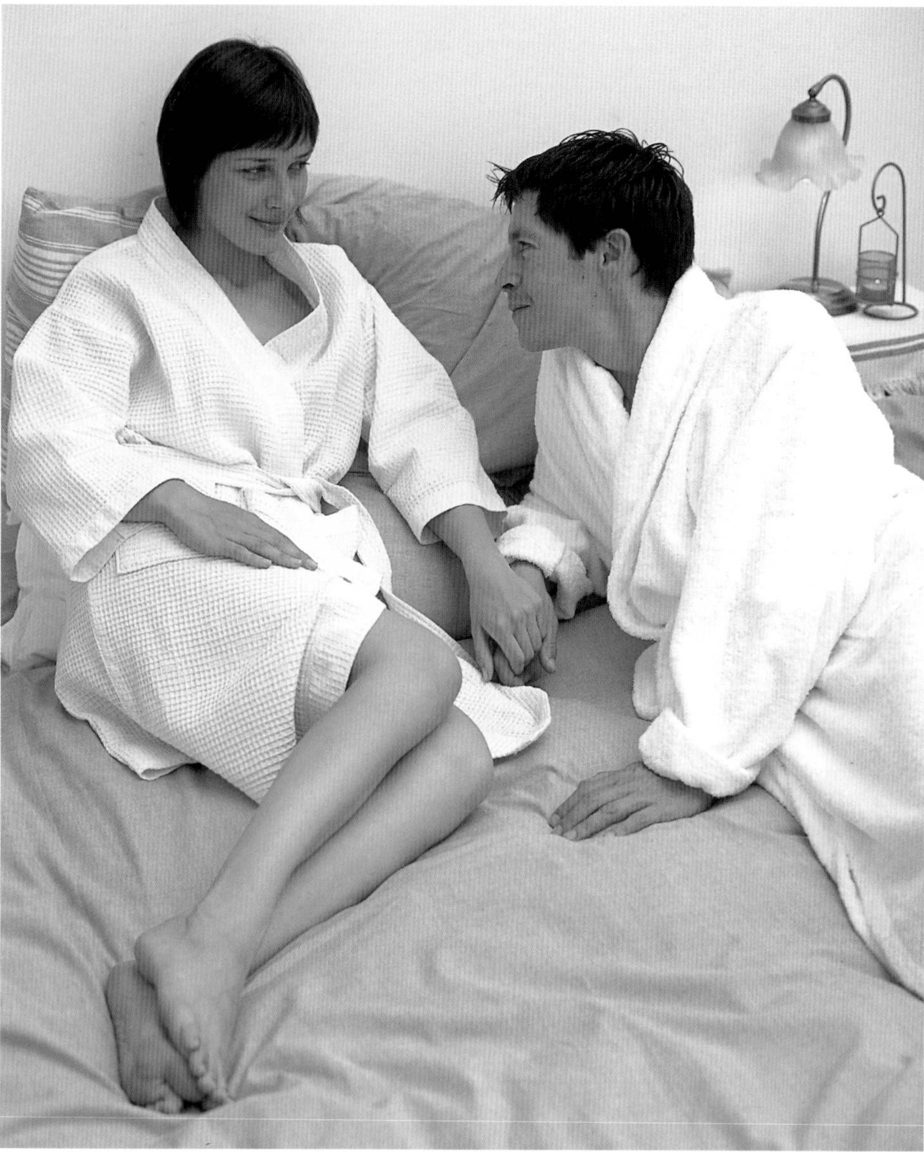

◁ This is a lovely massage to do in the bedroom, perhaps after a warm, relaxing bath or shower. Arrange plenty of cushions or pillows at the head of the bed, so that your partner can lean back and enjoy the massage.

aphrodisiac bath oil

The warm and spicy aroma of this sensual bath oil blend will linger seductively on the skin for some time after your bath – the perfect prelude to an intimate foot massage.

ingredients

- 100ml/3½fl oz almond oil
- 20ml/4 tsp wheatgerm oil
- 15 drops rose essential oil
- 10 drops sandalwood essential oil

Pour the almond and wheatgerm oils into a bottle with a screwtop or tight stopper, then add the essential oils. Shake well.

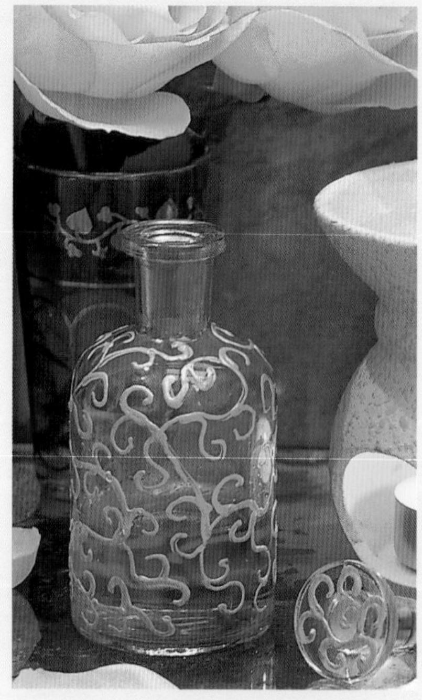

△ Storing oils in pretty bottles helps set the mood, but bottles like this are not ideal. Choose dark glass to keep the oils' aroma for as long as possible.

Sometimes, our days seem to be so filled with work and other commitments that it can be hard to make space for our most important relationship. Massage gives you an opportunity to spend some quiet time with your partner, without the TV, radio or other distractions.

A foot massage is a wonderful way of treating your partner, and for him or her to treat you. It allows you to touch each other in a loving, gentle way that is not necessarily always sexual. As well as soothing and calming the body, foot massage offers a quick route to reconnecting with each other, and re-establishing intimacy.

creating the right mood

When sharing massage with your partner, take a few moments to create an ambience of warmth and intimacy. Make sure that your bedroom is tidy, and that any clutter is cleared away. Have plenty of cushions on the bed so that you can lie back and relax. Use soft lighting – turn off overhead lights and use lamps or candles instead.

You might like to have music playing while you massage. Use the aroma of intoxicatingly-scented essential oils to add sensuality to the experience if you wish. Sandalwood is a warm, heady oil that is said to have genuine aphrodisiac qualities.

sensual foot massage

Try this routine with a relaxing or sensual essential oil, such as geranium or sandalwood, diluted in almond or another carrier oil. Place a towel over the bedcover to protect it from the oil.

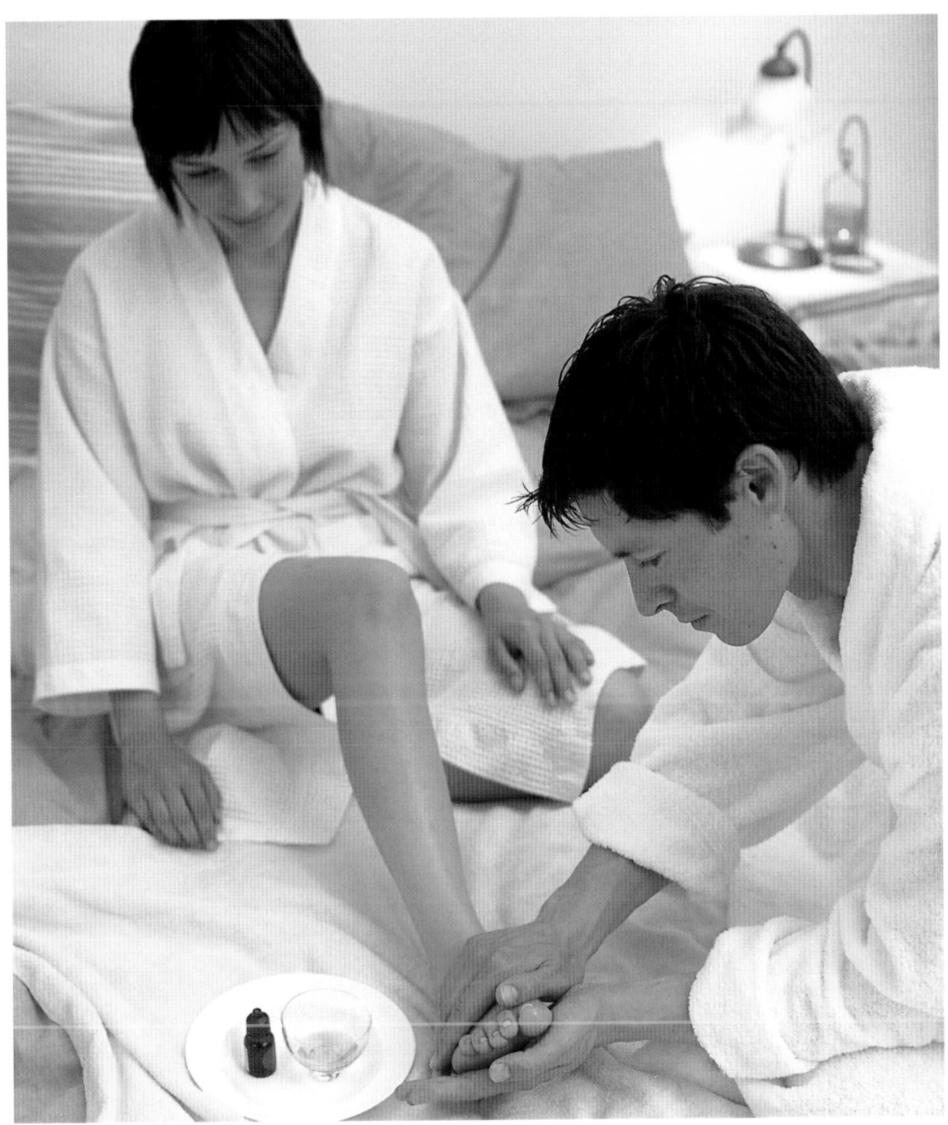

△ **1** Put three or four drops of massage oil in your hand, then lightly rub the palms together to spread it evenly. Take the right foot in a sandwich hold, with one hand across the top of the foot and the other across the sole. Hold for a minute or two, breathing quietly as you maintain contact.

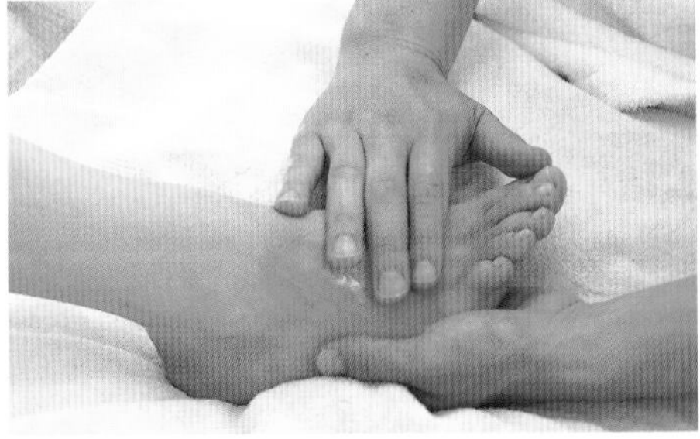

△ **2** Keeping the same hand position as Step 1, stroke the hands down the foot, towards the ankle, then slide back to the toes.The pressure should be firm, but pleasurable. Do this movement three times.

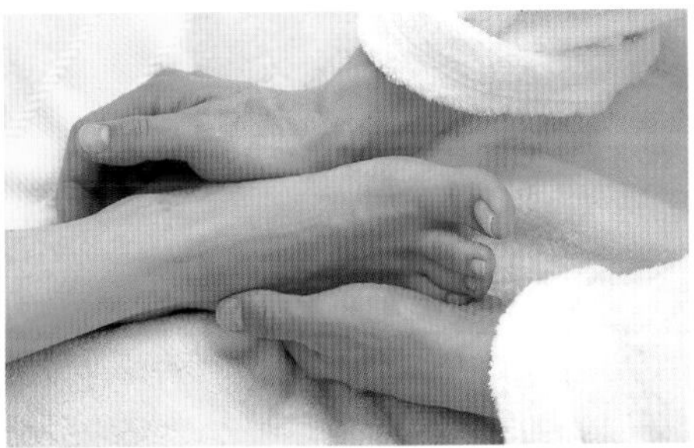

△ **3** Support the outside edge of the foot, so that the toes rest on the heel of your hand. Use the heel of the other hand to stroke down the inside edge of the foot from the big toe to the base of the heel. Work slowly and smoothly. Return the hand to the toe, and fan the inside edge in the same way twice more.

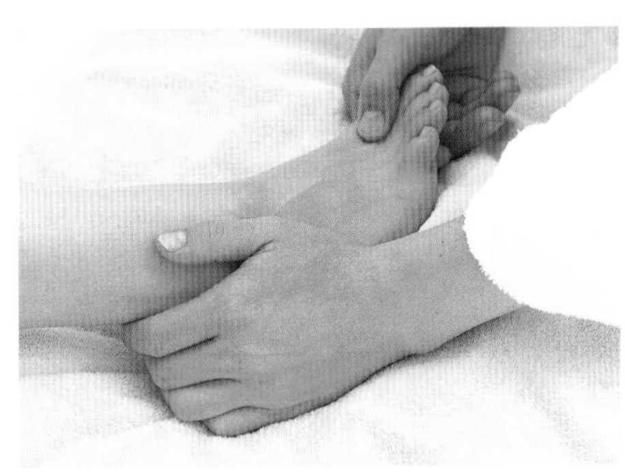

△ **4** Now support the inside edge of the foot, by holding your partner's toes quite firmly. Use the other hand to stroke down the outside edge of the foot, from the little toe to the base of the heel. Stroke back down to the little toe, working slowly and smoothly. Repeat this action two more times.

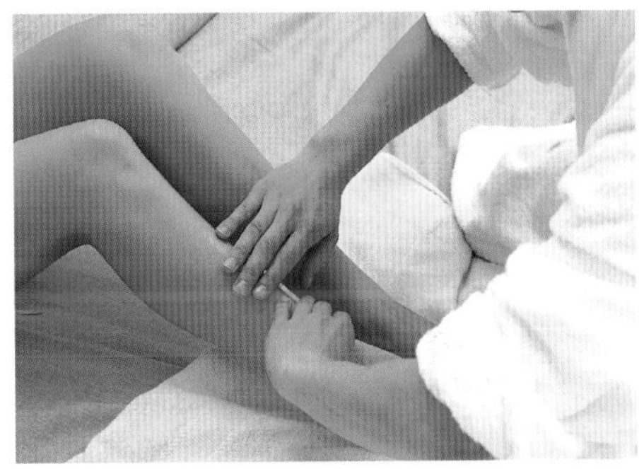

△ **5** Ask your partner to bend his or her knee, so that the foot rests flat on the bed. Apply a little more oil to your hands, then place both hands on the top of the foot – one slightly higher than the other. Stroke down the foot from the toes, and continue to stroke up the leg to the knee, using light pressure. Slide back down to the toes, using no pressure. Repeat twice more.

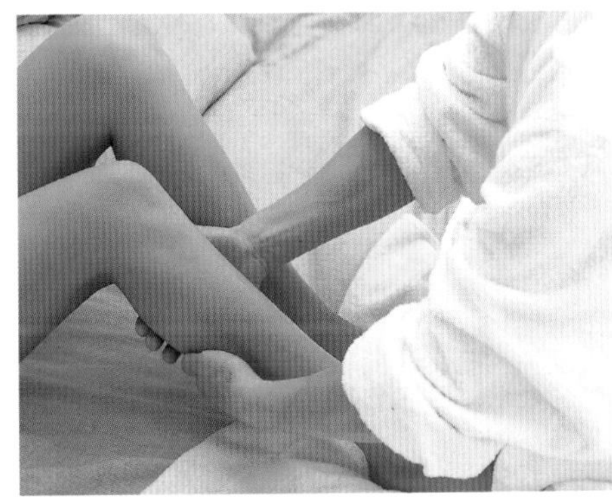

△ **6** Cup both hands around the heel, so that they point in opposite directions and one is higher than the other. Slide the hands up the lower leg to the knee: this helps release stored tension, so keep the pressure reasonably heavy. Slide down to the heel area, using no pressure, and repeat twice more. To finish, use alternate hands to stroke over the top and sole of the foot. Repeat the sequence on the left foot.

Maintaining Well-being

Everyday life can prove to be a strain for our bodies. There are many ways in which you can manipulate your feet and so help yourself through the stresses and strains of work, long-distance travel, or tough physical activity. Slip off your shoes, and try these routines.

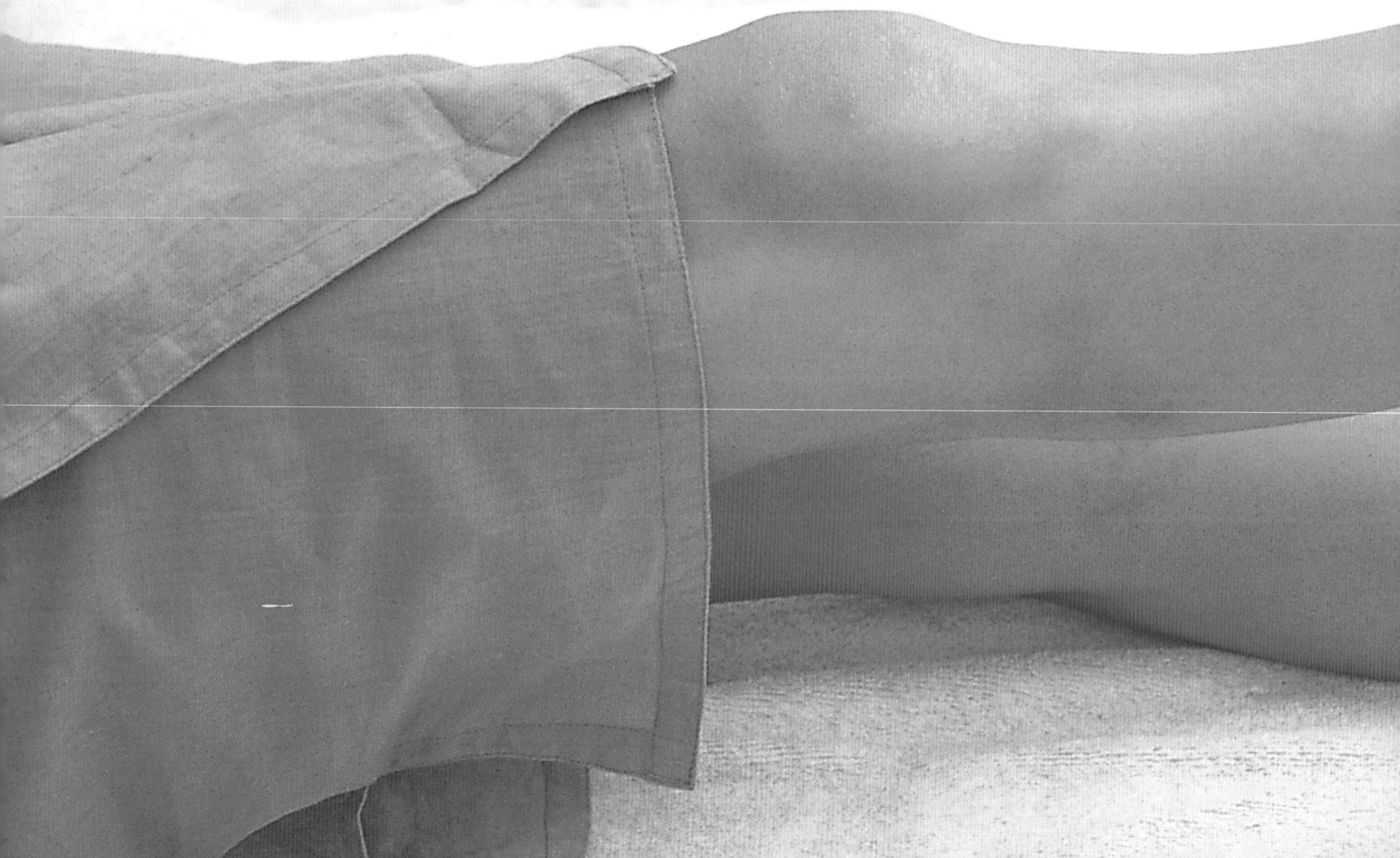

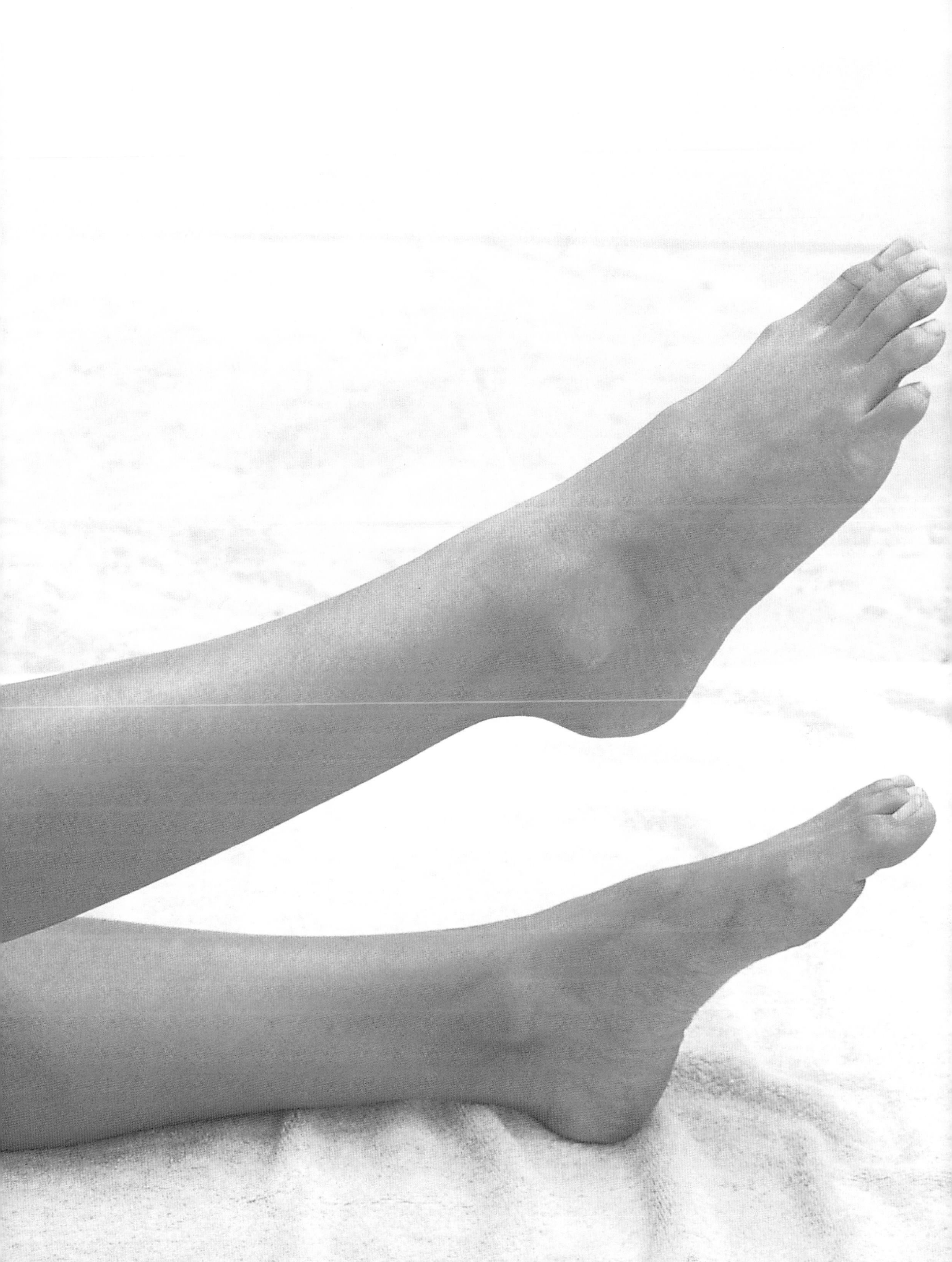

Detox treatment

Fast foods, sugary or salty snacks, alcohol, coffee and tea all contain toxins, which can build up in the body and cause us to feel lethargic and unhealthy. Even if you have a healthy lifestyle, you are still exposed to poisonous substances in the atmosphere. The air that we breathe contains chemicals, gases and dust particles, and it can pollute our land, water and food.

The body is a highly efficient machine, and it is constantly working to remove toxins from the circulation. However, an unhealthy diet, stress or late nights all put the body under pressure, and can affect how well its elimination systems work. Regular exercise supported by a healthy diet and a weekly detox massage regime will help improve your circulation, eliminate waste from the muscles and keep the detoxifying organs in good working order.

It is also important that you drink plenty of water. We lose fluid daily through the natural elimination processes of urination, defecation and sweat. This fluid needs to be replaced. To maintain good health and an efficient detox system we should drink at least three large glasses of water each day.

the role of the feet

The feet are the most distant part of the body – that is, they are furthest away from the heart, the main circulation organ. Toxins and wastes therefore tend to collect in the feet, particularly around the joints. Regular foot massage helps to break down and eliminate these toxins, and also to mobilize the joints. At the same time, it improves the circulation. This has a knock-on effect throughout the body, aiding the natural purification processes.

cleansing routine

It takes only a few minutes to do this simple routine, but it can have a highly beneficial effect on your general well-being. Use gentle strokes at first, to help relax the foot, then increase the pressure as you go on. If you like, use a massage cream or an oil of your choice.

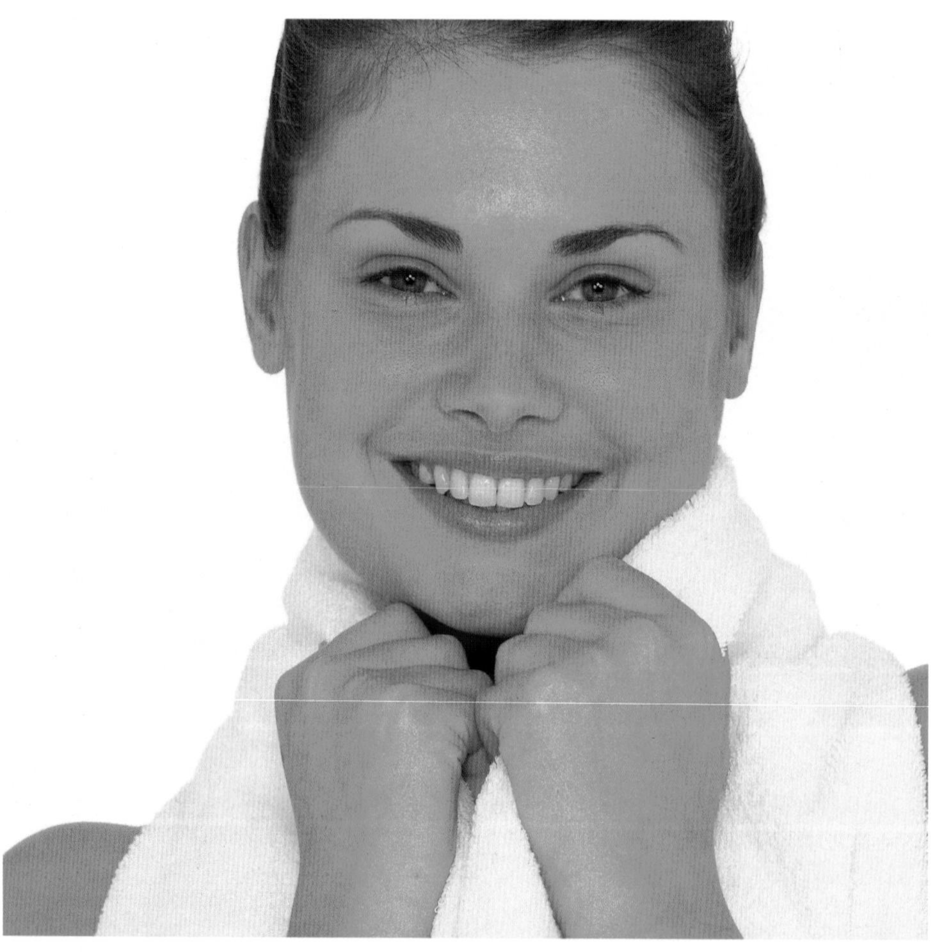

△ **You can include the foot detox routine in a fuller programme of cleansing and relaxing. Dedicate some time – perhaps a full day – to enhancing your well-being. Enjoy some brisk exercise, such as running or fast walking, as well as some gentle stretches. Drink plenty of water and eat small, healthy meals consisting of whole grains, fresh vegetables and fruit.**

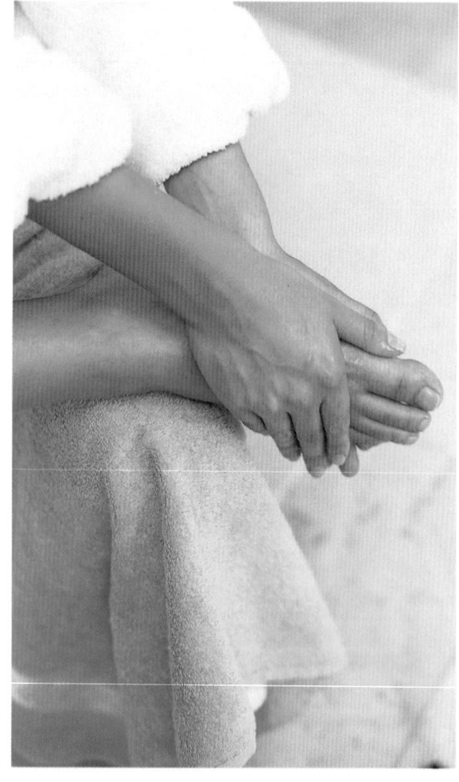

△ **1** Bring your right foot to rest on your left knee. Place your right hand across the top of the toes and your left hand underneath them, with the fingers of both hands pointing towards the outside edge. Gripping the foot between the hands, in a sandwich-like hold, slide both hands down to the heel then back to the toes. Do the movement three times in each direction. Repeat on the left foot.

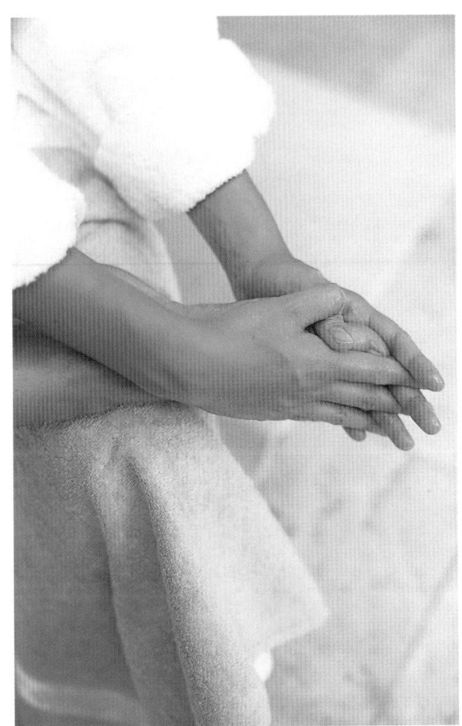

△ **2** Put your left hand on the right sole, fingers towards the toes. Place your right hand on the top of the foot in a similar position. Link the fingers of both hands across the tops of the toes. Now gently pull the hands apart, sliding one down the sole and the other down the top. Do this three times. Then, repeat the movements on the left foot.

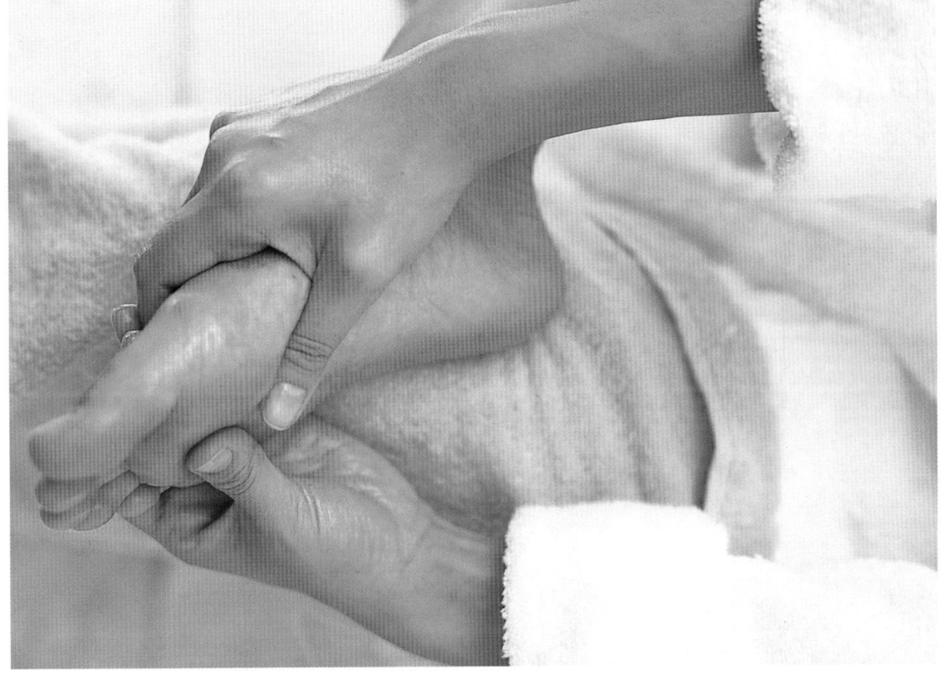

△ **4** Place the thumbs of each hand across the sole of the right foot, so that they point towards opposite sides of the foot. Start off as close to the toes as you can. Using a strong pressure, slide your thumbs backwards and forwards across the sole, pulling out to the edge of the foot each time. In this way, work down the foot to the heel, then back up to the toes. Do this three times; this movement helps to improve circulation and eliminate waste. Repeat the whole movement on your left foot.

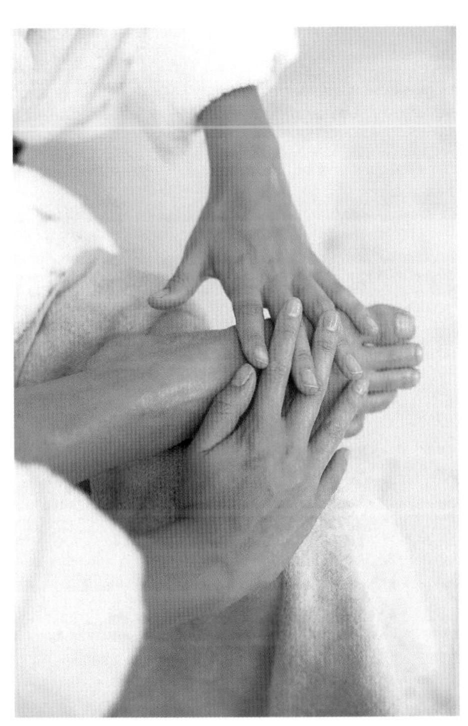

△ **3** Link your fingers together over the top of the right foot. Keep pressing down into the foot at the same time as you pull your fingers apart and draw them towards the edges of the foot. Work in this way from toes to ankle, then work back to the toes; this helps to eliminate waste. Repeat on the left foot.

what is detoxing?

Toxins can build up in the body, causing us to feel tired and drained. Detoxing is a way of cleansing the body of these impurities by helping the body's natural elimination processes. Most people benefit from the occasional detox – having a healthy day once a month can be a great way to keep energy levels up. It will also benefit your skin, hair, nails and general well-being.

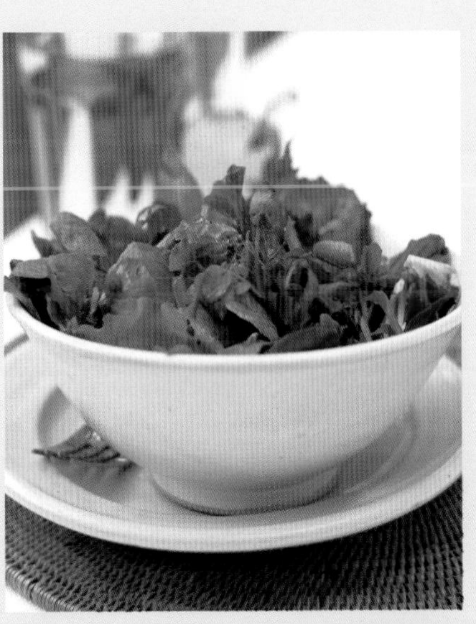

△ **Raw, fresh foods play a vital role in any body-cleansing programme.**

how to detox

There are different approaches to detoxing. The most extreme one is fasting – abstaining from all foods and drinking only water, herbal tea and juices over a short period.

Fasting tends to slow the digestive system, so it can be counter-productive and is not recommended for most people. Your body is more likely to benefit from a gentle programme that does not place it under pressure. A detox is best done over a day or two. During this time eat little and often, having only fibre-rich, healthy foods such as raw or lightly cooked fruits, vegetables and grains. Do several sessions of gentle exercise and get lots of rest. Drink plenty of water to help flush toxins away. You can also drink fresh juices, and herbal teas. Massage speeds the detox process, and brings a pleasurable, relaxing element to the day.

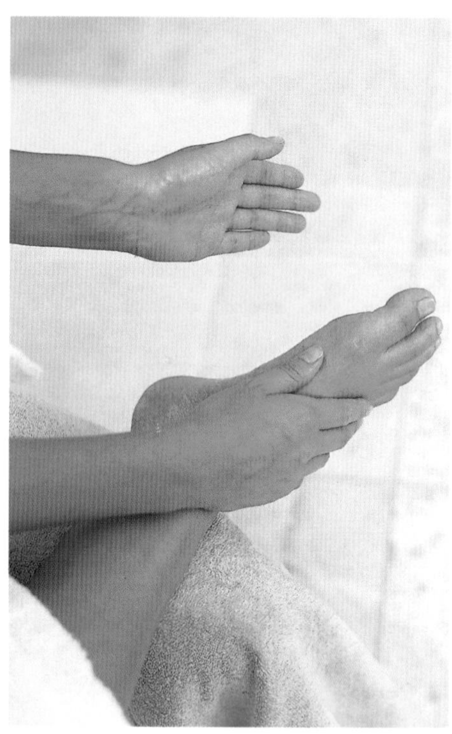

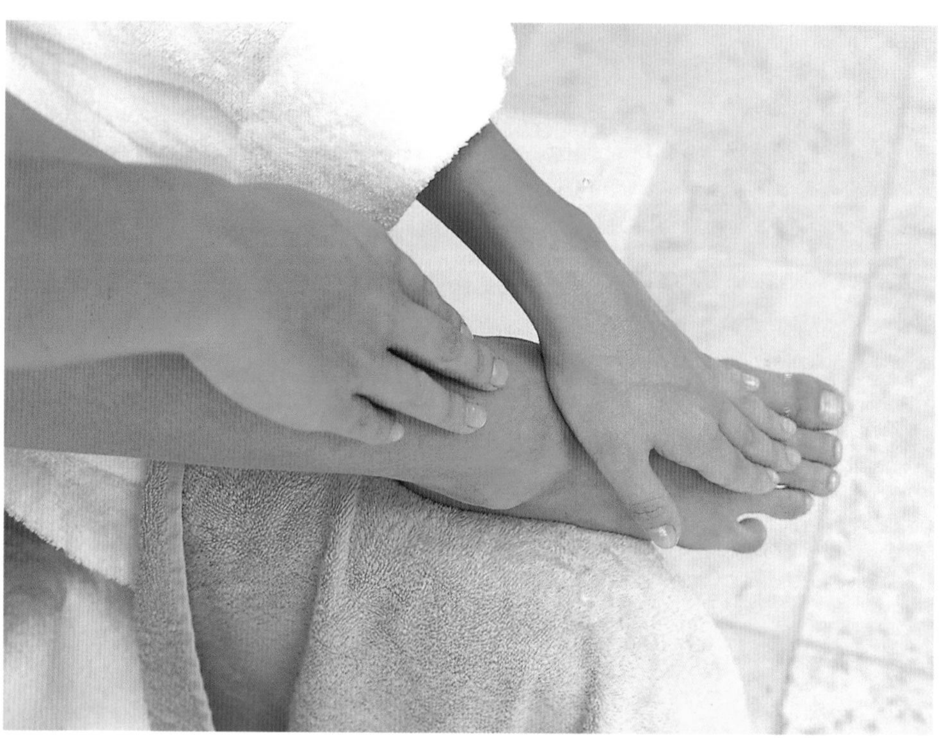

△ 5 Put the right hand on the top of the right foot, fingers pointing towards the toes. Put the left hand in a similar position on the sole. Using alternate hands slap the foot all over, moving up and down between the heel and toe to boost the circulation. Pressure should be harder on areas where the skin is thick. Slap all over four times, then repeat on the left foot.

△ 7 With alternate hands, make light strokes from toes to ankle. Do ten strokes with each hand, using the whole palm. Now stroke five times with each hand, making the pressure as firm as is bearable. Finally, start with the fingers interlaced between the toes. Do five medium-pressure strokes with each hand. Repeat on the left.

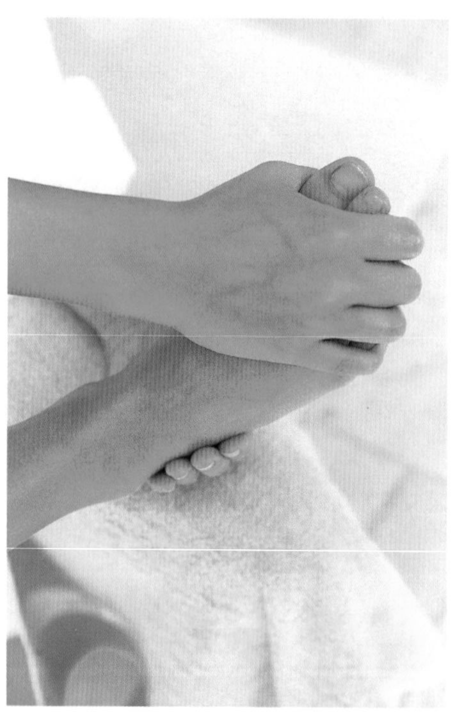

△ 6 Hold the toes of the right foot in your right hand and cup the heel in your left hand. Circle the foot, rotating it from the ankle three times clockwise, then three times anticlockwise. This action helps to mobilize the joints. Rest then repeat. Do not force the ankle beyond its limits. Repeat on the left.

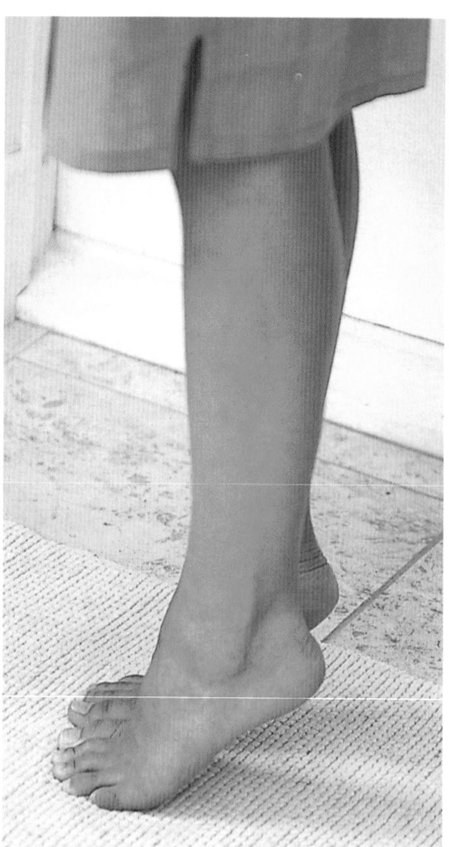

△ 8 Stand up straight. Keep breathing as you lift both heels off the ground and hold them there for a slow count of ten. Return the heels to the floor and count to five. Do this muscle stretch three or four times, depending on your fitness level. You can rest your hands on a chair back if you feel unsteady.

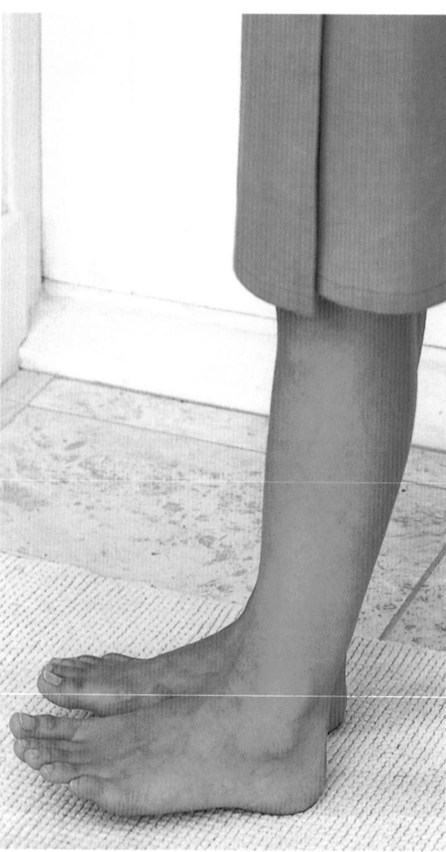

△ 9 This movement stretches the tendons as well as the muscles. Standing upright, firmly press your heels into the floor as you lift the forefoot and toes off the ground. Hold to a count of five, return feet to start point. Rest to a count of five. Do the movement three times. Again, use a chair if you find this difficult.

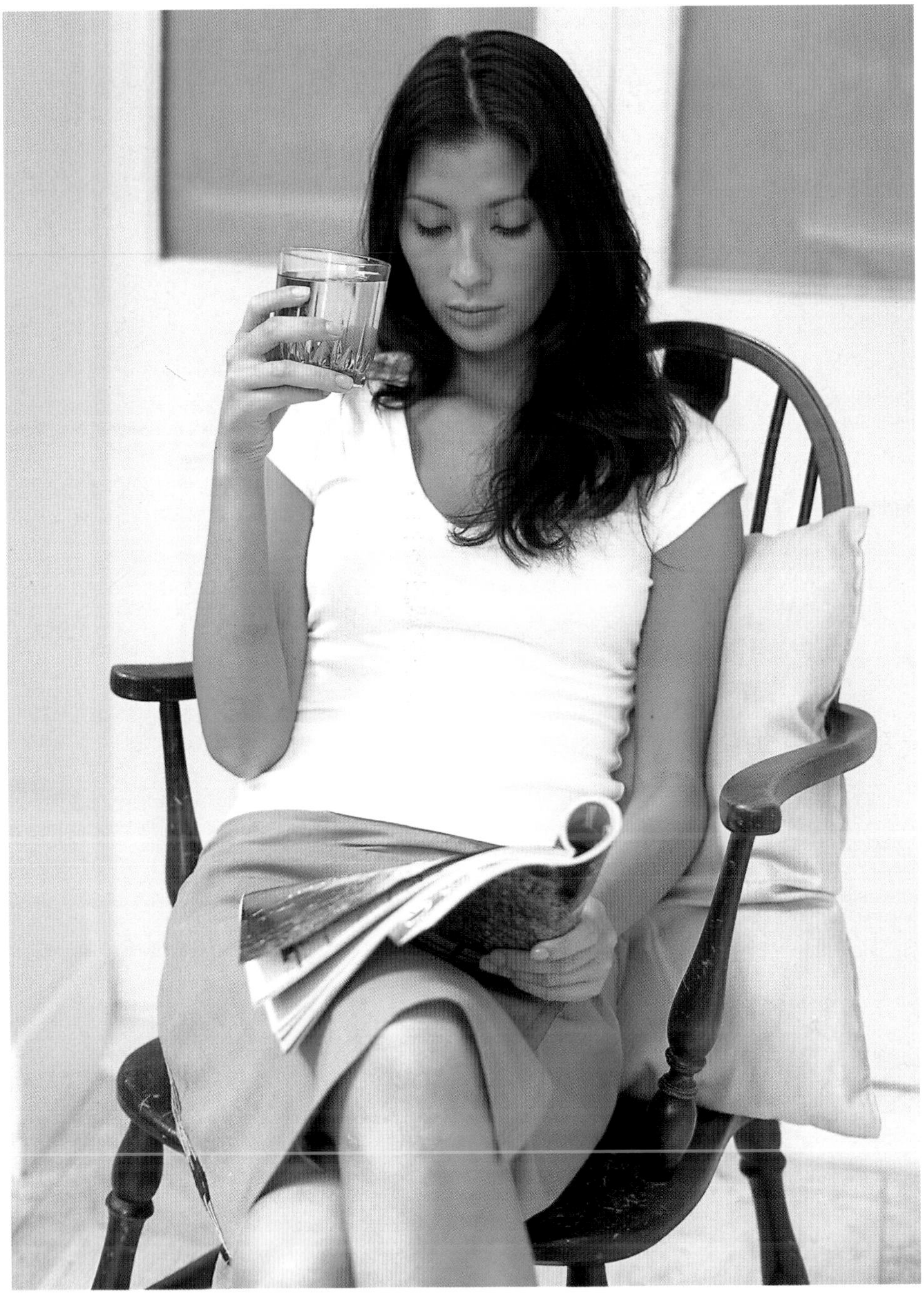

◁ **10** When the massage is over, sit down quietly. Enjoy some peaceful time on your own or read a magazine or book. Spend at least 20 minutes relaxing. During this time, drink a large glass of water or fruit juice. This will help the elimination processes started by the massage routine.

after the routine

If possible, you should try not to do too much after doing the detox routine. If you have time, it is a good idea to combine this treatment with other health-enhancing activities. For example, you may like to do some gentle exercise – such as swimming, walking, yoga or Pilates. You could also go for a sauna; impurities are passed out of the body in sweat.

Make sure that you drink plenty of water. If you like, add a slice of lemon to zing up the taste; lemon has cleansing properties so this will aid the detoxifying process. Try not to eat any sugary, salty or processed foods, at least for the rest of the day. The best foods to help the body get rid of wastes are those that contain plenty of fibre. Eat fresh fruit and vegetables, in the form of juices, soups and salads, together with whole grains such as wholemeal bread, wholewheat pasta or wholegrain rice.

For the best results, you should do this detox routine every week or so. Combined with regular exercise, a healthy diet and drinking plenty of water, it will help to keep your system working well, and prevent the build-up of toxins in the body.

vitamin-packed juicing

Drinking freshly made juices is an easy way to up your nutrient intake and boost your energy levels without placing the digestion under any strain. Here are some good juices to try when you are detoxing, or at any time.

- Apple, orange and carrot: packed with vitamin C and energizing fruit sugars to give you a lift.
- Papaya, melon and grapes: papaya is soothing on the stomach, and this juice can also help the liver and kidneys.
- Carrot, beetroot and celery: a good juice to kickstart the system in the morning. Try using 100g ($3\frac{1}{2}$ oz) beetroot to three carrots and two celery sticks.
- Cabbage, fennel and apple: a cleansing juice with antibacterial properties. Use $\frac{1}{2}$ a small red cabbage, $\frac{1}{2}$ a fennel bulb, 2 apples and a spoonful of lime juice.

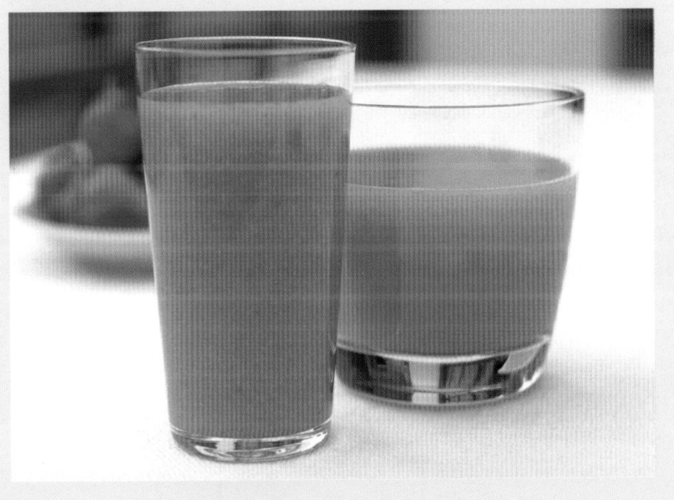

△ **Fruits and vegetables are packed with vitamins and nutrients. Use the freshest produce, and buy organic whenever you can.**

De-stress and unwind

The modern world presents us with more opportunities and choices than we have ever had before. With these new opportunities come new challenges, responsibilities and the need to make an ever-increasing number of decisions. Our everyday life now involves a multiplicity of claims on our time, involvement, commitment and energy.

It is not surprising, then, that we all feel overwhelmed occasionally. Stress has become one of the biggest health problems in the western world, and most of us are affected by it at some point in our lives. Sometimes, a little stress can be helpful; it may galvanize us into action, for example, or motivate us to finish a necessary task. All too often, though, it is counterproductive, and leaves us feeling exhausted, anxious and less effective than we might otherwise be.

the need for rest

The best antidote to stress is rest. However, when you are feeling tense, it can be hard to relax. The solution is to slow yourself down so that your mind becomes quieter and the tension drains out of your body.

There are many ways to do this, but giving yourself a foot massage is probably the quickest. Not only does it require you to focus on what you are doing, which always helps to clear the mind, but you are working on one of the body's most sensitive areas. It is almost impossible not to relax when your feet are being stroked and pummelled.

Do this routine in a quiet place where you won't be disturbed; close the door and switch off the phone. After the treatment, give yourself a few minutes simply to sit and listen to the sound of your breathing.

essential oils for de-stressing

Using an essential oil that has soothing and uplifting properties will heighten the relaxing effects of this routine. Add a few drops of your chosen oil to a carrier and massage into the feet at the start of the routine, or heat in a burner. Good stress-relieving oils include geranium, lavender, bergamot, jasmine, camomile, neroli and rose. Choose one with an aroma that really appeals to you.

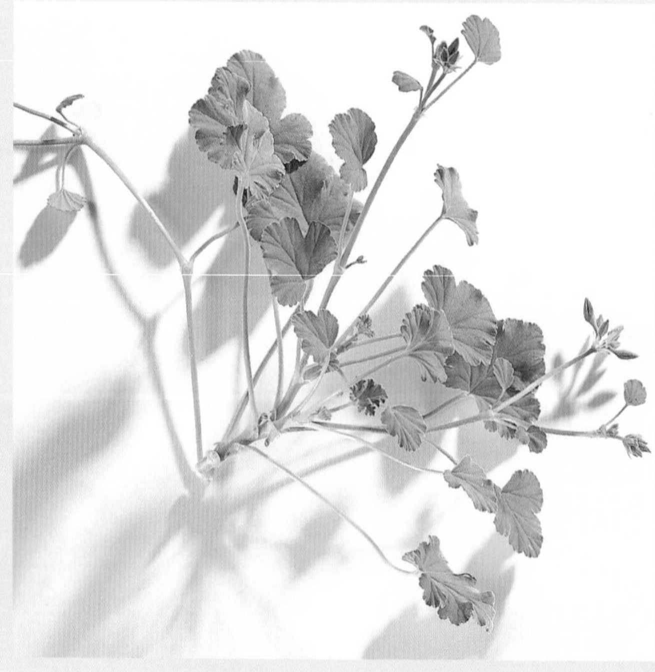

▷ **Geranium is a sweet-smelling oil that has a soothing effect on the nervous system. It can also be helpful for PMT. Use it on its own or combine with rose or lavender.**

releasing tension routine

This de-stressing routine has been designed to help you to let go of strain and tension. Try to relax your whole body as you do it; this will enhance the effects. The routine could be practised each day – perhaps after work – but a one-off at any time will bring rewards.

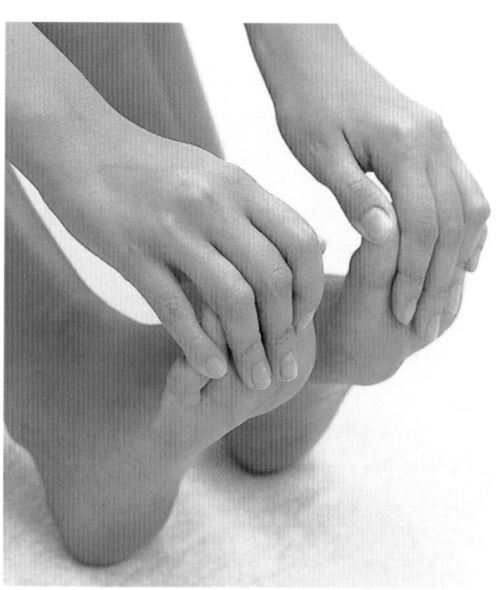

△ **1** Stretch both feet out in front of you, toes pointing upwards. Bend forwards and bring your fingers to rest on the ball of the foot, then pull your feet gently back towards you.

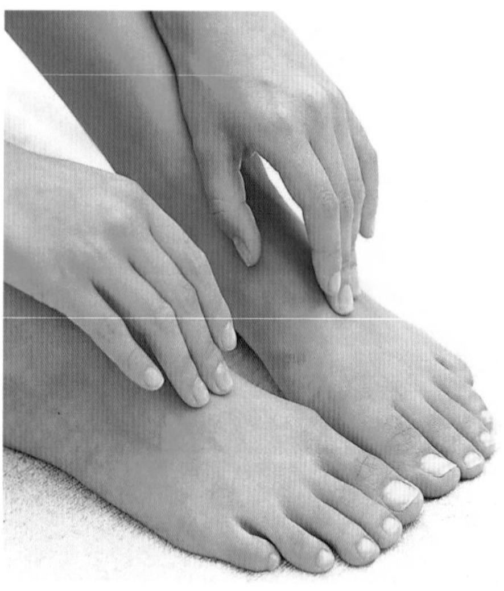

△ **2** Massage the grooves that start between the toes and run up the foot: use the two middle fingers of each hand to make small circles. Start between the two biggest toes, then do the others in turn. Repeat.

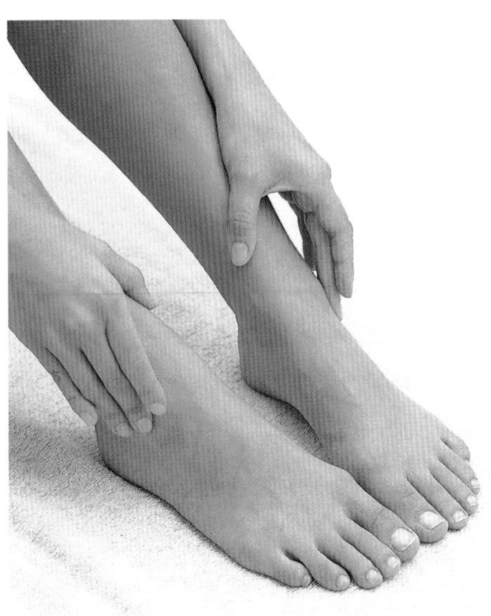

△ **3** Massage around both outer ankle bones at the same time, using the two middle fingers of each hand. Massage first in a clockwise direction, then in an anticlockwise direction. If an area feels tender or tight, repeat the movement in both directions. Do the same on the inner ankles.

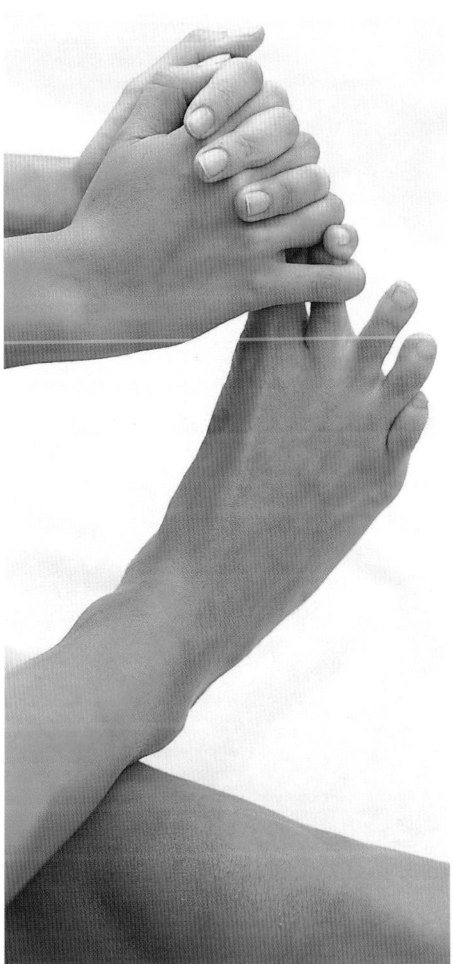

△ **4** Place one hand on the sole and the other on the top of the right foot. Cup your hands together, interlocking your fingers. Slide the hands over the tips of your toes, pulling and separating each one as you go. Repeat on the left foot.

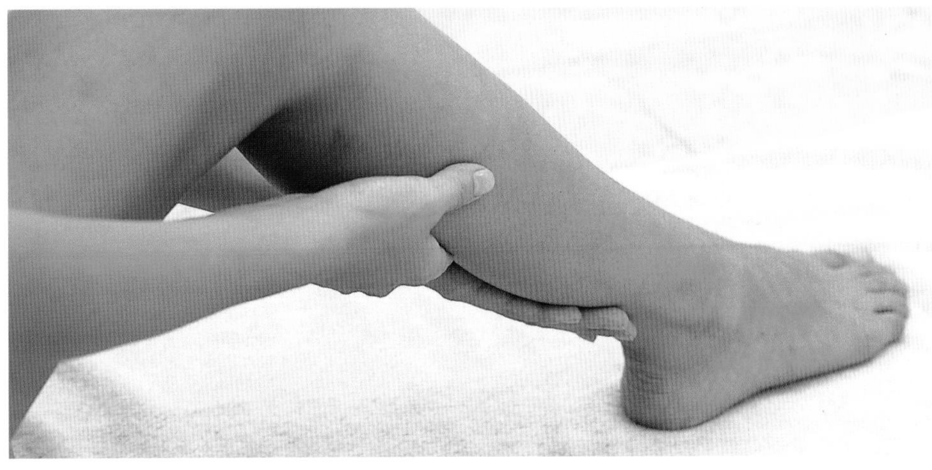

△ **5** The next step is to massage the Achilles tendon and muscles of the lower leg. This helps to relieve tension in the feet and legs; it works best if you oil your hands first. Begin the massage on the right leg. Use alternate palms to work up from the back of the heel to behind the knee. Massage the area twice. Repeat on the left leg.

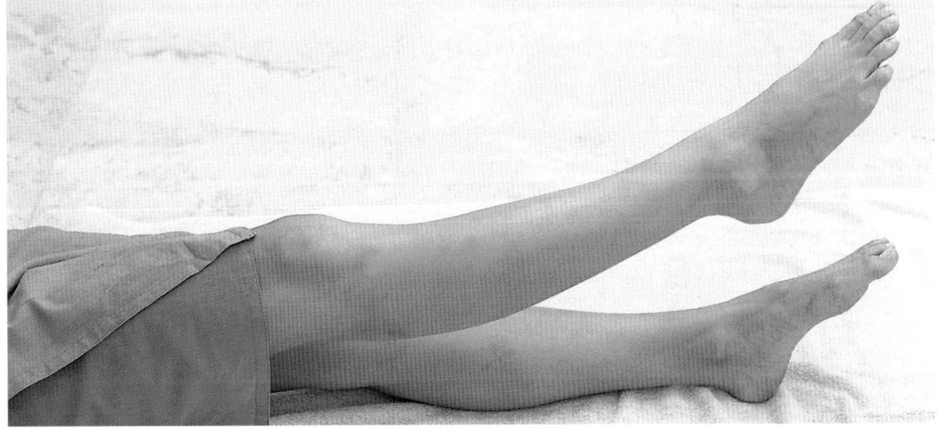

△ **6** Lie on the floor or sit on a chair. Stretch both feet out in front of you. Make scissor movements by crossing the right foot over the left, then the left over the right. Keep your feet and toes pointing straight up towards the ceiling. Work each leg ten times. Rest for a few moments, then repeat the exercise.

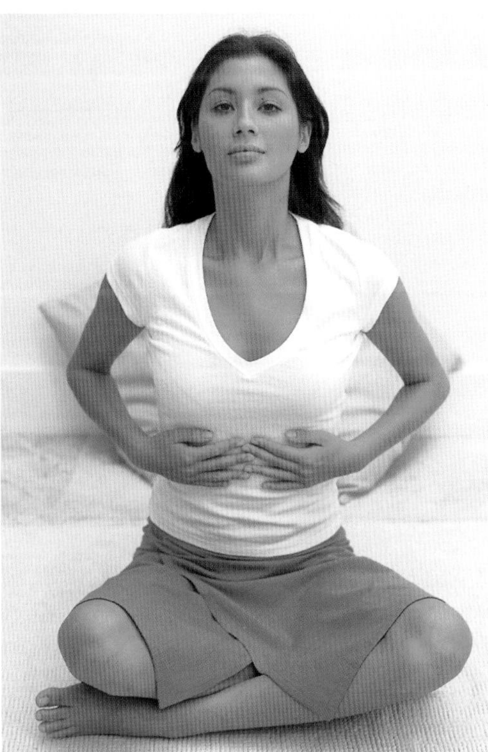

◁ **7** Sit in a comfortable position, eyes closed, fingers resting on your solar plexus. Allow your breathing to follow its own rhythm. Quietly repeat to yourself a meaningful two-syllable word, such as re-lax or hea-vy. This helps to soothe your mind while simultaneously encouraging your body to unwind and de-stress. Don't worry if you feel a little awkward or find this difficult at first. With practice, your voice will become calm and low, and your breathing deep and slow.

ports routine

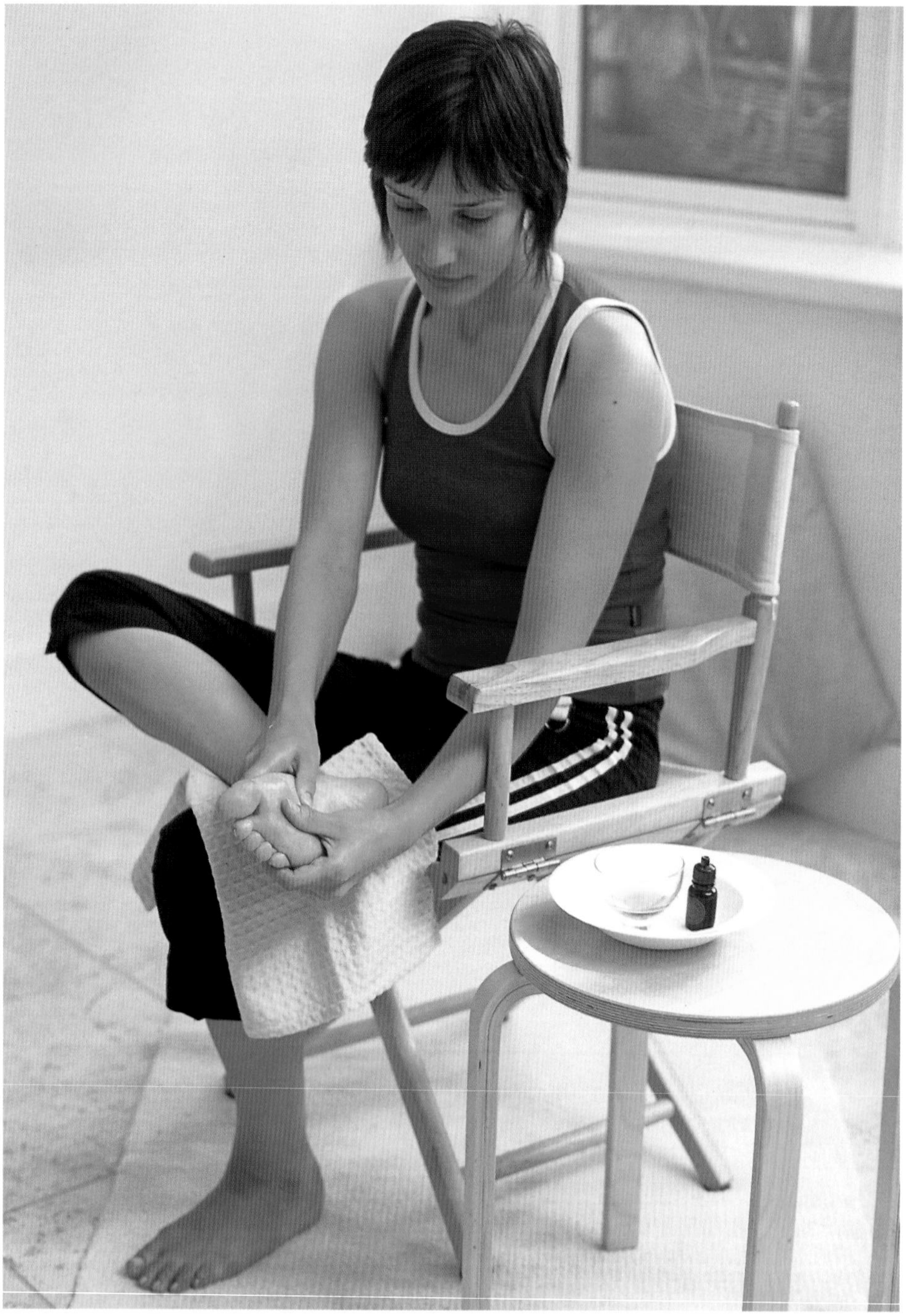

◁ **If you wish to use oil for this routine, add a few drops to your palm. Rub the hands together to distribute the oil, then briskly rub all over the right foot and lower leg – you should add enough oil to create a light sheen but not so much that the skin becomes greasy. Oil the left side when you are ready to massage it. Afterwards, wipe off any excess with a towel before putting your shoes back on.**

It is essential to warm up properly before doing any type of sport. Warming up helps to prevent cramp and reduces the possibility of aches and pains – you are much more likely to get injured if your muscles are cold.

Cool-down exercises after a work-out are also important. They give the body a chance to come back to a balanced state after its exertions. Warm-ups and cool-downs also help you to manage the transition between normal life and exercise and back again.

Massage is a valuable addition to your usual warm-up and cool-down routines. It is a good way of connecting with your body, and becoming aware of any held tension or awkwardness that you may be experiencing. It is also good to pay some attention to the feet, which bear the brunt of much of the exercise that we do.

soothing foot powder

This is a great powder to use before or after doing sports. It will help to keep the feet dry and fresh. Tea tree is a vital component because of its antiseptic qualities, but you could use rosemary or sandalwood instead of the lemon – choose whichever has the most appealing aroma.

ingredients

- 150g/5oz rice flour
- 150g/5oz orris root powder
- 150g/5oz bicarbonate of soda
- 1 tsp boric acid powder
- 6 drops each lemon and tea tree

Mix together the rice flour, orris root powder and bicarbonate of soda. Add the boric acid powder and mix well. Drop in the essential oils, and stir well until they are thoroughly absorbed. Now transfer your powder to a clean, plastic shaker.

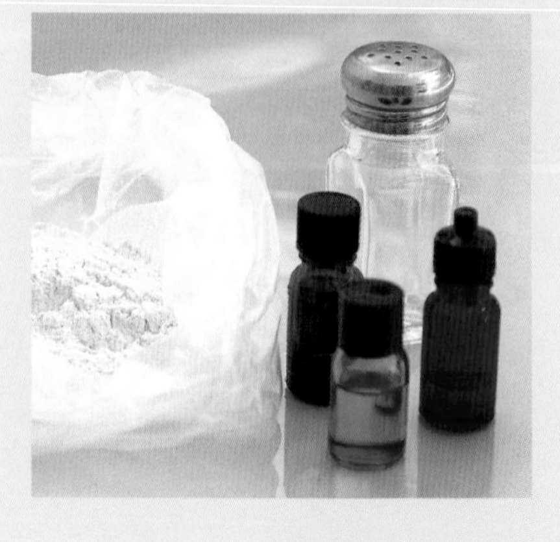

before a work-out

This short routine is easy to do in the gym or at home. Start on the right foot, and then do the left. For the first two moves, sit down and bring the foot you are working on to rest on your knee.

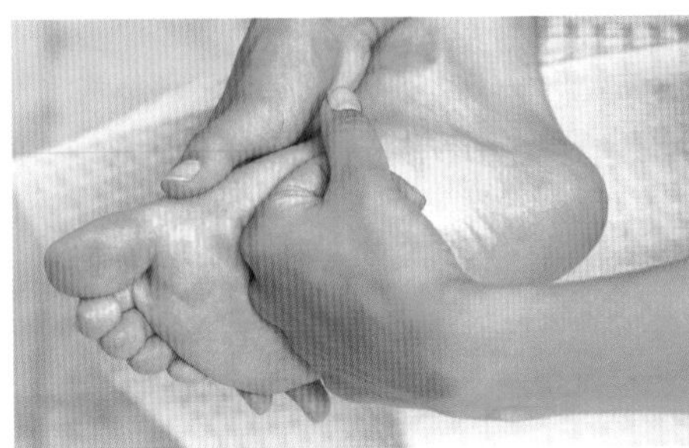

△ **1** Hold the top of your foot in your right hand and make the left hand into a loose fist. Use the flat area between the knuckle and first joint to knead the sole. Work all over the foot, starting at the heel. Use firmer pressure for the heel and ball, and light pressure on the arch. Massage the sole area three times.

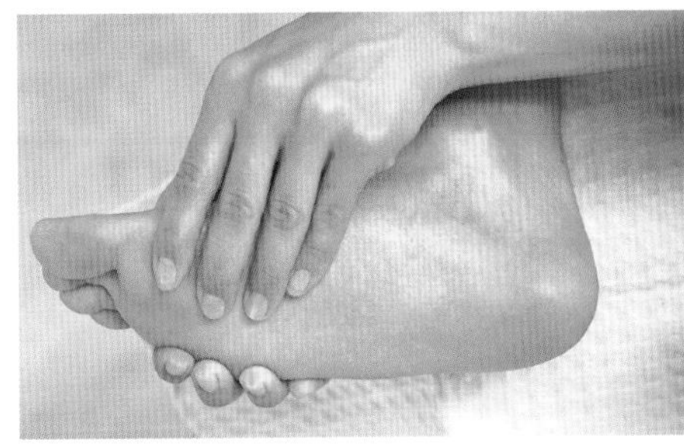

△ **2** Place the thumbs on top of your foot, near the toes, and let the fingers of both your hands curl round the foot to meet in the middle of the sole. Keep your thumbs in position and press the fingers in deeply, then pull them out to the edges to spread the sole. Slide the fingers back to the middle and work in this manner down the foot towards the heel. Repeat.

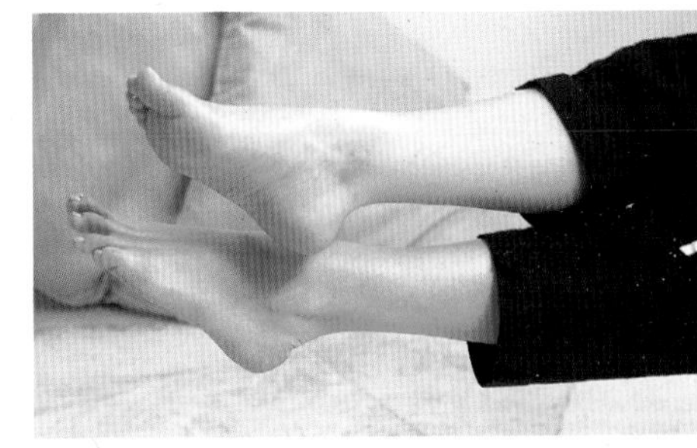

△ **3** Sit down on the floor or on a very stable chair with your legs stretched out in front of you. If on the floor, raise your feet up. Now cross them alternately and rapidly, one over the other in a scissor-like action. Keep the feet straight and the toes pointing upwards. Do the movement at least ten times with each leg.

after a work-out

After exercise or a sporting activity, have a warm shower to help relax your muscles. If you are at home, it is a nice idea to soak your feet in a large foot bowl half-filled with warm water. Add 10ml/2 tsp of almond oil blended with two drops each of rosemary and tea tree. Dry your feet thoroughly before the massage.

▷ **1** Start with the right foot. Use the thumb and index finger of your left hand to pull your big toe straight. Hold to the count of five. Gently rotate it in clockwise direction, then anticlockwise. Do the same to all the toes in turn, ending on the little one.

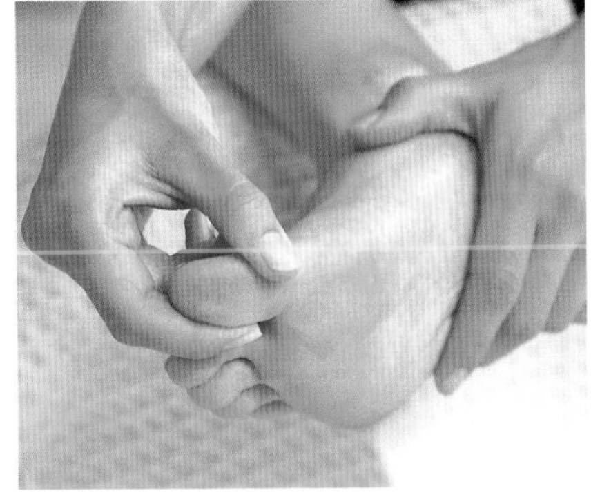

▷ **2** Using the back of the fingers, slap all over the foot. Start on the sole, then do the top of the foot. Repeat so that you cover the entire area twice. Make the slaps as heavy as is tolerable; they should be lighter on the top of the foot than on the sole. This is an excellent action for breaking down toxins.

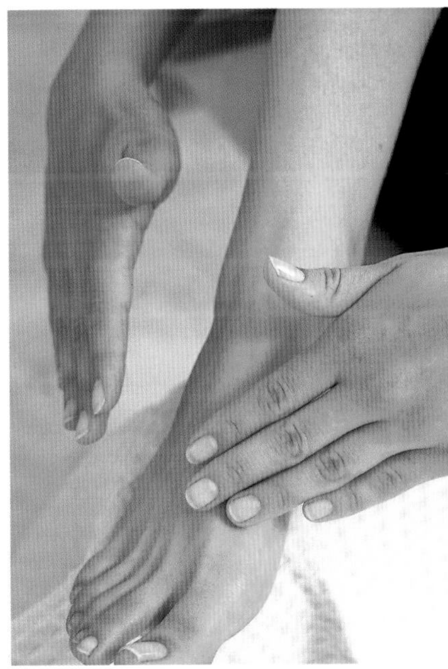

▷ **3** This movement is good for eliminating cramp in the calf. Put the first two fingers of the left hand on the Achilles tendon, then slide upwards to the base of the calf muscle. Press in and make deep circular movements on the spot. Continue to work in this way as you move up the leg, so that the entire muscle is treated. Slide your fingers back down to the Achilles tendon. Do the movement five times in total.

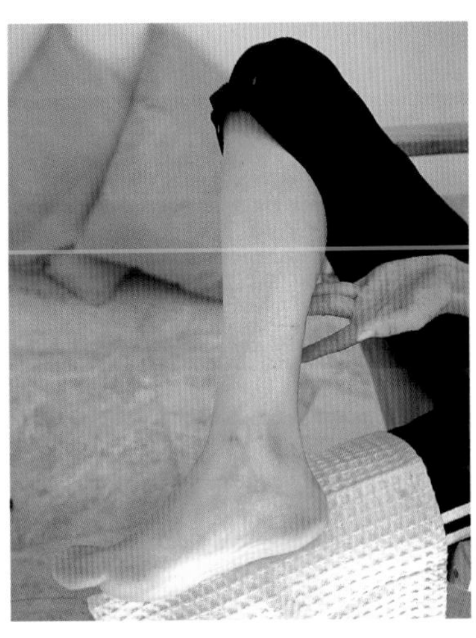

▷ **4** Finish off with some brisk stroking up the back of the leg, using both of your hands. Briskly stroke up the lower leg, from the ankle to the knee. Slide the hands down to the ankle and repeat twice more. Now repeat the whole sequence on the other leg.

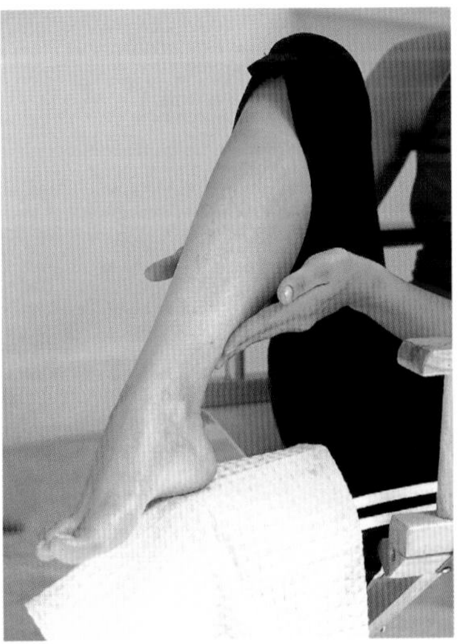

Take a **break**

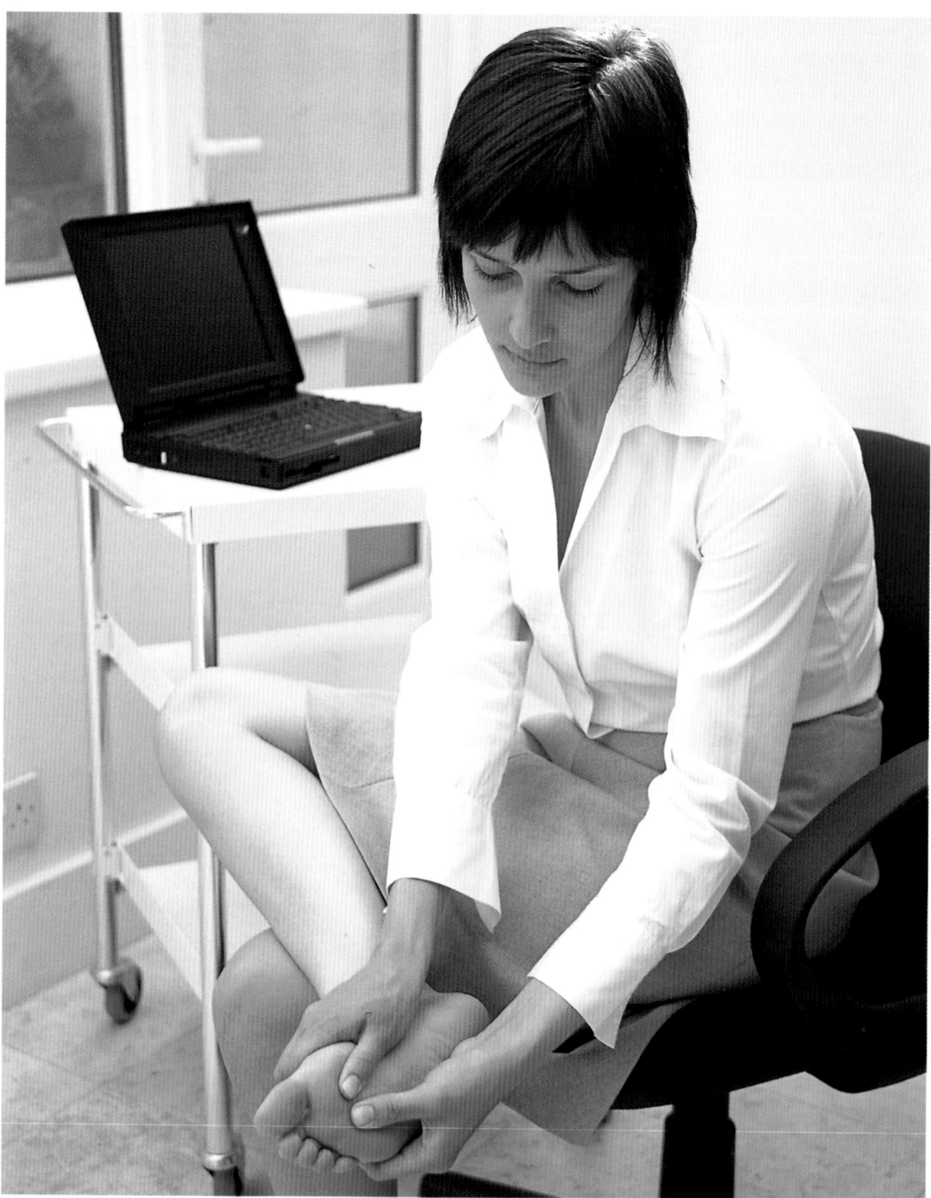

We often have to work or fulfil other obligations when we are feeling under par, because it just isn't possible to take a day out every time we feel a little unwell. Even on a good day, your energy will inevitably flag at various points.

Taking regular breaks from work is always beneficial – and, in the long run, will help you to work more efficiently. If possible, get some fresh air every day, perhaps taking a short walk during your lunch hour. Many office workers eat lunch at their desk, but it is important to get away and have a proper break. Make sure you have healthy food, such as fruit, to snack on at other times of day, too. This will stop you from relying on quick sugar fixes, such as chocolate and biscuits, to keep your energy up. You should also drink plenty of water – have a litre bottle to hand, and top up regularly.

Giving yourself a quick treatment can be a great way to revitalize body and mind. The treatments given here are easy to do in the office, or in a quiet area of any workplace.

◁ If you work in one place all day, such as an office, you may find that you feel low at certain times. If you also work on a computer, you are likely to develop tension in the shoulders and neck. Giving yourself a quick self-treatment will make you feel cared for, and will help to release tightness in the back of the body.

quick cure-all

The reflexology points that treat the spine also have an effect on the whole nervous system. Working these points may help to shift a headache, backache or shoulder tension, and it is a great way to give yourself a general boost.

Remove your shoe and bring one foot to rest on your left knee. Turn the foot to expose the inner edge. Starting at the base of the big toe, walk your thumb along the bone and down to the heel, using a caterpillar-like crawling motion. Now thumb-walk back towards the toes, but this time press up into the bone as you go. Repeat the movements on the other foot.

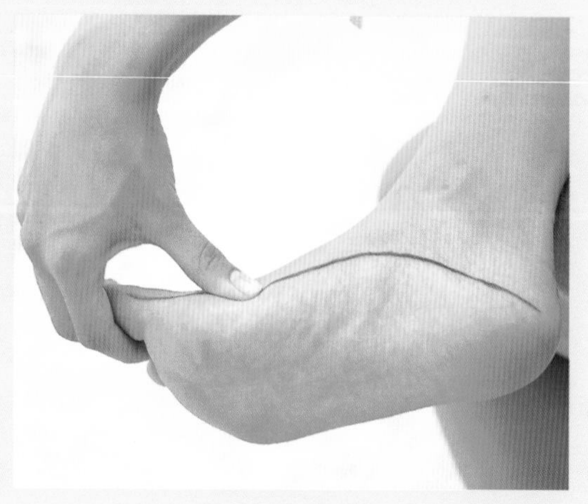

▷ The spine reflexes run along the inner edge of each foot. As you work the points, try to be aware of any areas of tenderness, and give them a gentle massage.

general pep-up

This easy revitalizing routine uses a combination of massage and reflexology. It's easy to do at your desk or in any quiet corner. Start with the right foot, then repeat on the left.

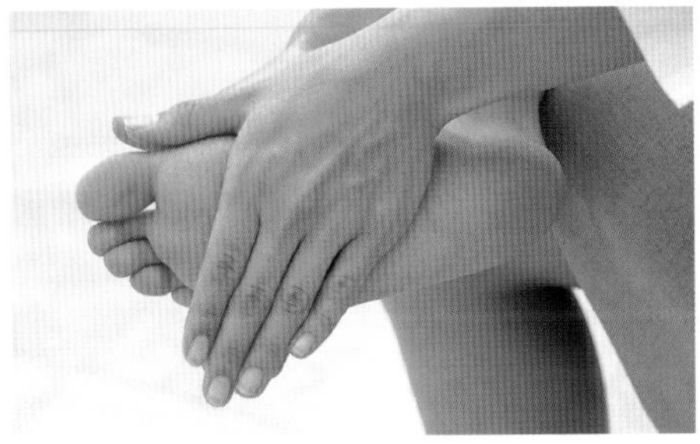

△ **1** Place your right hand over the top of the foot and your left hand on the base, in a sandwich hold. Gently slide your hands up from toe to heel and back again. Press the lower hand in so that the pressure is firmer on the sole. Do this three times, or more.

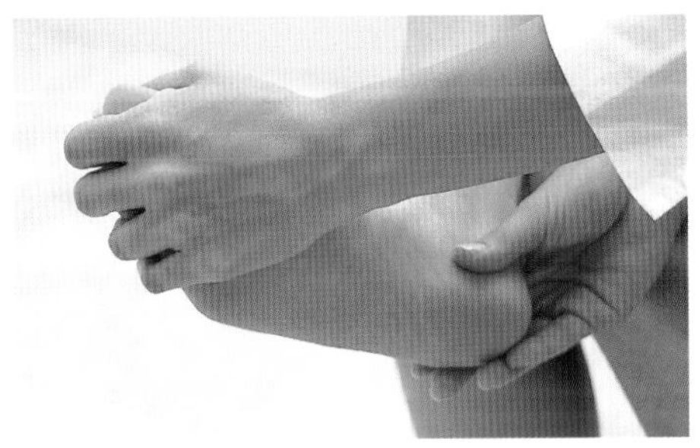

△ **2** Cup your heel in your right hand for support. Hold the top of your toes with your left hand and rotate the ankle gently. Do this first in a clockwise direction, then circle it anticlockwise. Repeat until you have done three circles in each direction.

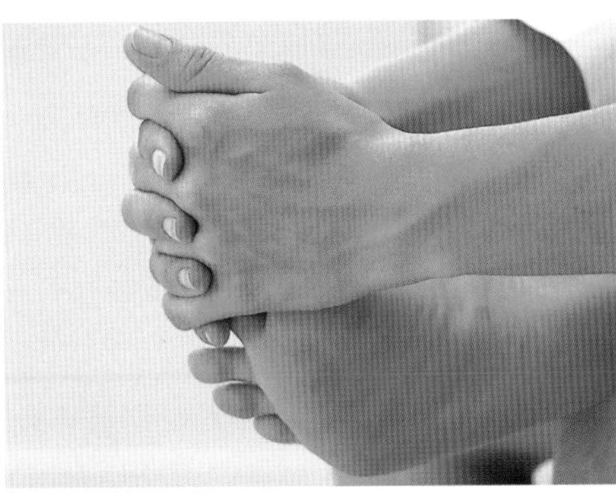

△ **3** Clasp your hands over the toes, so that they join directly over the little toe. Slowly pull along the top of the toes, allowing each one to open out as you go. This releases tension in the head area.

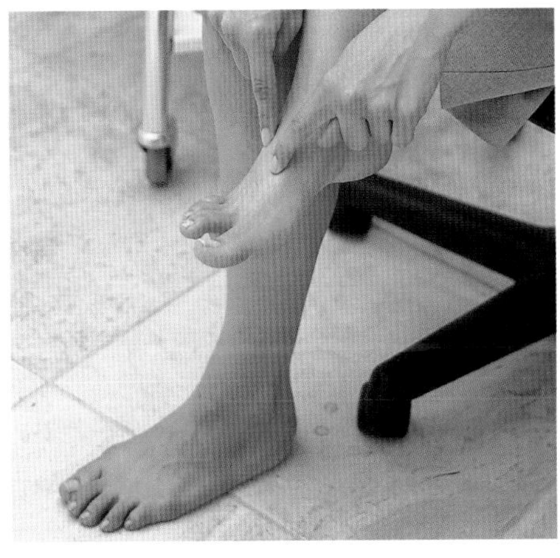

△ **4** Move your foot so that you can reach the top easily; you may like to rest it on a stool. Use both index fingers to make tiny circles all over the top of the foot. Work from the base of the toes up to the ankles. Vary the pressure depending on how you are feeling; light pressure is very relaxing, heavier pressure will have an energizing effect.

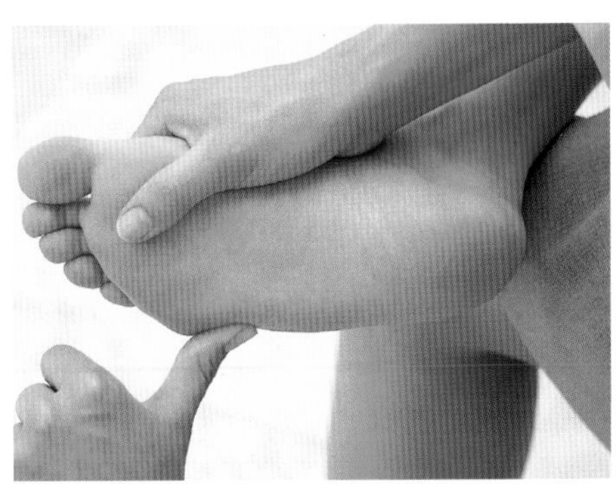

△ **5** Support the inner edge with your right hand, and use your left thumb to crawl down the outside edge. This works on the shoulder, hip and knee, relaxing the muscles in these areas.

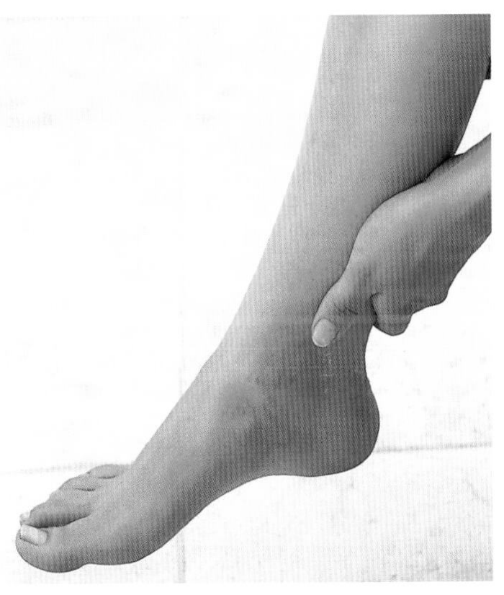

△ **6** Massage the back of the leg, using alternate palms to stroke briskly from the top of the ankle to just behind the knee. This is a good energizing movement to end the routine. Now repeat the whole sequence on the left foot and leg.

relieving headaches, sore throats and neck tension

Here is a excellent treatment for headaches or sore throats that are related to tiredness, stress and tension. This will also help if you have tension in the neck. Do it on both feet.

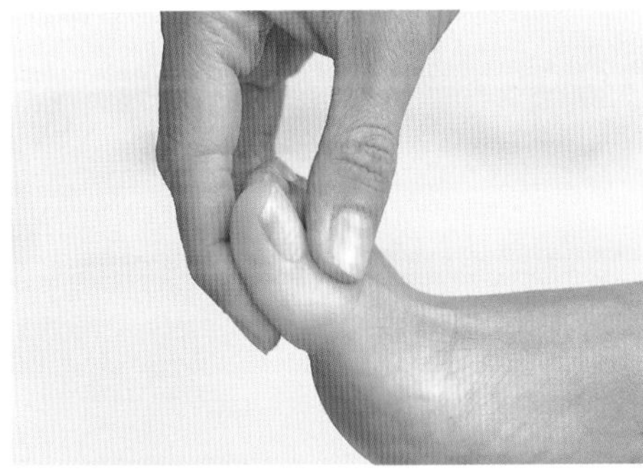

△ **1** Take off your shoes and raise up your right foot. Using your thumb and index finger, pinch your big toe all over. Do the sides, back and top. This action is good for the head and neck.

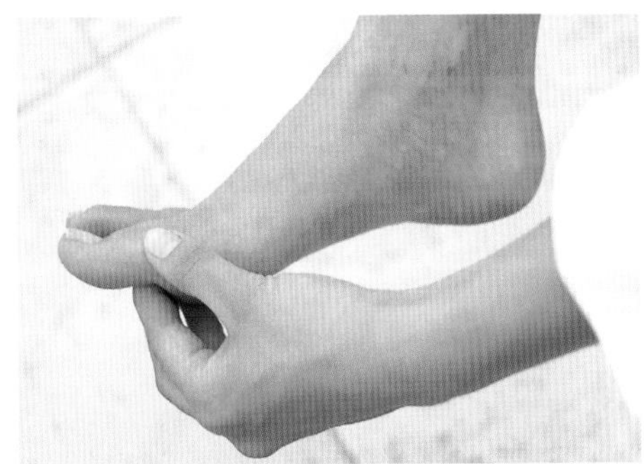

△ **2** Use your thumb to walk around the top of the big toe from the outside to the inside. This is a reflexology technique used to relax the throat area.

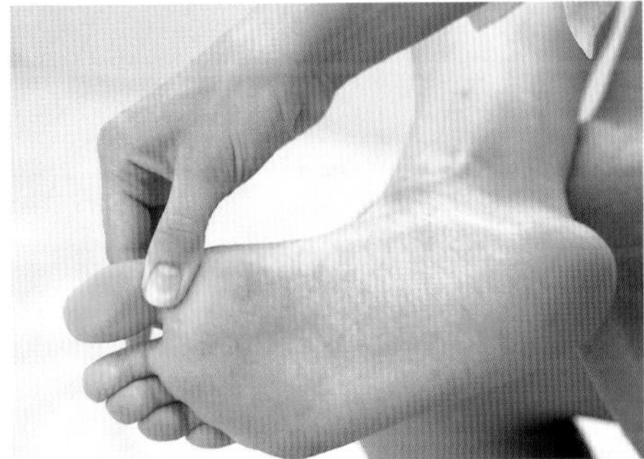

△ **3** Use your thumb to walk from the outside to the inside of the big toe, along the base. This helps relax the muscles at the back of the neck and base of the skull, which may be implicated in a tension headache.

Tonic for tired legs

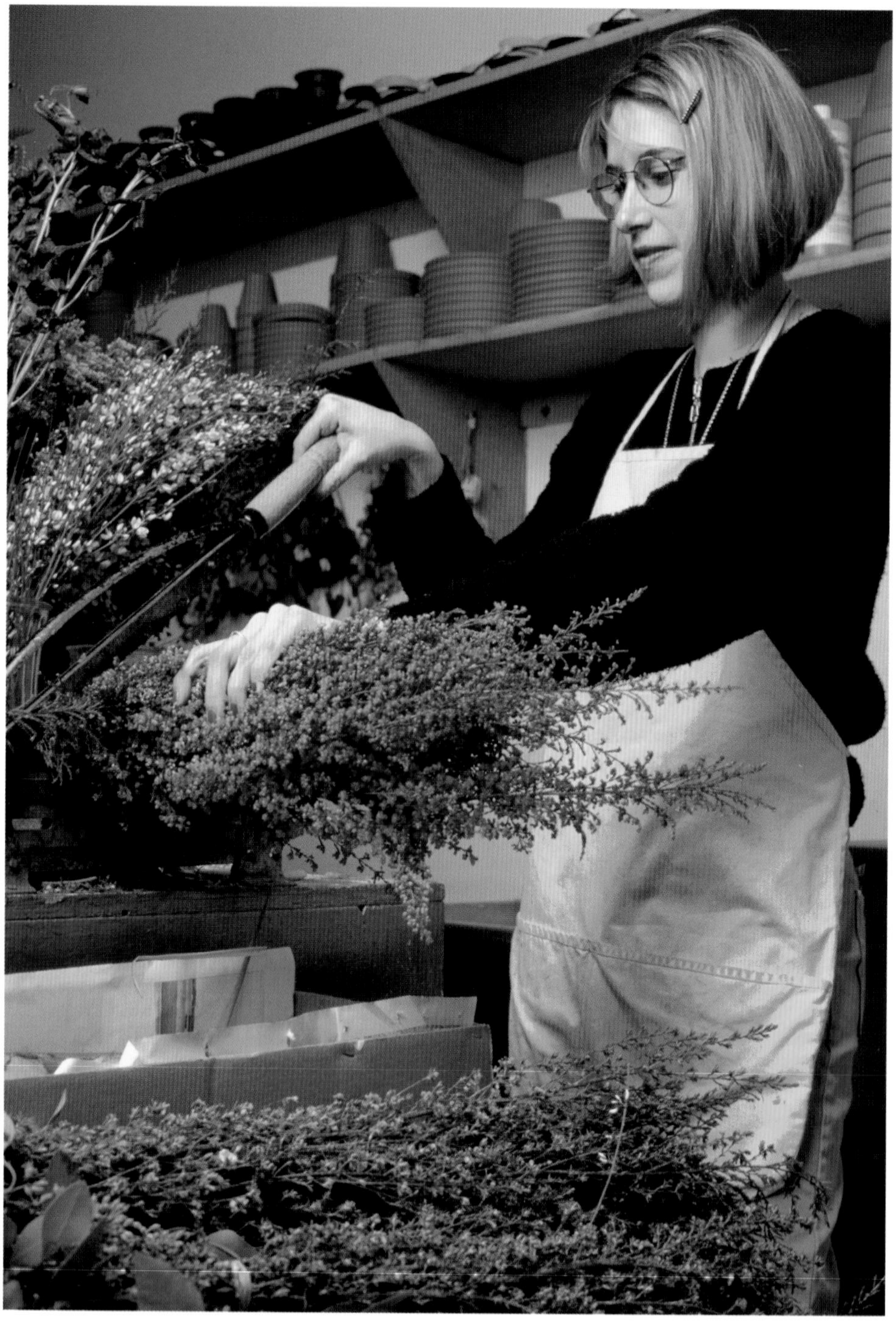

◁ **All kinds of occupations, particularly those in the service industry, require people to be on their feet for much of the day. Taking a quick break every so often to practise some simple exercises will relieve aching and heaviness, and may prevent long-term problems from developing.**

Standing on your feet all day long is not good for your circulation. The force of gravity means that fluid tends to pool in the ankle and feet area.

Muscles do not get a good supply of oxygen and nutrients unless they are moving. If you stand still for a long time, there will also be build-up of waste, which can make the muscle feel tired and achy. A sluggish circulation is the main cause of varicose veins. It also tends to make your skin very dry.

If you need to be standing for long periods, take regular breaks so that you can sit down. You should also keep your feet moving from time to time – walk on the spot, or go up on to the balls of your feet for a few seconds, then release.

quick rejuvenating routine

These simple foot-and-leg exercises will help to keep your circulation moving and should be done at regular intervals. They are particularly effective at the end of the day.

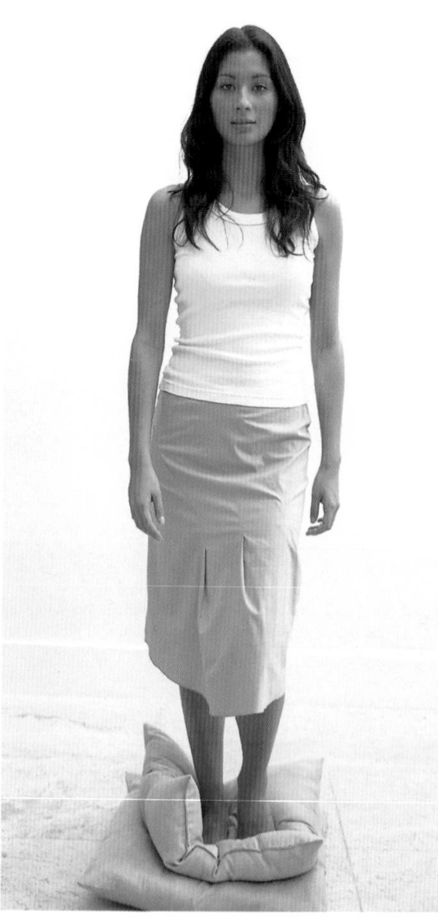

△ **1** Stand on a beanbag, or a couple of cushions if nothing else is available (the many tiny beans used in a bean bag have a pleasurable massaging effect). Try to balance for a few moments. Move your feet one at a time, in a walking motion. This gets all the leg muscles working, and kick-starts the circulation. Have a chair or wall nearby in case you feel unsteady.

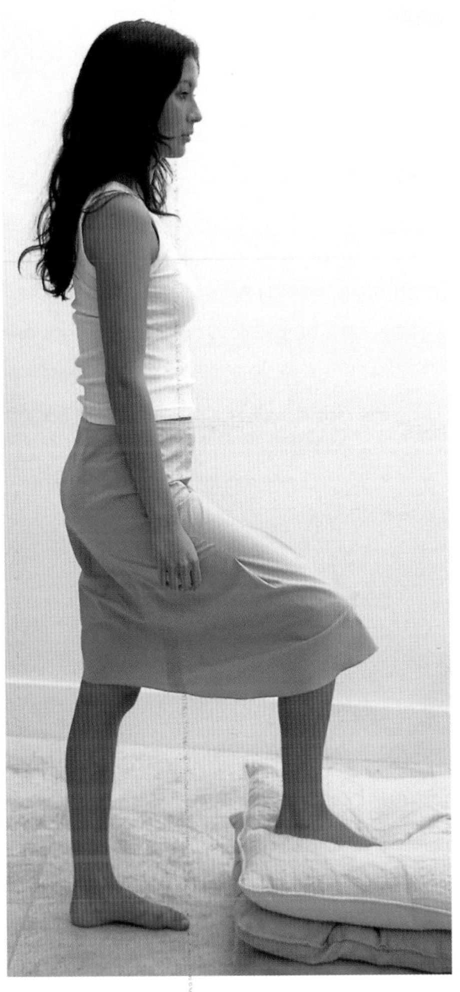

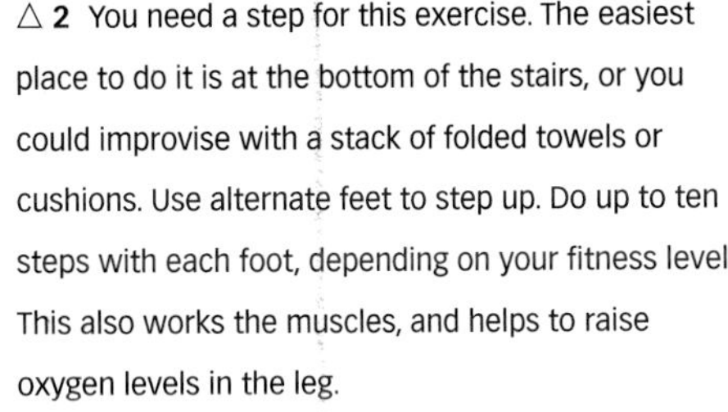

△ **2** You need a step for this exercise. The easiest place to do it is at the bottom of the stairs, or you could improvise with a stack of folded towels or cushions. Use alternate feet to step up. Do up to ten steps with each foot, depending on your fitness level. This also works the muscles, and helps to raise oxygen levels in the leg.

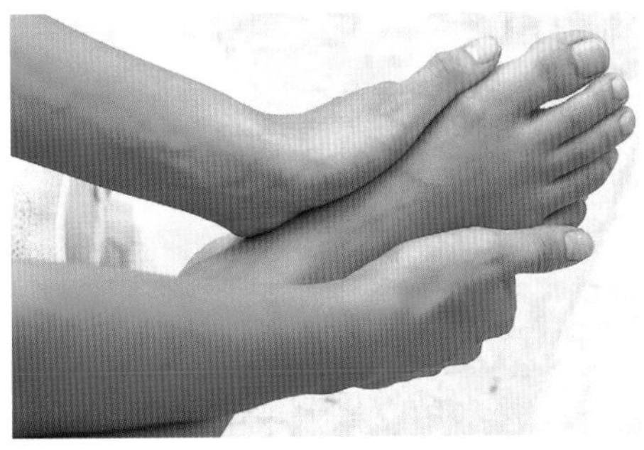

△ **3** Sit down, and rest the right foot on your knee. Place the thumbs on top of the foot, pointing towards the toes, and wrap the fingers round the sole. Draw the thumbs out to the edges of the foot. Return to the start position, and draw the fingers to the edges of the sole. Do this alternate spreading movement all along the foot, starting at the toes and ending at the ankle.

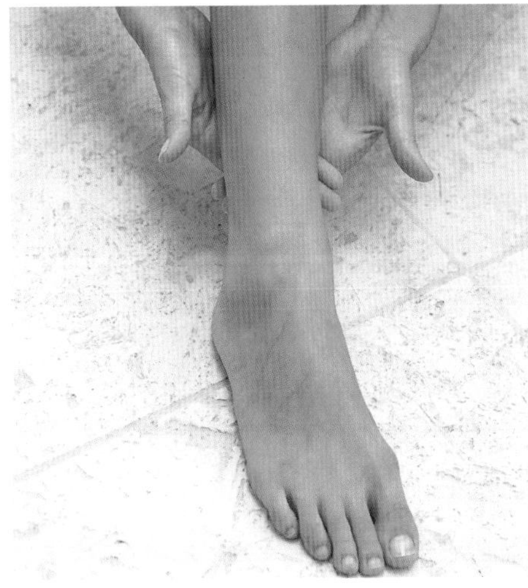

△ **4** Place your hands on the calf above the ankle area. Cross the back of one hand over the palm of the other, as shown, ready for the following step.

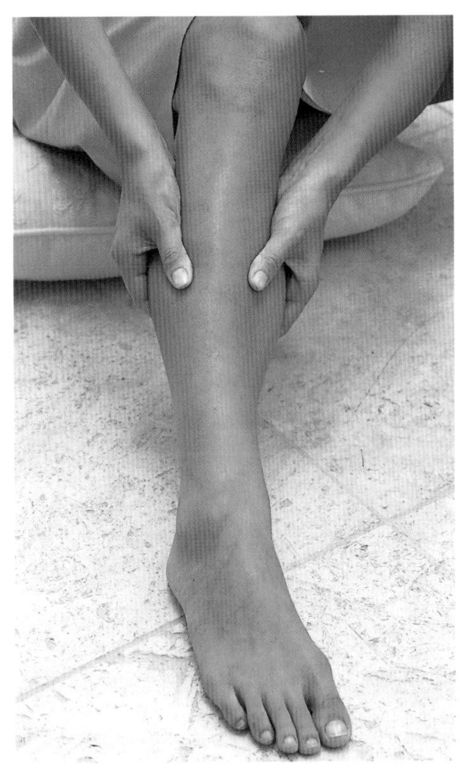

△ **5** Now grasp the sides of the calf muscle with your thumbs. Pull back the thumbs to squeeze the muscle between thumbs and fingers. Work up your entire calf muscle to just below the knee. Repeat.

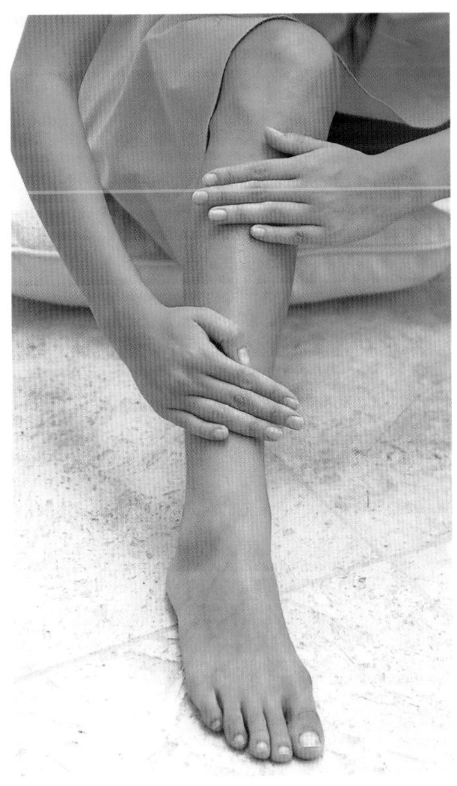

△ **6** Stroke up the front of the leg from ankle to knee, using alternate palms. Use soft pressure. If you wish, stroke a diluted essential oil into the leg in step 6 of the routine, shown here. Good oils to help the circulation and aid relaxation include a blend of geranium and rosemary. Repeat on the other leg.

at the end of the day...

It is an excellent idea to rest with your feet above hip level for at least 15 minutes at the end of the day. A good way of doing this is to use the following modified yoga pose. Find a place next to a wall and put a folded blanket, rug or mat on the floor. Sit on the mat with the side of one buttock against the wall. Lie down and at the same time bring your legs up against the wall, then move onto your back. The backs of your legs should be flat against the wall, your buttocks should touch the base of the wall, and your body should be straight. Stay like this for 15 minutes.

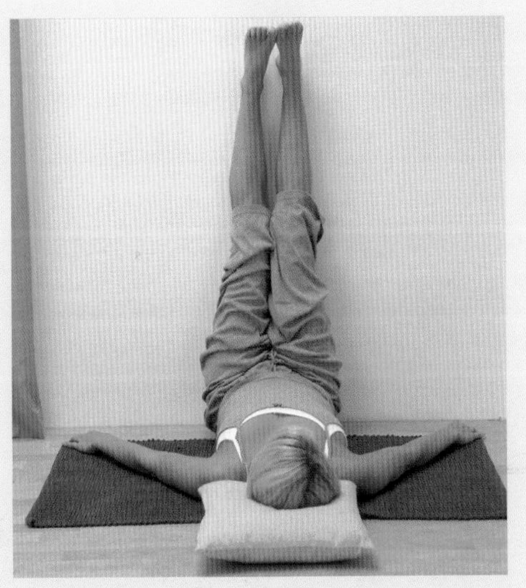

△ **As you rest in this circulation-restoring position, relax your arms and close your eyes.**

Travel tips

Travelling is hard on the body. Whether in a car, train or aeroplane, we tend to sit in cramped conditions and often need to maintain the same posture for many hours.

A few simple techniques can make travelling more pleasurable, and reduce any negative effects on the body. First of all, make sure that your clothes are comfortable and do not restrict your movements.

If you are travelling by car, stop the vehicle and get out at regular intervals. Walk around for a few minutes; stretch your arms above your head and out to the sides and drop your neck towards each shoulder in turn. Raise and drop the shoulders a few times to relieve tension here.

On a plane or train, get up and walk down the aisle from time to time. Every half an hour or so, do some foot and leg exercises to keep the circulation moving.

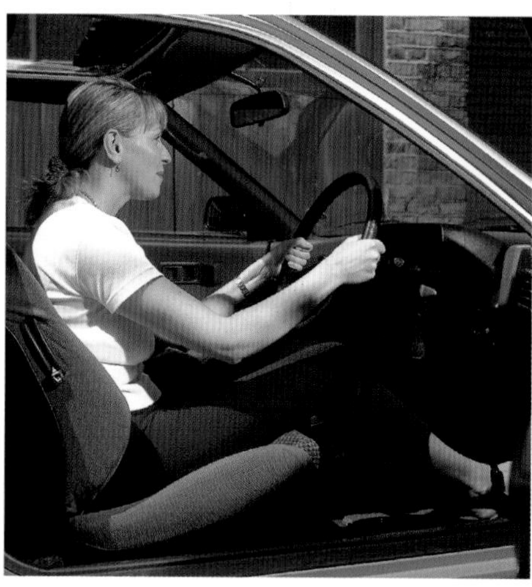

◁ **Travelling often involves sitting in fixed positions in a cramped space for long periods of time. This is bad for all of the body, and it takes a heavy toll on the legs and feet. Make sure that you don't slump forwards, like this woman, but sit up straight. It may help to place a wedge-shaped cushion under the buttocks.**

On aeroplanes, the air is dry and your feet and ankles can swell. If you are flying, it is important to wear comfortable shoes with laces so that they can expand with your feet. You should also wear loose socks – or compression socks as advised by the airline or your doctor. If you take your shoes off, put them back on a few hours before landing so that your feet have a chance to get used to them. Drink lots of water during the flight, and take no alcohol, since it has a dramatic dehydrating effect.

foot exercises in transit

Keeping the feet moving during a long air, bus or train journey minimizes swelling and helps to reduce the risk of deep-vein thrombosis (DVT), a potentially life-threatening condition. You should also do any exercises that are recommended by the airline. You will need an inflatable travel neck cushion to do the following routine.

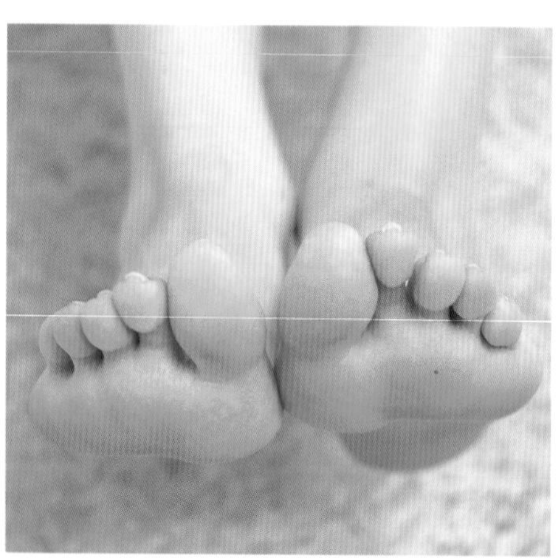

△ **1** Take off your shoes (and socks if you wish). Press the heels into the floor and lift your toes. Pull your toes towards your shins as far as you can; feel the stretch in the front of the lower leg. Then stretch them the opposite way, by pressing the toes into the floor.

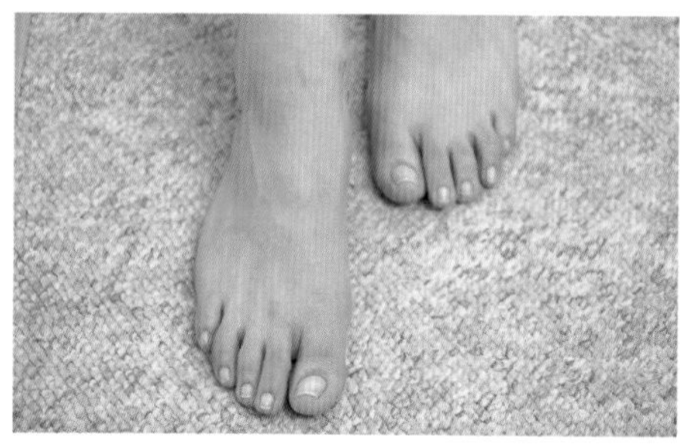

△ **2** Slide one foot forwards, then slide it back as you slide the other one forwards. Repeat this alternate action many times, starting off slowly and increasing the speed. If doing the exercise in bare feet, do not press too hard or you will get carpet burns.

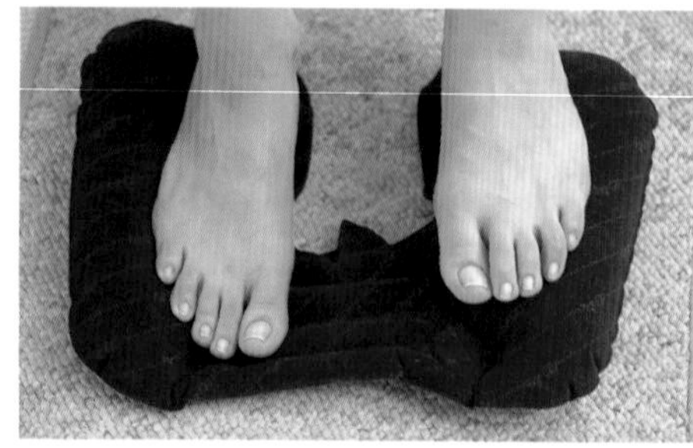

△ **3** Inflate a neck cushion to about three-quarters capacity. Place under the feet, then press alternate feet down as though you are walking. Push down hard enough to move the air from side to side.

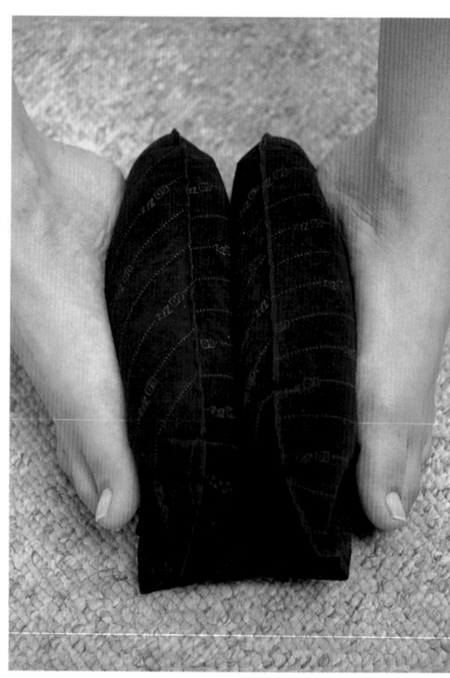

△ **4** Now fold the cushion in two and place it between the soles of your feet. Keeping the cushion in position, try to push your feet together. The partially inflated cushion provides resistance, giving a good workout for the thigh and buttock muscles. You will also feel the stretch in the abdomen. Relax, then push again a few times. Do the whole routine at regular intervals – twice an hour – during the flight.

jetlag routine

These steps will specifically help to relieve the symptoms of jetlag. They are an excellent way of keeping yourself going so that you can go to bed at the correct time.

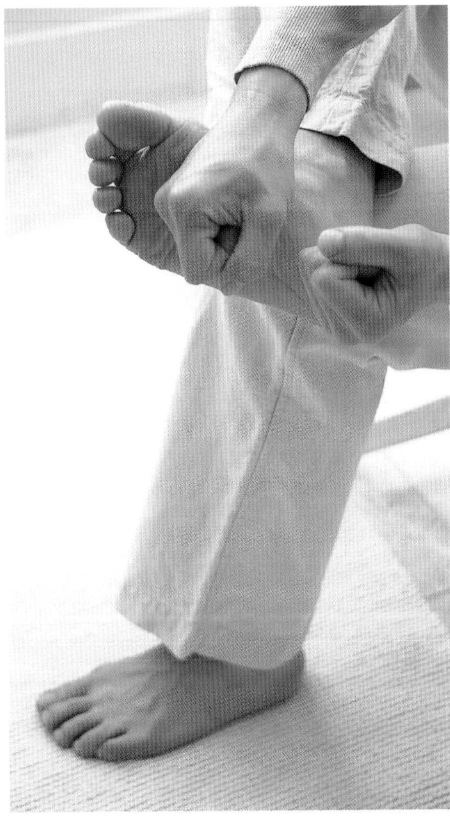

△ **1** Curl your hands into loose fists. Use the flat edge on the little finger side to strike the sole of the foot. Strike all over, working from toe to heel, then back to the heel.

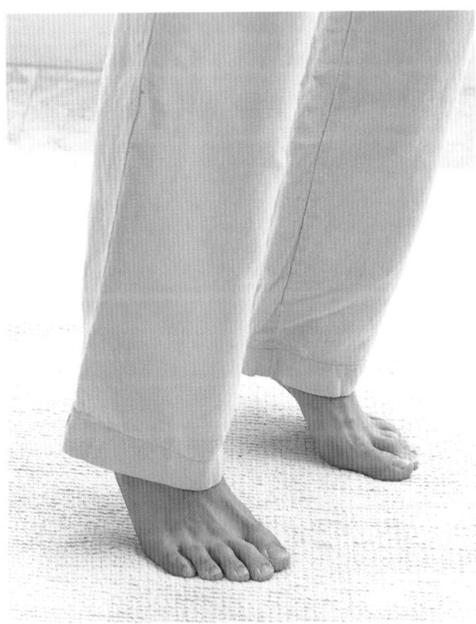

△ **2** Stand up. Stand on the balls of your feet to the count of ten – hold on to a chair or wall if you feel at all unsteady. Relax, then repeat.

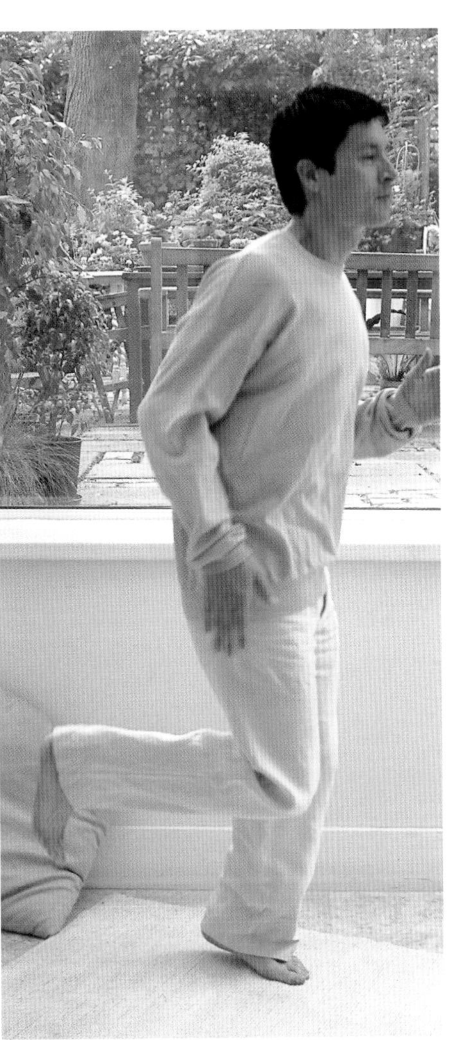

△ **3** Run on the spot to a count of 30. Relax for a count of 10, then run again. Do this about five times, depending on your fitness level.

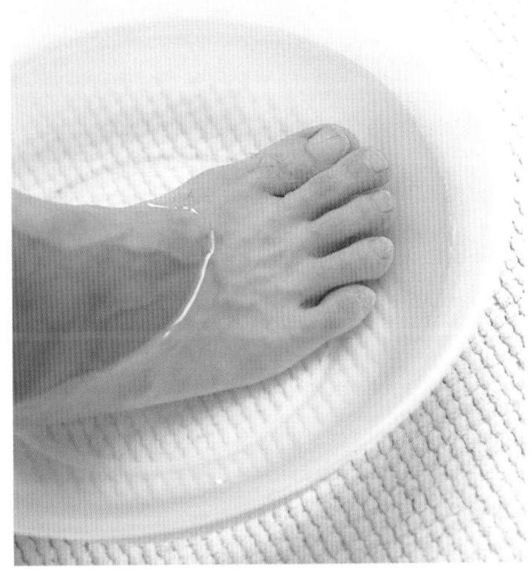

△ **4** Fill a large bowl with cool water (not too hot or cold), or run a very shallow, cool bath. Now place your feet in the bowl or bath. Lift up the toes, then the heels a few times. Rotate your right foot from the ankle, ten times clockwise, ten times anticlockwise. Do the same with the left foot. Repeat the rotation on both feet.

travel beads

Wearing an anklet or bracelet of wooden beads soaked in appropriate oils is a great way of staying fresh and relaxed in crowded places. It also helps to keep germs at bay, as you jostle with fellow travellers.

ingredients

- 5ml/1 tsp almond oil
- 1 drop lavender oil
- 1 drop tea tree or niaouli oil

Mix all the oils. Roll some unpainted, unvarnished wooden beads (you could just use a few) in the oils, leave for five or six hours, then thread onto a cord. Wear on the wrist or ankle (loosely) during a long journey.

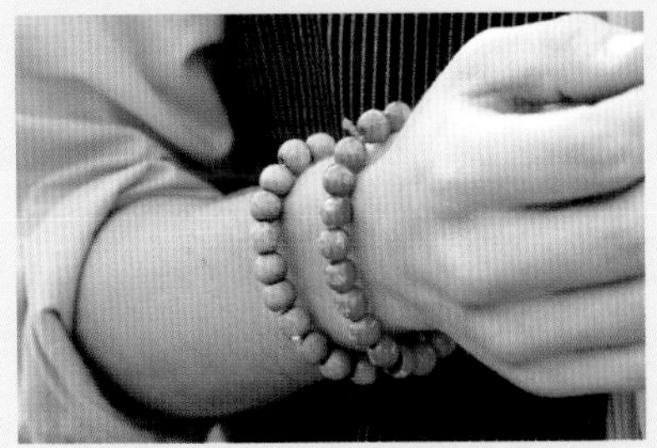

△ **A bracelet of wooden beads soaked in healing oil makes a natural travel talisman.**

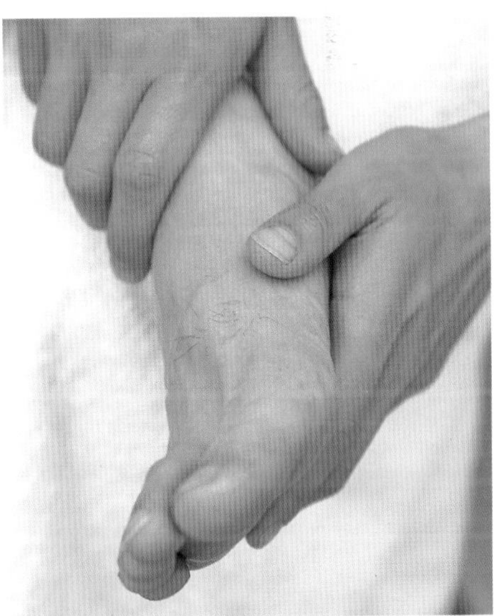

△ **5** Dry your feet. If you like, apply a tonic spray or some talcum powder, or stroke some revitalizing oil into your feet: rosemary is a good uplifting oil to use. Stroke the foot gently to warm up the muscles again.

Circulation booster for the later years

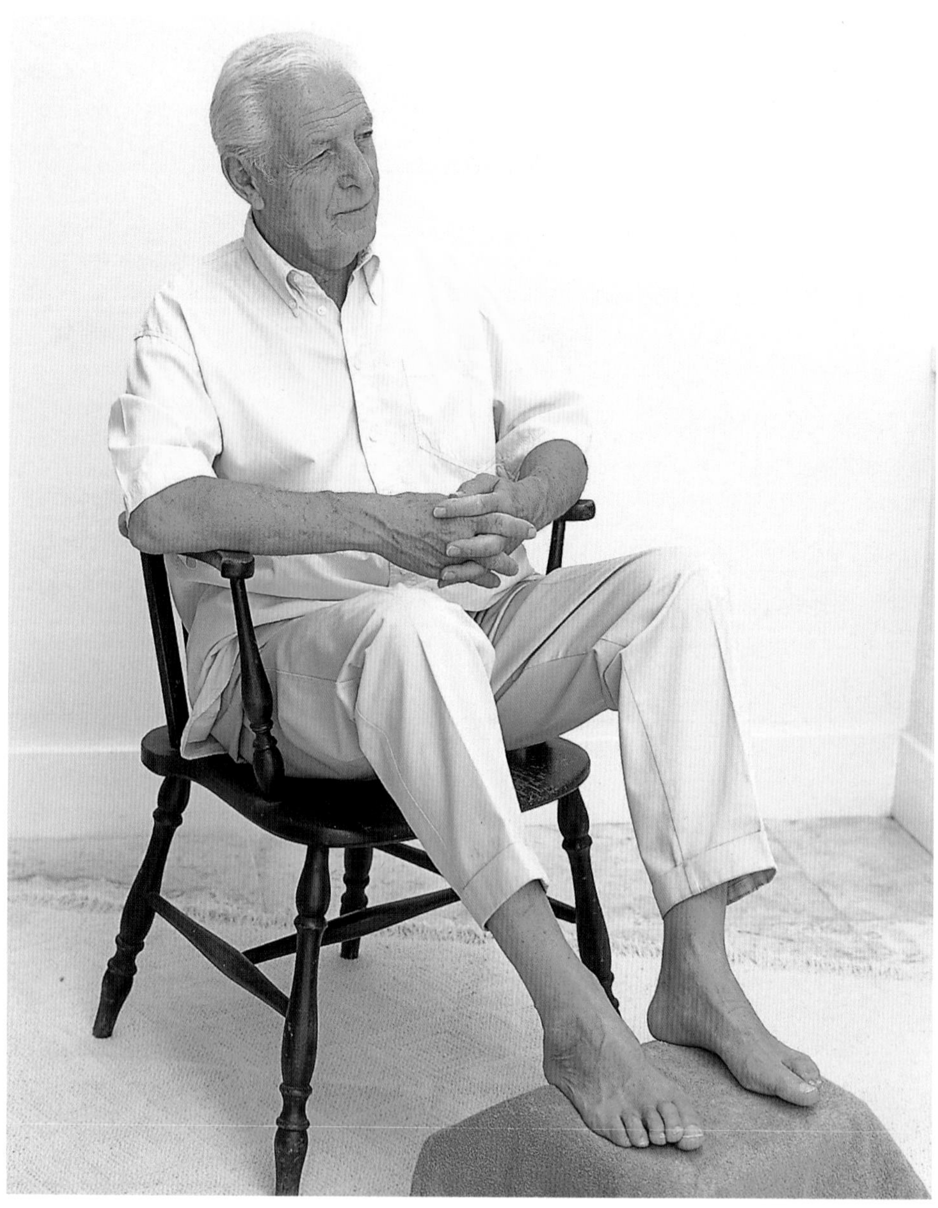

Everyone can benefit from foot massage. Older people, in particular, will benefit from the increase in blood flow that massage brings. We tend to become less active as we age, with the result that our circulation becomes less efficient. Self-treatment once a day will help to keep the feet healthy, bringing oxygen and nutrients to the area and boosting the circulation throughout the body. It will also help to keep the ankles and toes as mobile as possible.

The skin often becomes dehydrated when we are older; using a massage cream in this routine will help keep it moisturized.

△ **Self-massaging the feet once a day will help keep your circulation flowing. Always sit down to treat yourself. Rest your feet on a low stool so that you do not have to bend as far to reach them. Cover the stool with a towel to protect it from any foot spray or oil.**

safe for all

This treatment is very safe; it is fine to do if you have varicose veins, arthritis or other age-related complaints. The routine featured here is designed for self-treatment, but it can also be given by another person if you find that easier.

self-treatment routine

You need a towelling strap with loops for this routine, or you can improvise with a long folded towel, as shown. You also need some empty cotton reels threaded through some strong cord. At the start of the routine, it is good to use a light spray on the feet. You can make your own (plenty of light carrier oil, a little rosewater and glycerine and some of the essential oils listed below). Otherwise, use a ready-made spray.

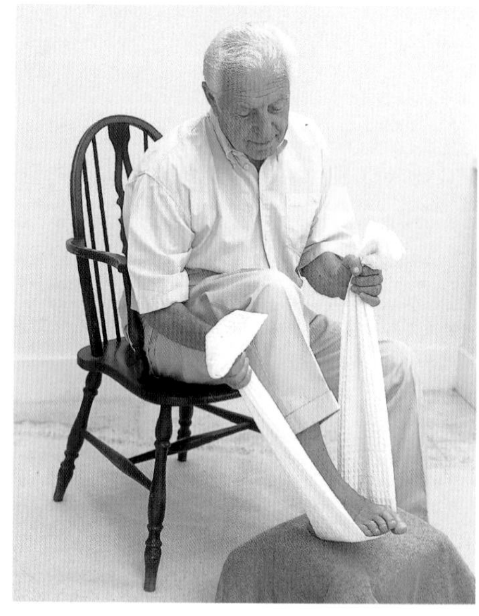

△ **1** Rest your feet on a footrest, covered with a towel. If using a spray, turn the right foot on to its edge to spray the sole, then straighten it up to spray the top. Drop a tissue on to the foot and rub with your left foot to blot excess spray. Now rub your soles over the towel on the footrest until they feel warm. Put the strap under your right foot and pull from side to side. Work all over the sole, from toe to heel, three times.

good oils for older skin

Try using one of these oils in a foot spray, or add a few drops to a carrier and smooth into the skin.

- Sandalwood, which is relaxing
- Cypress, which is stimulating
- Clary sage, which has pain-relieving properties

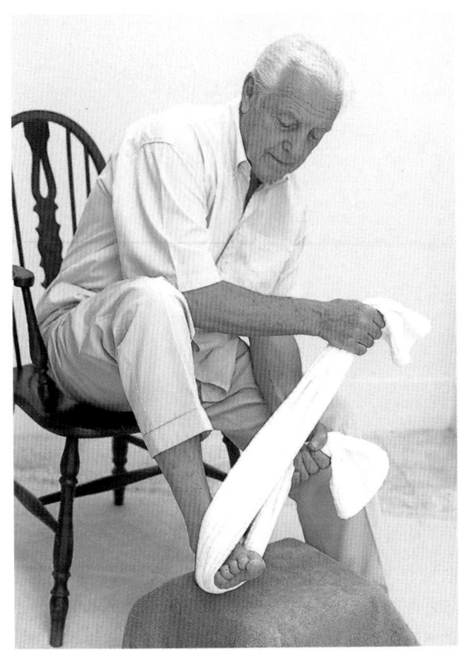

△ **2** Now turn the foot back on to its outside edge. Holding the strap out to one side, pull it back and forth so that you are gently rubbing the top of the foot as you did the sole. Again, work over the area three times, from toe to heel.

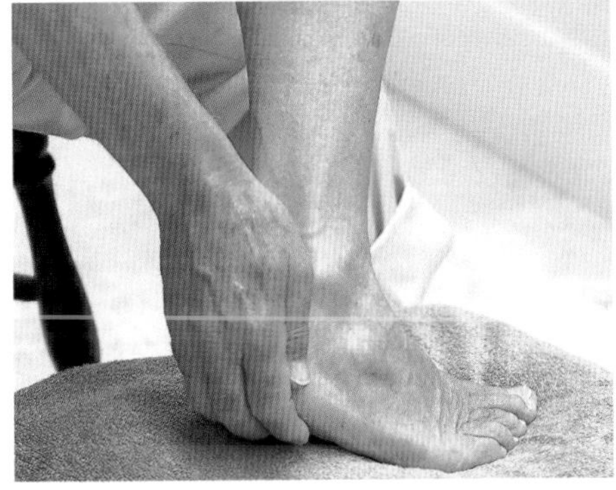

△ **3** Place the middle fingers of your right hand at the base of your heel. Draw them slowly up the back of the heel, using as firm a pressure as you can comfortably tolerate.

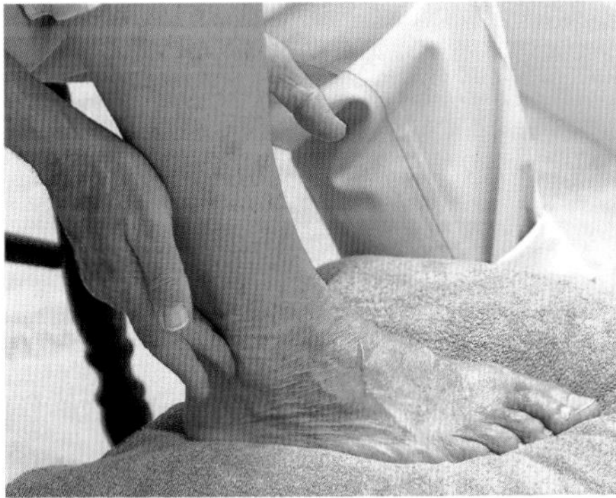

△ **4** Use the fingers of both hands to circle round the inner and outer ankle at the same time. Do steps 3 and 4 once again.

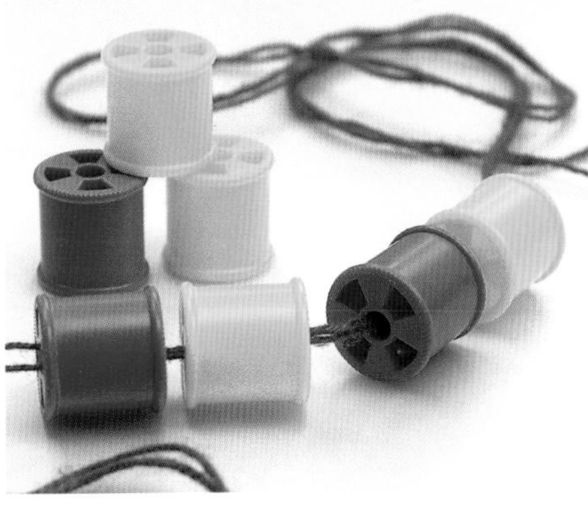

△ This routine involves using a home-made massage aid consisting of several cotton reels threaded on to a strong piece of cord or string. The string should be roughly the length of your leg. Devices such as these can be very helpful if you have difficulty bending down, or if it feels uncomfortable to rest your foot on your knee.

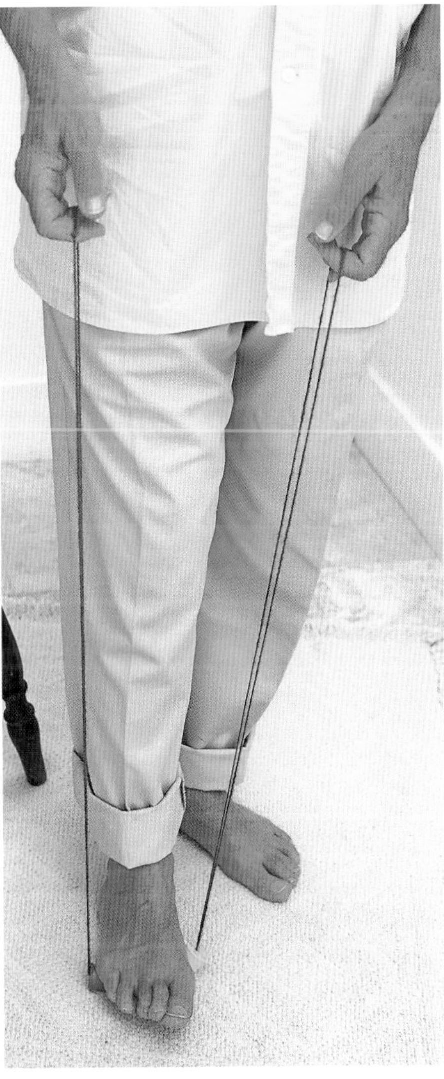

△ **5** Stand up (stay seated if you are unsteady). Place the threaded cotton reels under your right foot and hold the ends of the cord. Roll your foot backwards and forwards on the reels from heel to toe. Do five complete rolls in each direction.

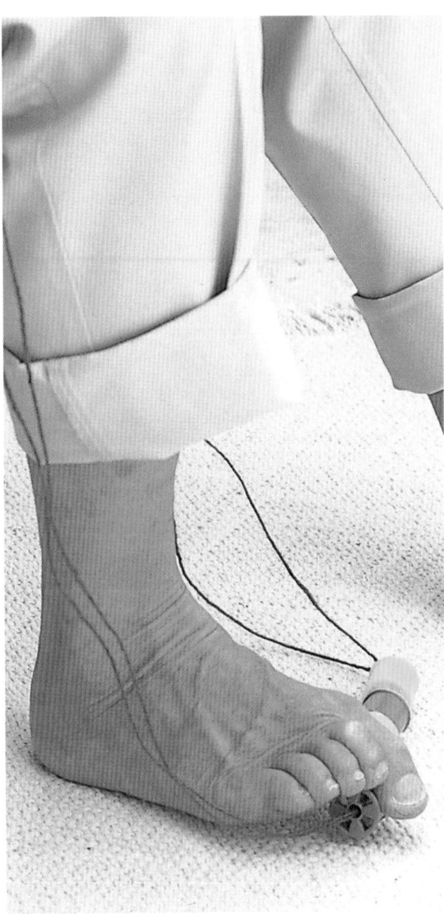

△ **6** Sit back down again, keeping the cotton reels under your right foot. Now try to pick up one or two of the reels with your toes. Practise this lifting exercise five times, making sure that you get all of your toes working.

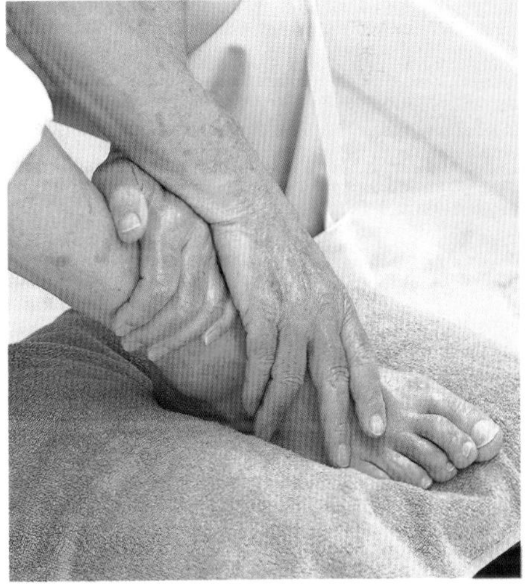

△ **7** Place a little nourishing oil in your hands and rub the palms together to distribute evenly. Using alternate hands, stroke over the top, then the sole, of the right foot. Continue stroking until there is no oil residue left on the top or bottom of your foot. Now repeat the whole routine on your left foot. Make sure there is no oil on the soles of your feet before you get up, so that you don't slip.

Feet treat for mothers-to-be

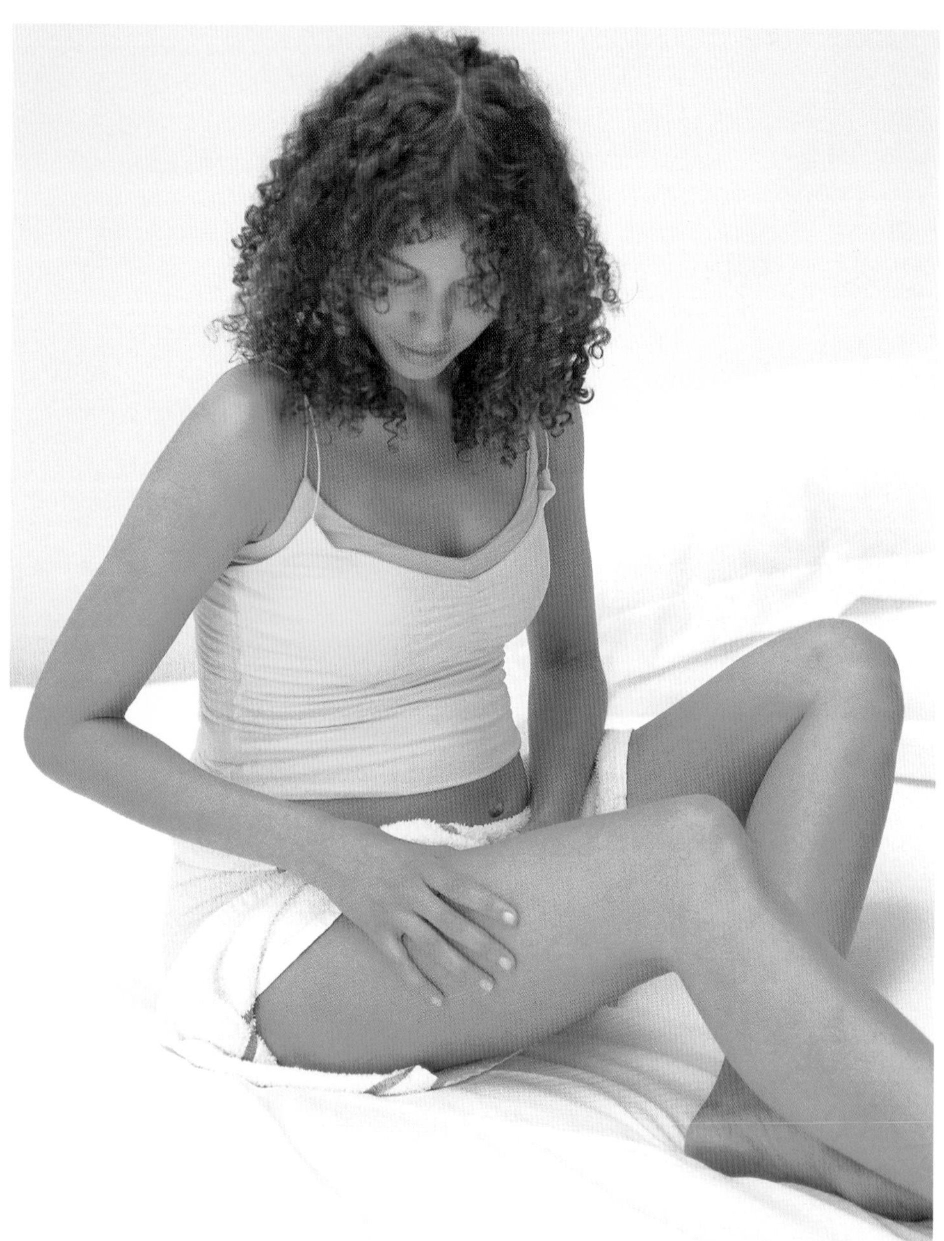

△ In early pregnancy, it is easy to self-massage your legs and feet, and it is extremely helpful for the circulation. However as your pregnancy advances, and the baby grows larger, you are likely to need props, such as marbles in a bowl, or a long-handled brush.

Some women sail through pregnancy with ease, but most will experience minor discomforts of one kind or another. Almost all women feel uncomfortable in the weeks before the birth, and may need some extra support at this time.

Massage has a feel-good factor, which may be particularly welcome in late pregnancy when the woman is likely to feel heavy and tired. Massage is also a good way of oiling the skin, which can get very dry in pregnancy. Working on the feet and lower legs will also help to shift the fluid that tends to collect in these areas during pregnancy. In addition, putting your feet up above heart level regularly will encourage fluid to drain out of the legs, which may prevent varicose veins and reduce feelings of heaviness and aching in the area.

soothing pregnancy routine

This is a gentle and calming routine for pregnant women, which can be adapted for self-treatment (see box). Let the feet soak in the aromatic water for at least five minutes. It's a good idea to put your feet up for 15 minutes after receiving this treatment; enjoy a cup of herbal tea at the same time.

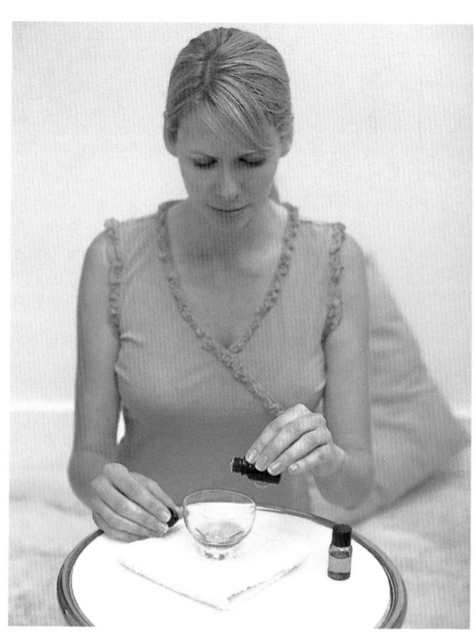

△ **1** Mix 2 drops of essential oil such as mandarin in 20ml/4 tsp of carrier oil – you need a lighter dilution than normal when treating in pregnancy.

safe oils in pregnancy

You should be careful about the essential oils that you use in pregnancy; many are not suitable because they may have an adverse effect. It is best not to use any essential oils other than citrus oils such as mandarin and tangerine during the first three months of pregnancy. Thereafter, always check that any oil is safe for use during pregnancy: camomile, geranium, lavender and sandalwood are good oils for most women, but should only be used well-diluted.

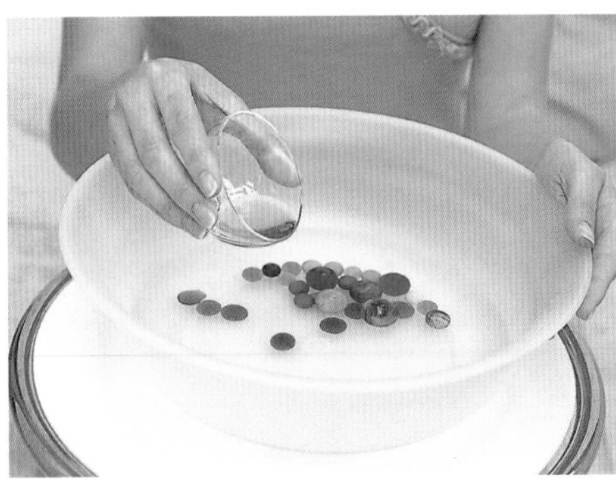

△ **2** Half-fill a foot bowl with warm water, then add a layer of marbles of different sizes. Pour in 5ml/1 tsp of the blended oil.

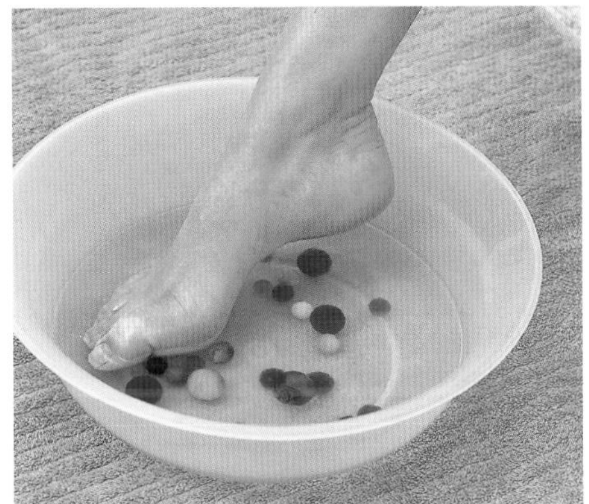

△ **3** Place the feet in the bowl, and push them backwards and forwards over the marbles: this gives a massage-like effect. Move the toes between the marbles. Stretch the feet by lifting up the heels and then placing them flat on the base of the bowl. Now raise up the toes. All these movements will help to open up the feet and to stimulate the circulation in the feet and lower legs. Remove the feet from the bowl and dry thoroughly.

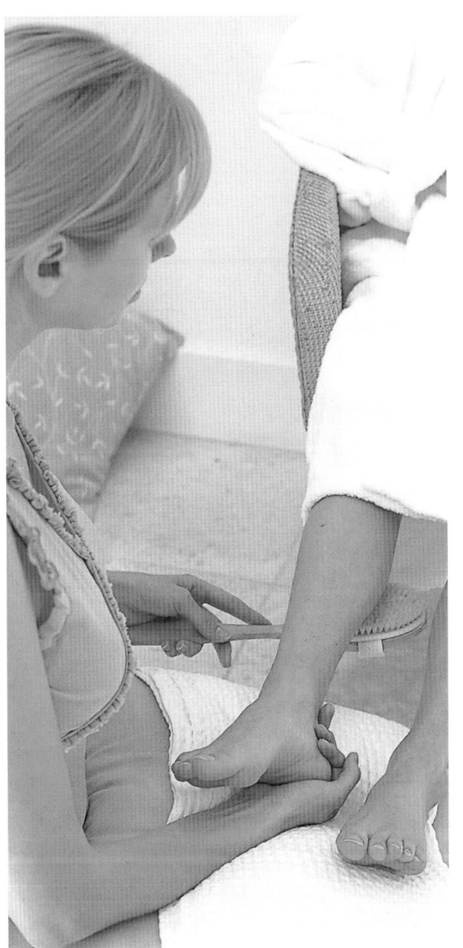

△ **4** Dampen a soft-bristled brush with warm water. Then pour about 5ml (1 tsp) of the oil over the bristles. Rub the brush over the top of the foot, using upward strokes. Cover the area three times, adding more oil if necessary. Rub up the heel and around the ankle area, followed by the front, and then the back, of the lower leg, using upward strokes. Again, cover the area three times. This helps to remove dead skin cells and will also stimulate the circulation.

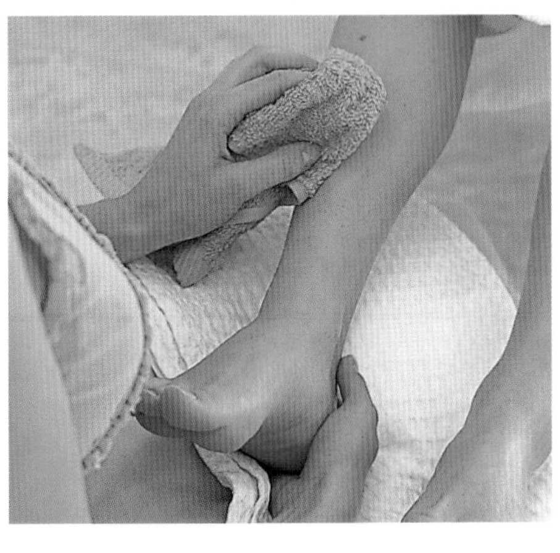

△ **5** Wipe off any excess oil with a cloth. Then use the cloth to stroke gently all over the top of the foot and the front of the lower leg. Once this area feels dry and comfortable, wipe the back of the leg.

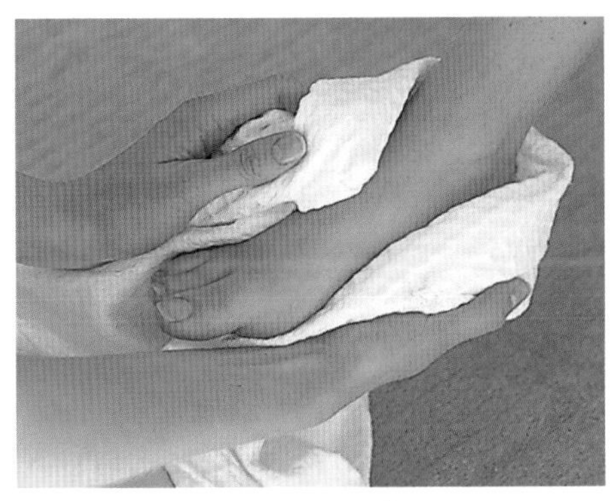

△ **6** Take a small hand towel and fold into a long strip. Holding either end, pass the towel backwards and forwards across the back of the leg. Start just above the ankle and work up the leg to just below the knee. As in step 4, this helps to activate the circulatory system. Now repeat steps 4 to 6 on the left foot and leg.

adapting the routine

Ideally, you should receive this treatment from someone else. However, if this is not possible, the routine works almost as well as a self-treatment. First of all, enjoy soaking your feet, rolling them backwards and forwards on the marbles and lifting the toes up and down – you may wish to spend longer than five minutes doing this. If so, have a kettle filled with boiled water nearby, so that you can top up the footbath when it starts to cool (take care near hot kettles).

It should be easy to apply the oil to your feet using a long-handled brush, as in step 4. To wipe off the excess oil (step 5), simply wrap a soft flannel around the brush, tucking in the edges at the top. Using this means that you do not have to bend down, which can be very uncomfortable in pregnancy. You can try step 6 using a longer towel. However, if this is too difficult for you to manage, simply skip this step. After the massage, make sure that you put your feet up and enjoy at least 15 minutes of peaceful and enjoyable relaxation.

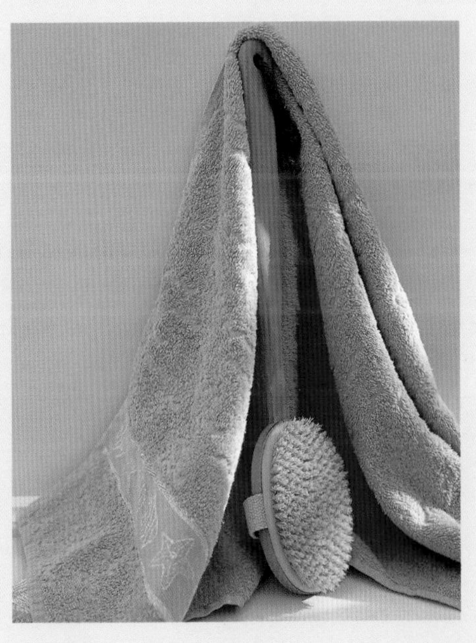

▷ **If you are treating yourself, wrap the head of the brush in a flannel or small towel so that you can remove oil from your feet easily.**

Tackling Common Complaints

Most of us experience minor ailments from time to time, and many people suffer recurrent symptoms. In this section you will find some quick footwork that you can use to alleviate common and repetitive problems such as tension headaches, menstrual pain and insomnia.

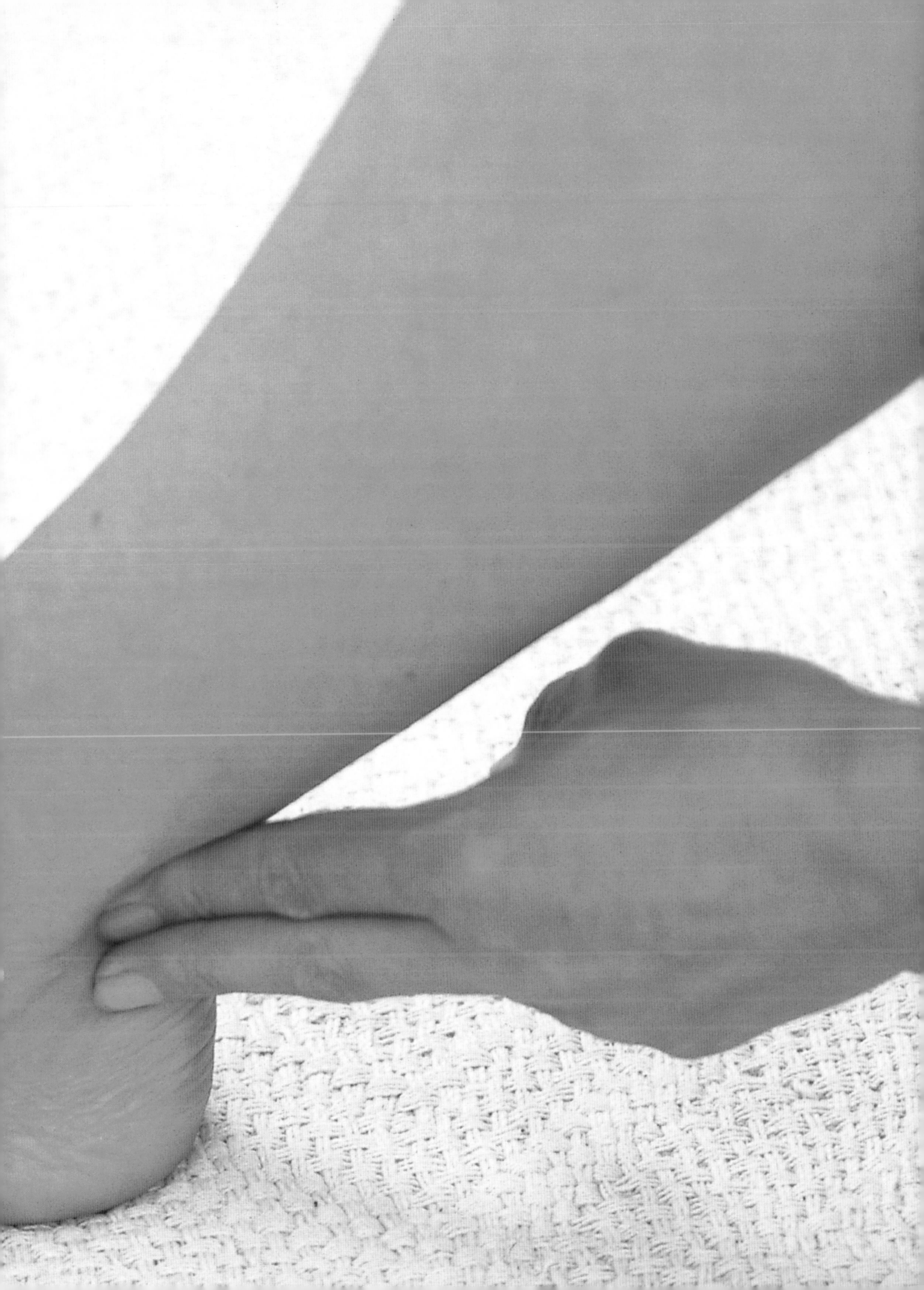

Arthritis

Arthritis is inflammation in the joints, which causes stiffness and pain. There are many kinds of arthritis: one of the most common forms is osteoarthritis, which is usually a result of wear and tear associated with age.

It is important for people with arthritis to take gentle exercise on a regular basis. This helps keep the joints mobile.

Massage can also be very helpful in encouraging mobility; the foot routine given here will help to loosen the ankle and toe joints. This treatment has a relaxing effect, and will improve the circulation of oxygen to the joints, which is also beneficial.

If you like, use massage oil or cream in the routine. Try adding a few drops of lavender and camomile essential oils, which are anti-inflammatories. Marjoram and black pepper are also helpful oils to use, for arthritis, since they can reduce stiffness.

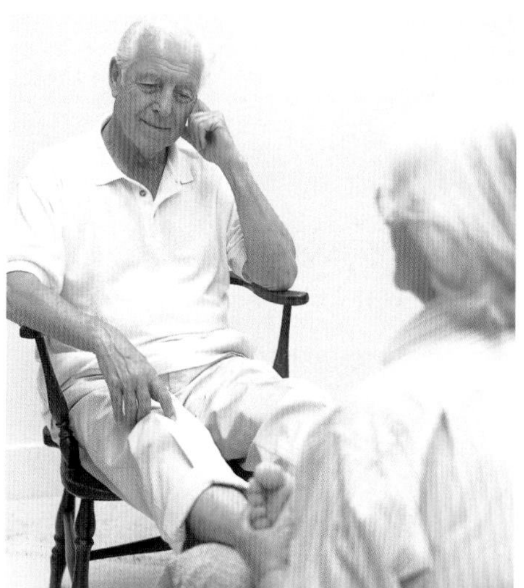

▷ **Mature skin can be very dry, so it is good to use a massage cream rather than oil when giving this treatment to an older person. Place a pillow on your lap, cover it with a towel and rest the person's feet on top. Apply some cream to your hands, then rub the palms together to distribute it. Stroke the medium all over the feet.**

mobility-improving routine

Do this short routine as often as possible – a daily treatment gives maximum benefit. You can do it in the garden or anywhere both giver and recipient can sit down. When treating someone with arthritis, always work gently; in particular, do not force the joints past their limits.

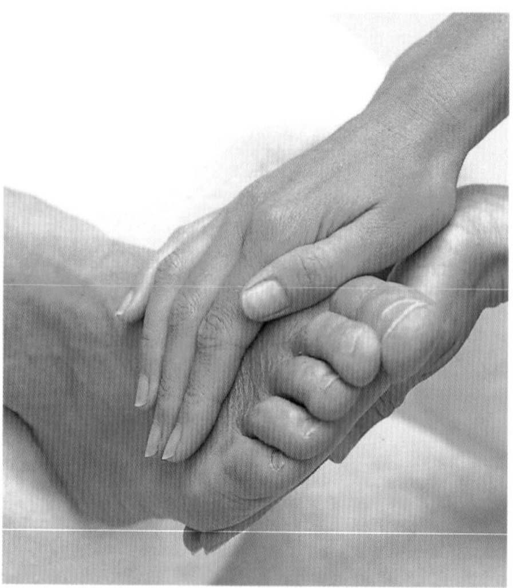

△ **1** Start with the receiver's right foot. Place one hand above and one hand below their foot, so that you are clasping it in a sandwich hold. Slide both hands down the foot from the toes to the heel, then slide them back. Press into the foot with the lower hand, so that you are applying firmer pressure here than on the more delicate top of the foot. Make sure that you ease the pressure when you are crossing the softer tissues of the arch.

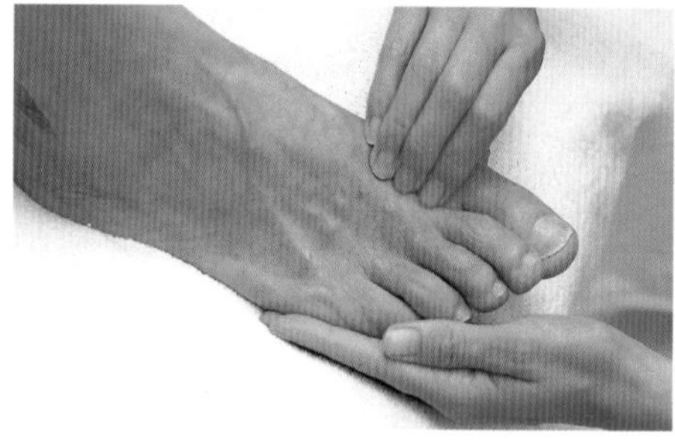

△ **2** Using the three middle fingers of your right hand, make small circular movements down the grooves between the long bones of the foot. Start in the groove between the big and second toes, then work down to the one between the two smallest toes. Use firm but not heavy pressure. Rest the inner side of the foot against your left hand to keep it steady.

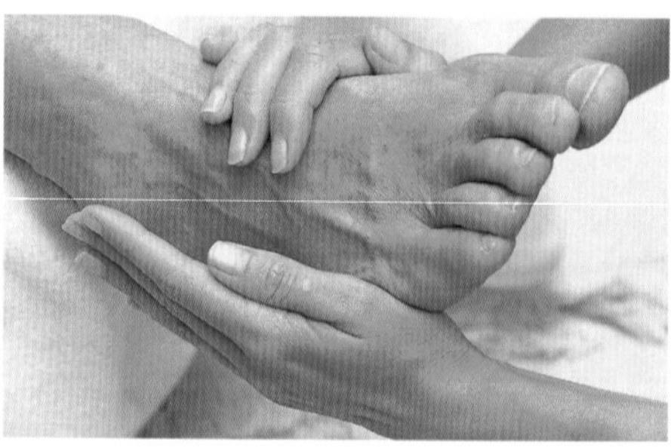

△ **3** Use the fleshy part at the base of the left thumb for this movement. Slide the pad down the outside of the foot, working from the base of the little toe to the heel. Use strong pressure, but keep it pleasurable. Steady the foot by wrapping the right hand around it, with the heel of the hand on the sole.

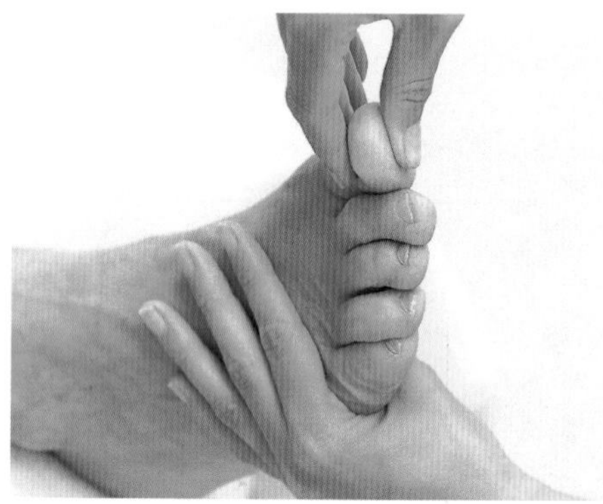

△ **4** Supporting the foot, hold the base of the big toe. Rotate it three times clockwise, and three times anticlockwise. Work gently. Repeat on all the toes.

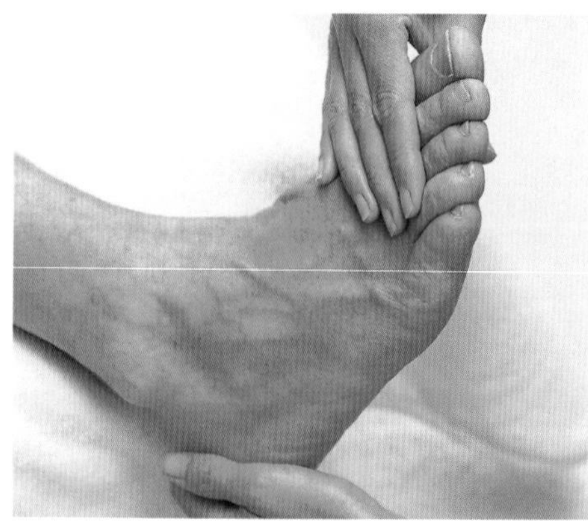

△ **5** Cup the heel for support and wrap the right hand around the foot, with your thumb on the ball. Slowly rotate the foot three times clockwise, and three times anticlockwise. Do not push the ankle beyond its limits. Repeat step 1, then repeat the routine on the left foot.

Muscle strain

It's easy to strain, or pull, a muscle. It happens when the muscle is put under excessive pressure - for example, if you lift a heavy object or make a quick, twisting movement. The muscle fibres may become overstretched, or even torn, and they can take several weeks to heal.

Muscle strain is more common where there is sudden movement or if the muscle is worked hard in a way that is unfamiliar. It is particularly likely to occur if you exercise without warming up the muscles properly, or if there is a burst of activity after a period of inactivity. For example, if you have taken no exercise for months and then do a long workout at the gym.

If you strain a muscle, you need to rest it to allow it to heal. Applying an ice pack or cold compress will help to reduce inflammation, while massage will keep the circulation going.

massaging a strained calf

This self-treatment helps to relieve pain and promote healing after a calf strain. Repeat several times a day, and combine with applying cold compression to the area.

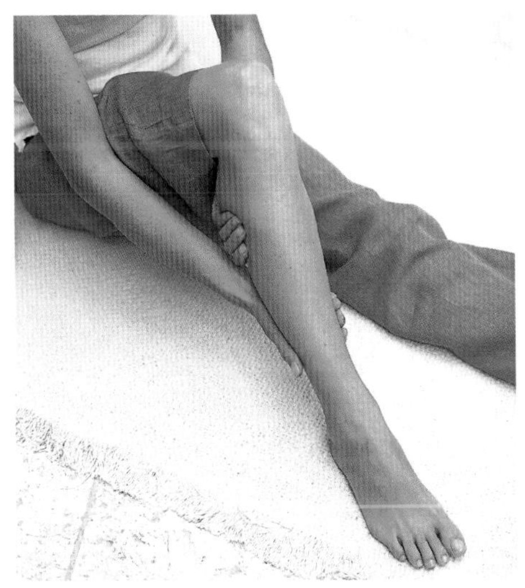

△ **1** Sit on the floor, or on a chair with your leg supported on a stool in front of you. Place your hands on the back of the lower leg, one above the other. Starting above the ankle, squeeze the calf muscle, then release. Work up the leg in the same way to just below the back of the knee. Slide your hands back down to the ankle, then repeat. Do this three times, making the pressure as hard as you can tolerate.

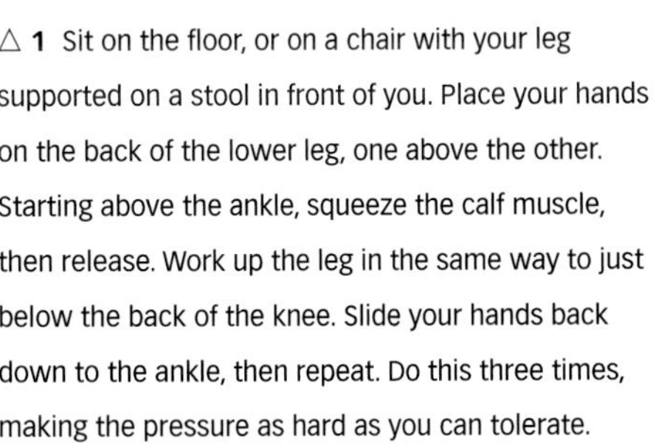

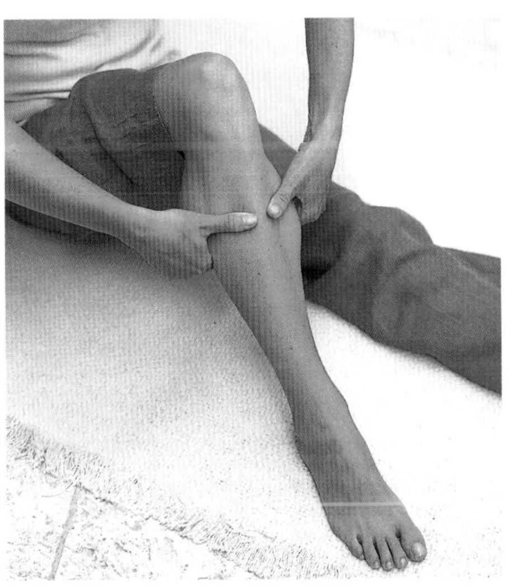

△ **2** Place your thumbs over the shinbone, curling your fingers around the back of the leg. Use your fingers to pull the muscle slowly out to each side, to give it a good stretch. Again, start just above the ankle and work up the leg to just below the back of the knee. Slide your hands back down to the ankle and repeat the action three or four times.

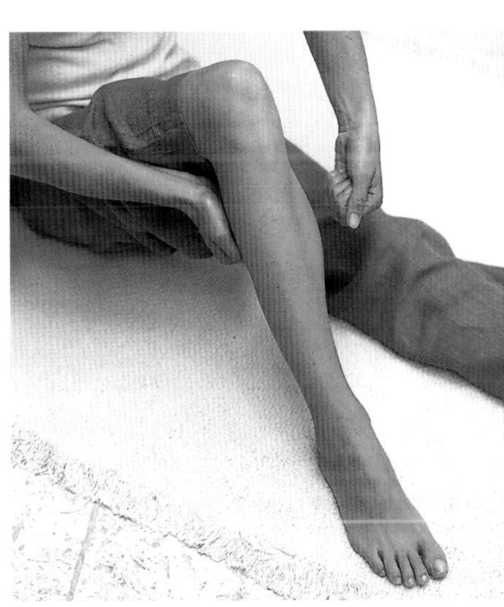

△ **3** Make your hands into fists. Push the calf muscle backwards and forwards from the sides, using alternate fists. Work from the top of the muscle to the bottom, then work back up again. Go up and down three more times (making eight times in total), increasing the speed as you progress. Keep the pressure comfortable at all times. Repeat on the other leg.

cold compress

ingredients

- 10ml/2 tsp grapeseed oil
- 4 drops geranium essential oil
- 3 drops each bergamot and clary sage oils

Fill a bowl with ice-cold water and mix in all the oils. Soak a cloth in the water, wring out and put on the affected area for 15 minutes.

treating a sprain

Sprained ankles are common in childhood. This soothing spray is a good one to have in your first aid kit.

ingredients

- 25ml alcohol or surgical spirit
- 5 drops geranium oil
- 5 drops camomile oil

Put the alcohol or surgical spirit into a 30ml (1fl oz) spray bottle. Use a plastic one if you are likely to be carrying it around. Now drop in the essential oils, then close the lid and shake vigorously to mix. Spray the affected area, then apply an ice pack to the area; to improvise an ice pack, wrap some ice cubes or a pack of frozen vegetables in clean cloth. Use the spray and ice pack treatment twice a day.

Headache and migraine

Most of us suffer headaches at some time or other. The most common cause is tension. A tension headache often feels like a tight band around the head, and it can last for many hours. There can be many different triggers for this type of headache, including stress, noise, tension in the neck and prolonged watching of television. Dehydration is another common cause.

Migraines can be very debilitating. They often manifest as a throbbing ache at the front of the head, which may be accompanied by flickering light, numbness or vomiting. A migraine can be brought on by certain foods, such as chocolate or red wine, by stress or by other triggers.

relieving symptoms

The foot treatments featured here may help alleviate a headache or migraine. If you develop a headache, you should try drinking some water, in case you are dehydrated. Eating a healthy snack and getting some fresh air or gentle exercise may also help. Many sufferers of migraines find it helpful to lie down in a dark quiet room until the attack passes.

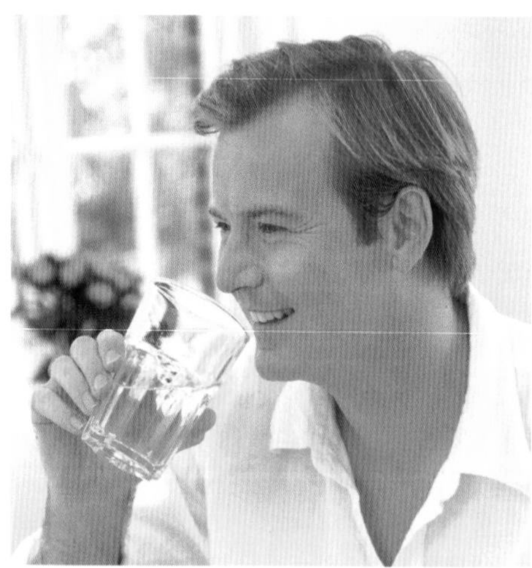

△ **Keep a check each day of how much water you are drinking. Many headaches are simply caused by dehydration, which is a common result of today's dry, centrally heated work and home environments.**

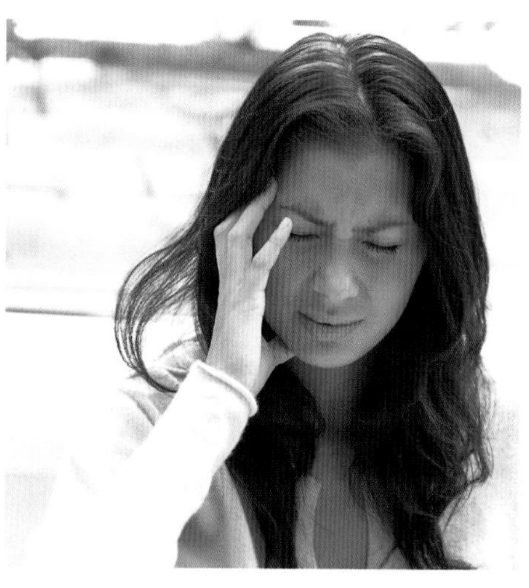

caution

You should see your doctor if you experience any unusual, very severe or persistent headaches.

◁ **If you suffer from recurrent headaches, you should try and identify possible triggers so that you can avoid them. It may help to discuss the problem with your doctor.**

reflexology routine

This routine is based on reflexology; you can use the techniques on yourself or on another person. Give a short foot massage before and after the treatment, to help with relaxation. Make sure that you treat both feet – the routine is shown here on the right foot. If you want to use oil, lavender and camomile are good choices. Juniper may help an allergy-related headache.

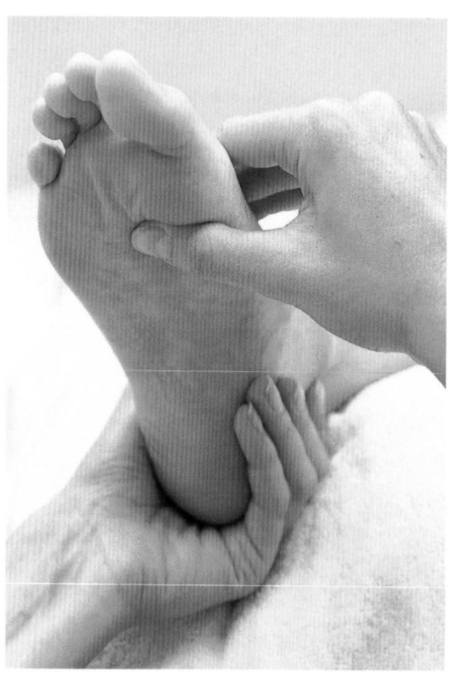

△ **1** Cup the heel with your left hand. Put your right thumb on the edge of the foot, just below the ball and in line with the big toe. It should point towards the inside edge. Thumb-walk across the sole, staying below the ball as you go, then repeat once more. This movement works on the diaphragm, which helps you to breathe deeply, sending oxygen and nutrients to all parts of the body.

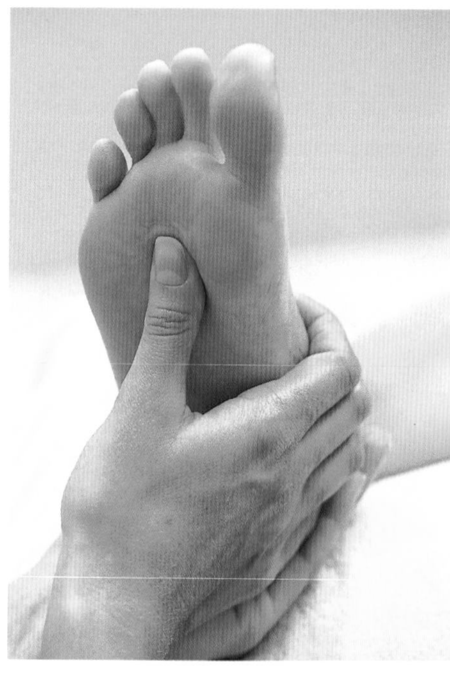

△ **2** Repeat the action described in step 1, but this time stop when you reach the point directly below toes two and three. Turn your thumb so it points up towards the toes, and give three distinct presses; this is the solar plexus point, which also helps with relaxation and breathing. Continue the crawl to the outer edge of the foot. Repeat the whole movement one more time.

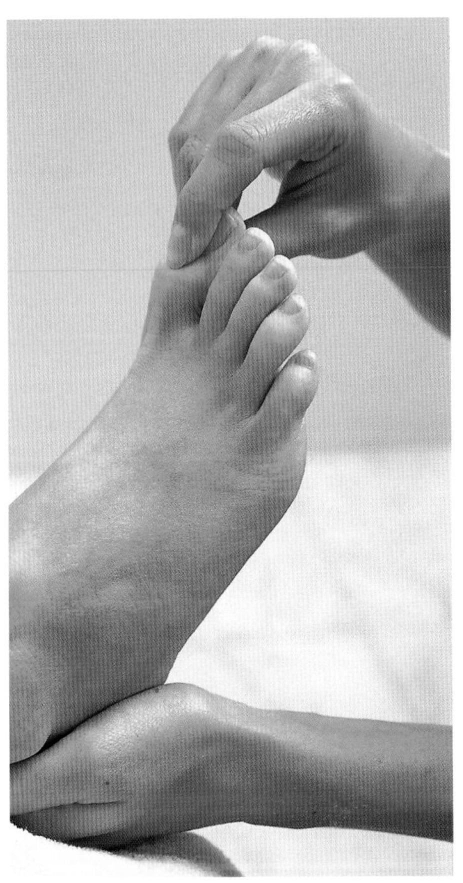

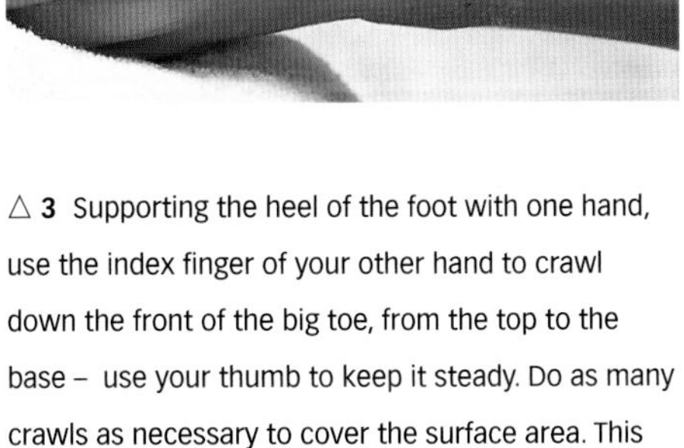

△ **3** Supporting the heel of the foot with one hand, use the index finger of your other hand to crawl down the front of the big toe, from the top to the base – use your thumb to keep it steady. Do as many crawls as necessary to cover the surface area. This action works on the front of the head.

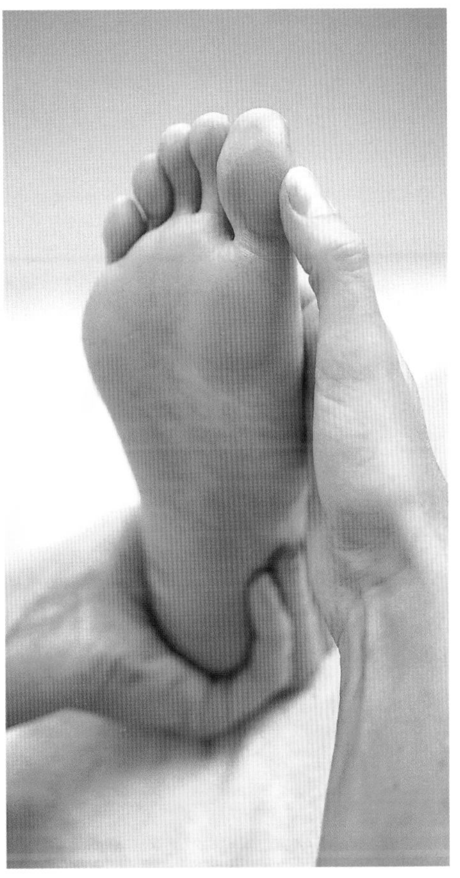

△ **4** Now, use the right thumb to crawl up the outside of the big toe, over the top and down the inner edge, making a horseshoe shape. Then crawl up the back of the big toe from the base to the top. Do as many crawls as it takes to cover the entire surface area. This helps to relax the head muscles and balance nerve functioning here.

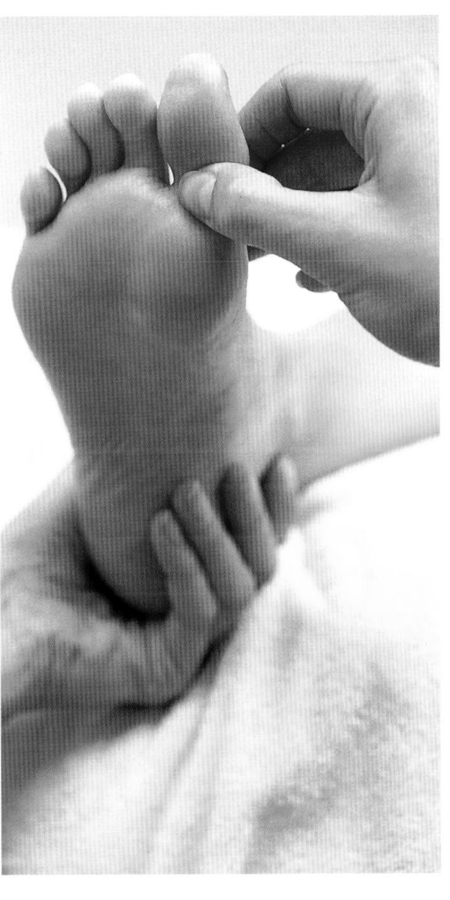

△ **5** Keeping the hold position, use your thumb to crawl around the base of the toe, from the outside of the foot to the webbing in-between the big toe and toe two. This works on the back of the neck, which may be a factor in a headache. Now repeat the whole sequence on the other foot.

quick acupressure routine

Although this is a short treatment, it is very soothing and can help to shift the discomfort of a headache surprisingly rapidly. Experiment with this and the reflexology routine to see which one works best for you.

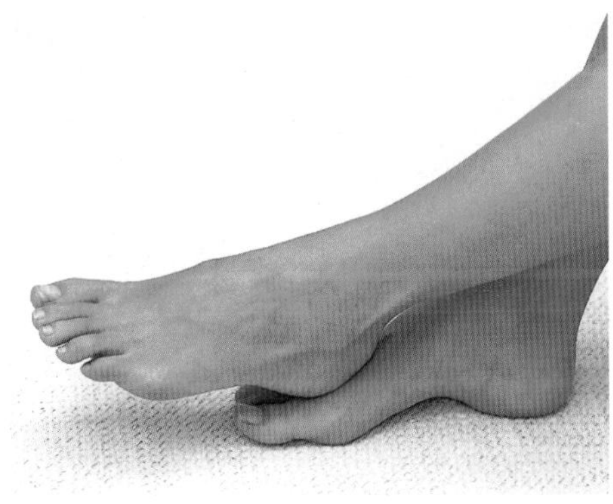

△ **1** Place your right foot flat on the floor. Use the outer edge of your left heel to rub the top of the right foot along the groove between the big and second toe. Rub back and forth from the base of the toes to halfway up the foot, to the count of 50. This soothing action at the Liver 3 point, helps to release tension. Change feet and do the other side.

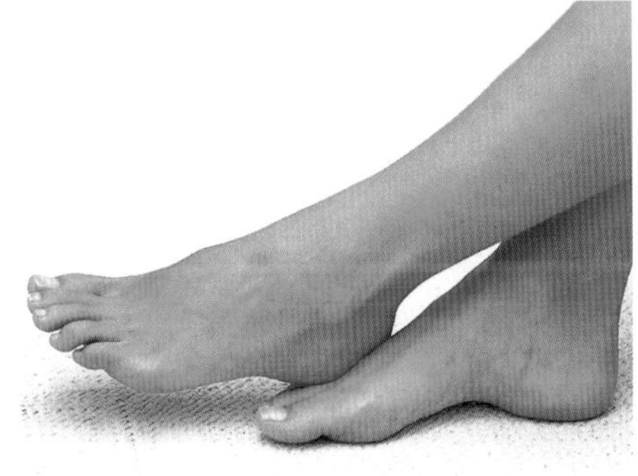

△ **2** Use the same action as described in Step 1, but this time rub the groove between the fourth and little toe. This activates Gallbladder 41, a point which is excellent for migraines, or one-sided headaches. Again, rub backwards and forwards to the count of 50, breathing deeply as you work. Then repeat on the other foot.

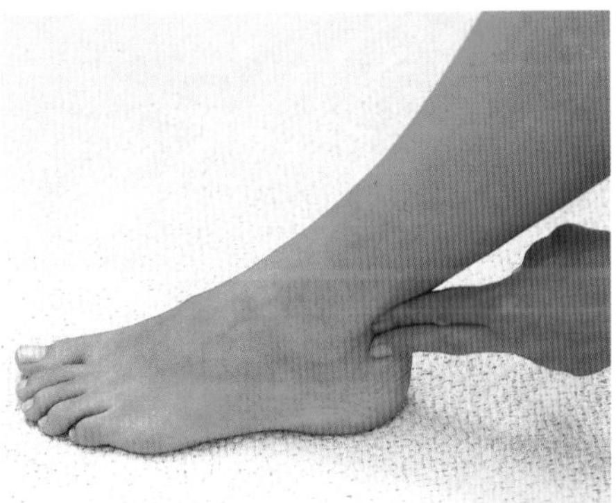

△ **3** Place your two middle fingers between the back edge of the heel and the Achilles tendon. Hold the pressure for the count of 30, release for a couple of seconds and then repeat. This point is Bladder 60, which may relieve headaches on the top or back of the head. It is also a good general relaxer. Now repeat on the other ankle.

Back and neck pain

Neck and back pain is part of everyday life for many people, and almost everyone experiences it at some point. Pain in this area of the body can be caused by certain disorders, but it also commonly occurs as a result of lifestyle factors – for example, office workers often spend long periods sitting in a slouched position, which puts pressure on the back.

Muscle strain can occur when people place excessive demands on the back – for example, if you spend hours digging the garden, make a sudden movement or do some unfamiliar exercises. Women often suffer back pain during menstruation or when they are pregnant.

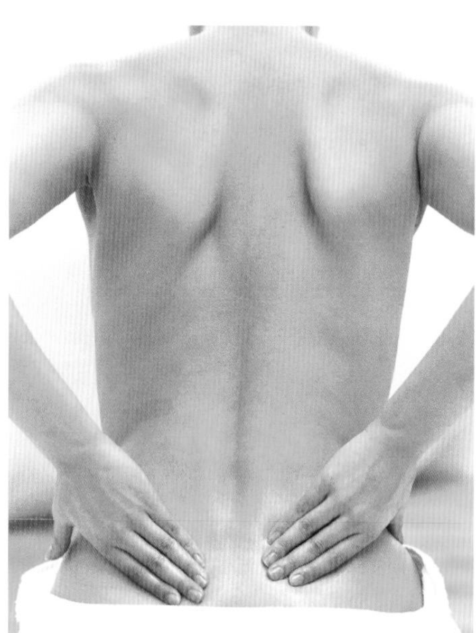

△ **Physical and emotional stresses and strains all too commonly gather in the neck and back.**

preventative measures

The best way to avoid back pain is by exercising regularly and improving your posture. Alexander technique, yoga and Pilates may all be of great help. Osteopathy and chiropractic can be excellent therapies for dealing with back pain and spinal misalignments. Reflexology is another good way to treat general back pain, and it is one of the easiest therapies to practise at home.

releasing upper back pain

This treatment helps to relieve discomfort and tension in the upper back and neck. It combines simple reflexology with massage techniques, and is very pleasurable to receive. If treating yourself, as shown here, sit on the floor or on a chair with the foot being treated resting in your lap. Do both feet – the right one is shown here.

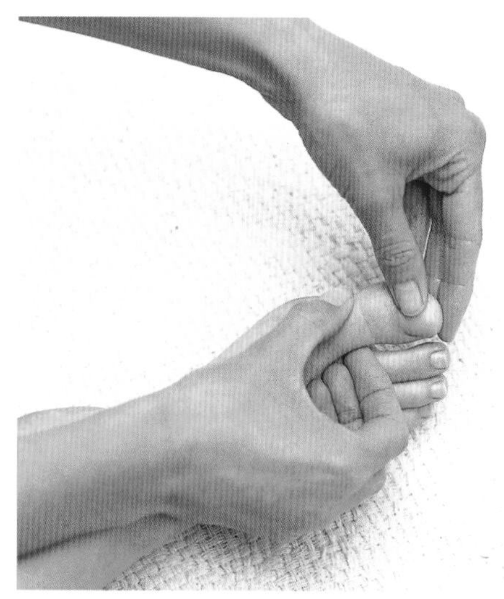

△ **1** Use one hand to support the big toe of the right foot at its base. Hold the big toe with the thumb and index finger of your other hand. Rotate gently three times in a clockwise direction, then three times in an anticlockwise direction.

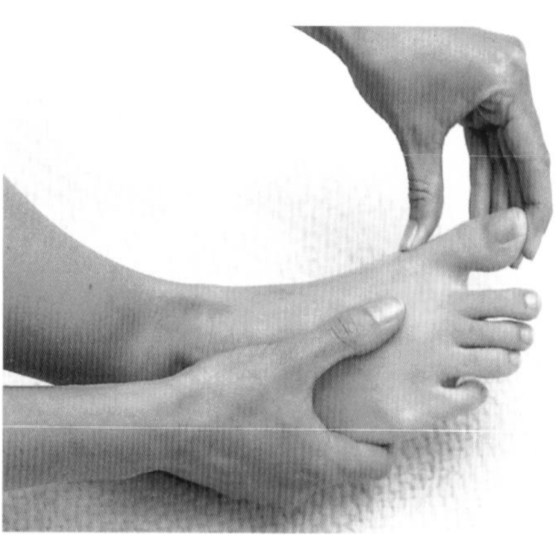

△ **2** Use one hand to support the right foot. With the index finger of the other hand, crawl around the front of the big toe. Start the movement at the edge of your foot, moving around to the webbing in-between the big toe and the second toe (not shown). Then use your thumb to crawl around the base of the toe, from the edge of the foot to between the big toe and toe two (shown here). This helps to mobilize the neck.

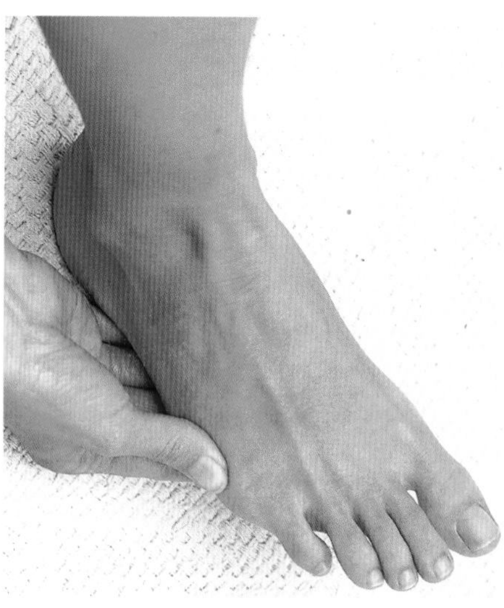

△ **3** Use the thumb-crawling technique to work down the outer edge of the foot, from the base of the little toe to the heel, and back up again. Walk up and down four times (eight walks in total). This helps to release tension from the shoulders.

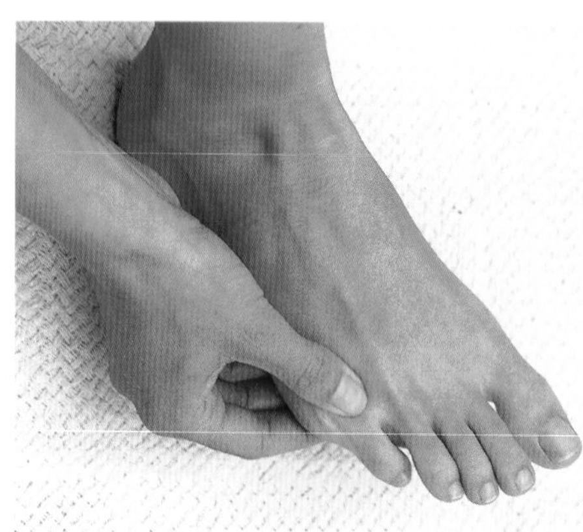

△ **4** Finally, pinch the ball of the foot just under the little toe; your thumb should be on top of the foot and your index finger underneath. Pinch the thumb and finger together, rotating the flesh in a clockwise direction as you do so. Do seven clockwise circles, then seven anticlockwise ones. If it is very painful, work more gently and just do the clockwise circles.

releasing lower back pain

Just a few reflex points are worked in this routine, which can also be done as self-help. They help to improve breathing and relaxation, and also work directly on the spine. It is a good idea to begin these routines with a short, general foot massage, which can make you more receptive to treatment. Make sure that you treat both feet – the right one is shown here.

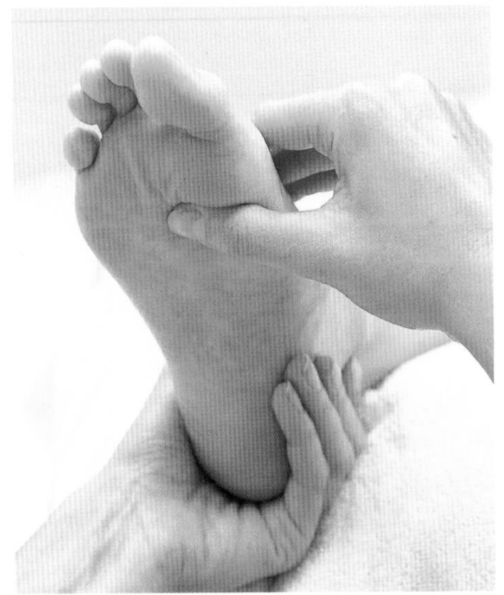

△ **1** Cup the heel of the receiver's foot with your left hand. Now place your right thumb on the edge of their foot, so that the thumb is positioned just below the ball of the foot. It should be pointing across the foot. Walk the thumb in a crawling movement across the sole, remaining just below the ball. Then, repeat once more. This action works on the diaphragm, which helps you to breathe deeply.

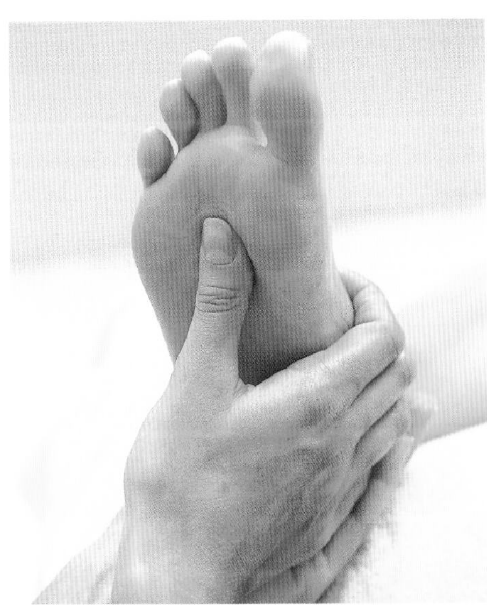

△ **2** Place your thumb in the same position as in step 1, then start to crawl across the foot again. When you are directly in line with toes two and three, turn your thumb to point towards the toes. Press here, on the solar plexus point, three times. Continue the crawl to the outer edge of the foot. Do this movement twice.

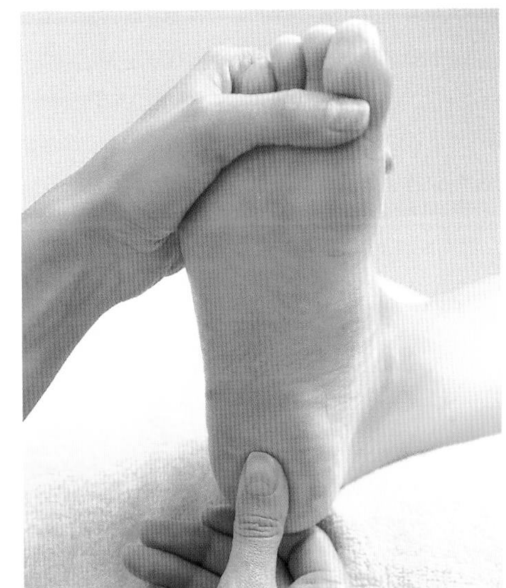

△ **3** Hold the toes with your left hand. Crawl your right thumb from the bottom to the top of the heel pad. Use as many crawls as is needed to cover the whole pad, always working from bottom to top. Now, crawl across the heel pad. Start with your thumb on the inner edge and crawl it to the outer edge. Do this as many times as it takes to cover the area. These movements work on the sciatic nerve, pelvis and lower back.

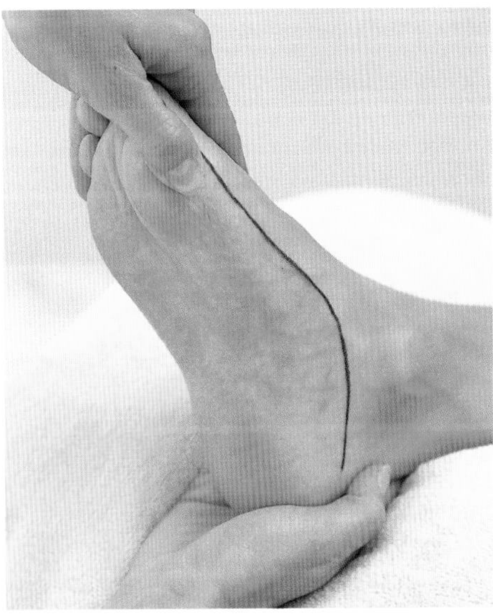

△ **4** Cup the heel in your right hand. Use your left thumb to crawl down the inner edge of the foot. Start from the first joint of the big toe and work to the heel, following the curve of the bone (as marked above). Change hands and crawl back, pressing upwards into the bone as you crawl. Repeat once more. This movement helps to loosen the spine.

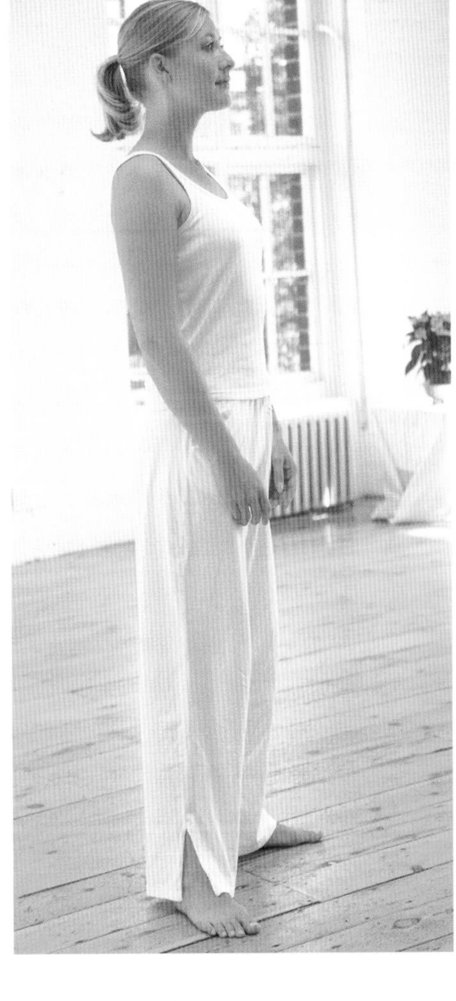

△ **Monitor your posture on a regular basis. Standing and walking tall will help allay countless back problems.**

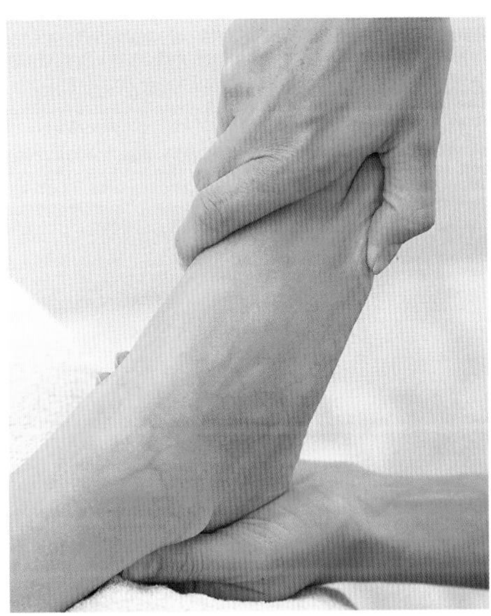

△ **5** Now cup the heel in your left hand. Use your thumb to crawl down the outside edge of the foot from the base of the little toe to the heel, and then work back up to the toe again. Do this once more, then repeat all the steps on the left foot.

Boost your immune system

The immune system is a collection of defences that the body uses to fight infection and disease. Organs such as the liver and kidneys contribute to the immune system, as do whole body systems such as the lymph network. Many illnesses can result from a poorly functioning immune system.

Your body's defences can be depleted by lack of sleep, stress or poor diet. This is why you are more likely to fall ill when you are tired or anxious: your ability to fight infection and to recover from illness is reduced. You can help to keep your immune system functioning efficiently by making sure that you get enough sleep, and that you follow a healthy balanced diet. This should include at least five helpings of fresh fruit and vegetables each day.

Exercising regularly will also help to boost the immune system, because physical exertion helps the circulation. You should also avoid drinking excessively and smoking. Alcoholic drinks and cigarettes introduce toxins into the body and put pressure on the organs that deal with waste.

Complementary therapies such as massage, reflexology and acupressure can all help the immune system. Like exercise, they aid the circulation and they also encourage relaxation, which in turn helps all the organs of the body to function well. Regular treatments are the best way to maintain good health, but you can also use reflexology and acupressure as quick fixes. These are particularly good to do if you feel depleted or as if you are catching a cold.

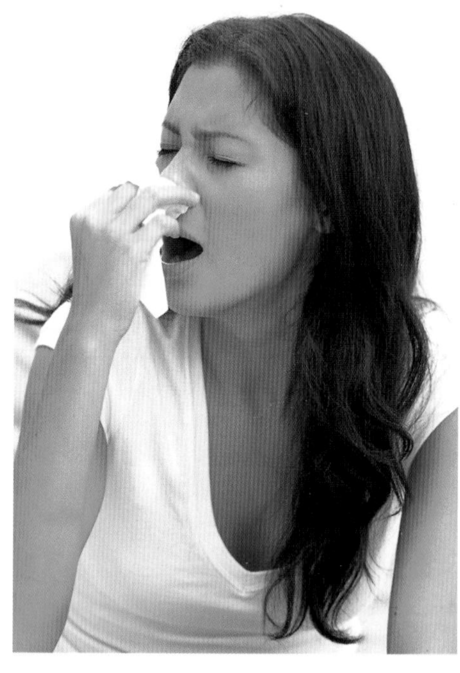

△ **Try the quick immune-boosting acupressure treatments on these pages whenever you feel that you are succumbing to a cold due to stress or overtiredness. They may help to stave it off, or reduce the severity of your symptoms. It can also be helpful to use these routines on a preventive basis, especially if you know you have had a number of late nights or are under a lot of pressure at work.**

useful essentials

Essential oils can enhance the effects of an immune-strengthening treatment. Eucalyptus oil is a good oil to use here. It has antibiotic qualities, and can be added to a steam inhalation to clear a cough or cold, as well as being used in a footbath or in massage. The oil is very strong, so use it sparingly – one drop per 10ml/2 tsp carrier.

Uplifting frankincense is another good oil for the immune system. It has anti-inflammatory properties, so it can help with chest infections, and it is also an antiseptic. If you do not want to use these oils in the foot treatments, try burning them in a vaporizer instead.

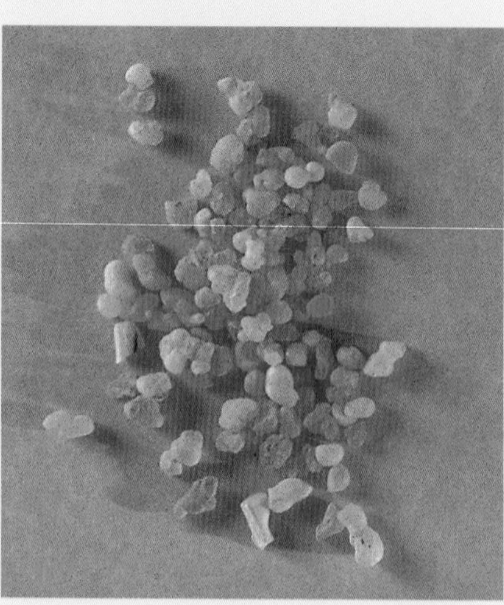

△ **Frankincense oil smells warm and spicy.**

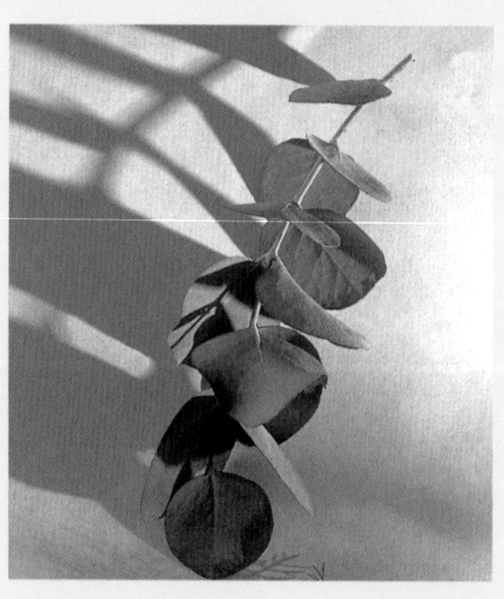

△ **Eucalyptus oil has a strong, lemony aroma.**

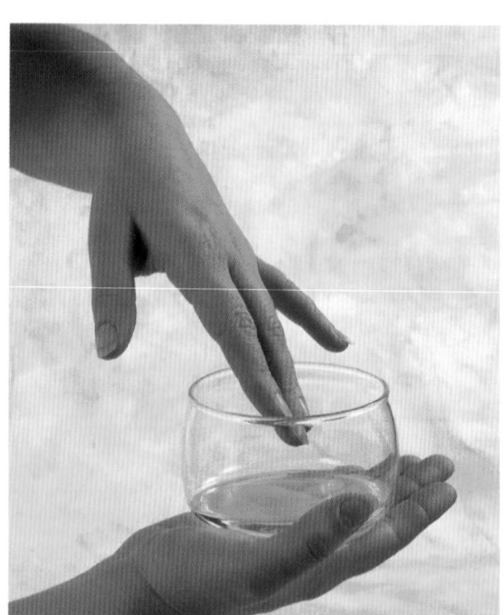

△ **Massaging essential oil into the feet enhances the effects of acupressure. Let the oil sink in.**

fighting infection with acupressure

This self-treatment uses several acupressure points. Acupressure works on the same principles as acupuncture; by pressing certain points you can direct healing energy to wherever it is needed. If you like, you can start the routine by giving a gentle foot massage. This helps to relax and open the foot, making it more receptive to treatment.

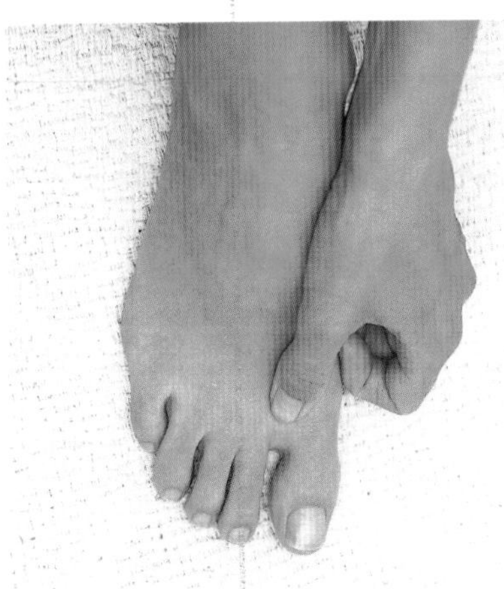

△ **1** Put your right foot flat on the floor. Place your thumb in the groove between the big and second toes. Slide the thumb up along this groove, then back down towards the base of the toe. Repeat a few times, applying firm pressure. This works on the acupressure point Liver 3, which helps to counteract the results of stress.

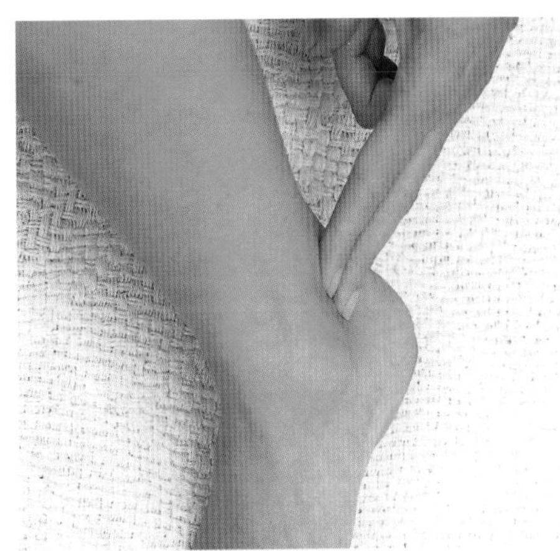

△ **2** Place your index and middle fingers between the inner ankle bone and the Achilles tendon. This is Kidney 3, which is good for when you are feeling depleted or have been overdoing things. Press for a count of 20, then release for a count of 30. Repeat twice more, so that you press the point three times in total. Now, repeat Steps 1 and 2 on the left foot. **Do not work these points during the first three months of pregnancy.**

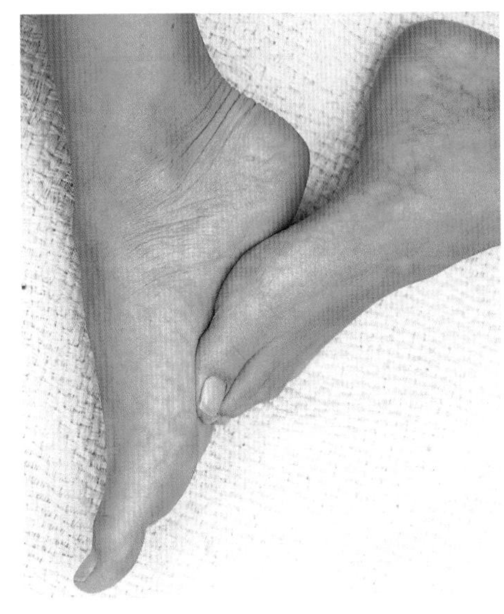

△ **3** Turn the right foot on its side, so that the inner edge points upwards. Use the toes of the left foot to massage along the edge, working from heel to toe. Now do the same on the left foot. This works on the liver and spleen; the spleen produces some of the body's natural antibodies, which fight infection.

reflexology strengthening treatment

When the immune system is functioning correctly, the body is able to fend off infections before they become established. This treatment uses several reflexoxlogy points to boost the immune system. Start on the right foot and repeat on the left.

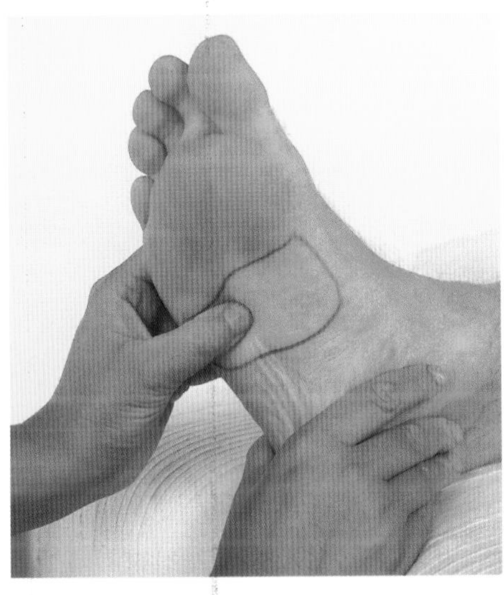

△ **1** Supporting the right foot with one hand, use the other thumb to crawl across the sole from the inner to outer edge. Repeat as needed to cover the area from the base of the ball to the centre of the arch (as marked above). Do this again. Now, crawl to the liver reflex area, where the thumb is positioned in the picture, and do three pressure circles.

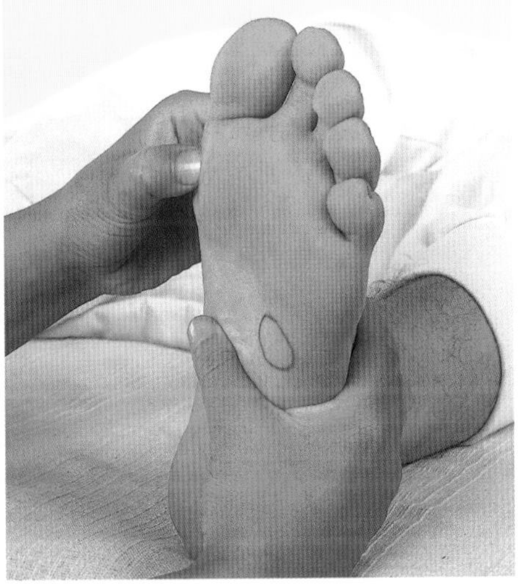

△ **2** Work the area in the same way as in step 1, but this time pause on the thymus point, where the left-hand thumb is positioned in the picture, and do three pressure circles before continuing. When you come to do the left foot, which is the one shown here, work both the thymus point and the spleen point (marked with a circle) in the same way.

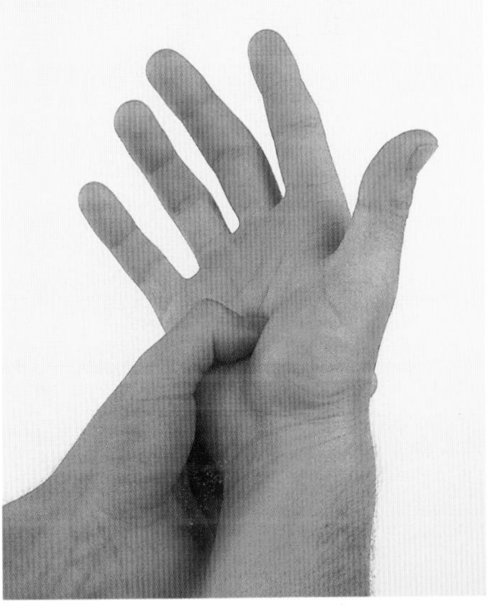

△ **Try a quick treatment on the hand if you are in a public place or cannot easily access the foot. Use thumb-walking to cover the area between the diaphragm and waist lines, which both run across the palm. The diaphragm line is a quarter of the way down; the waist line halfway down.**

Anxiety and insomnia

Everyone gets nervous, particularly before an important event. Knowing a few "emergency" treatments will enable you to soothe feelings of panic or nervousness as they arise. Stopping what you are doing and focusing on breathing deeply for a few minutes can also be very helpful.

Anxiety often affects people's sleep. Most of us will experience some kind of sleep problem at some stage in our lives. Often, this can be caused by changes in lifestyle – such as an increase of stress at work. Most people can cope well with one or two bad nights. However, if you are regularly having disturbed sleep, your general physical and mental health can suffer. If disturbed sleep continues longer than a few weeks, you should talk to your doctor about it.

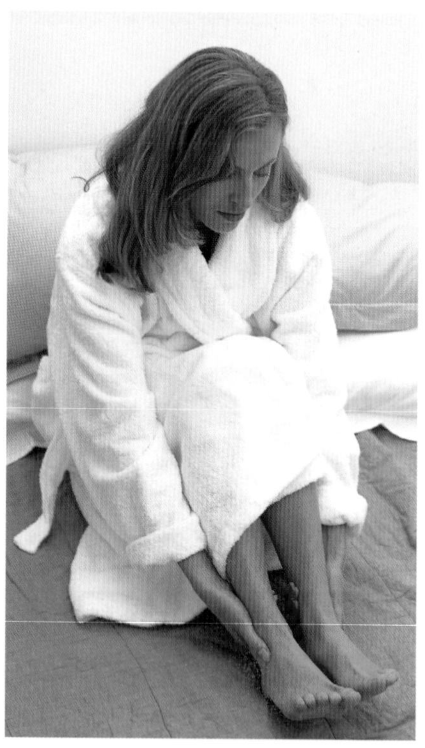

△ **Learning a few acupressure and reflexology points will give you access to immediate treatments for anxiety, exhaustion and insomnia. Breathe deeply when pressing any acupressure or reflexology point. This will help to make you receptive to the treatment, and also has a relaxing effect in itself.**

insomnia relief treatment

Acupressure can be very helpful for temporary sleeping problems. The two points used in this routine are excellent for promoting restful sleep and relieving stress-related insomnia. Sit on a low chair or the floor to work these points, or do the routine sitting up in bed.

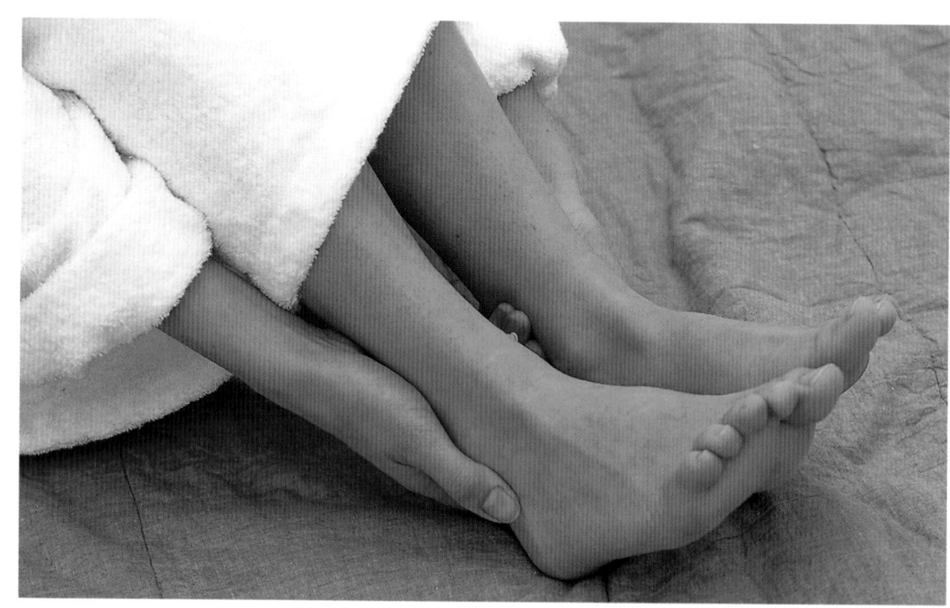

1 Put your feet close together on the floor. Place your thumbs directly below the inner ankle bones of both feet. This is Kidney 6, which is good for sleep problems. Press into the area and hold to a slow count of 30. Release the pressure for one minute, then repeat.

△ **2** Next, place your thumbs directly under the outer ankle bones. Press for the count of 30, release for a minute, then press again. Breathe deeply while your thumbs are pressing into the acupressure point. This point is Bladder 62 – also known as Joyful Sleep – and it has a very soothing effect on the spirit.

working the hand

When you feel anxious, press the solar plexus reflex in the centre of your hand. It encourages good deep breathing and also helps to calm feelings of panic or nervousness.

The solar plexus reflex is right in the centre of the hand, so it is easy to find. Working on a hand point is also much easier to do wherever you are, than working on your foot. To work the solar plexus point, press firmly (but not painfully) and then rotate your thumb in an anticlockwise direction. As you press, breathe deeply and relax your shoulders.

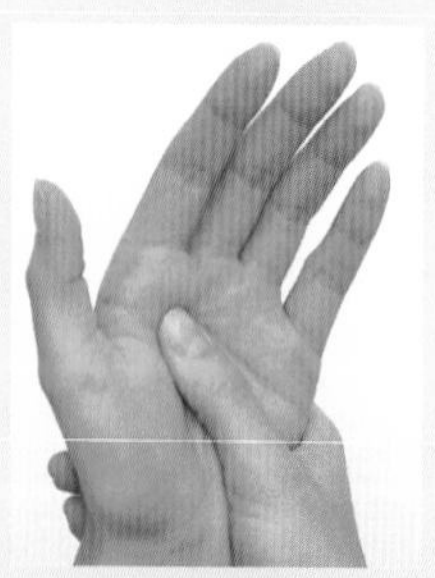

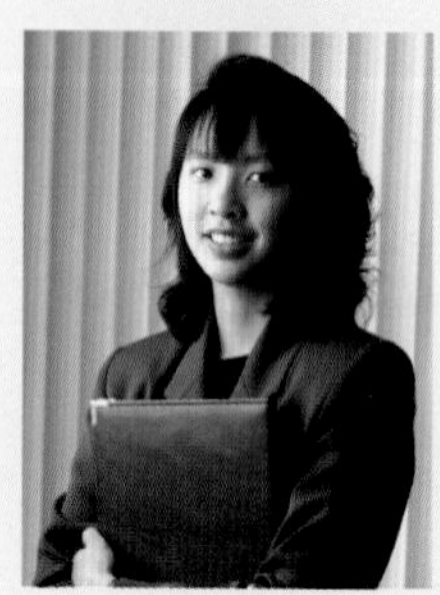

▷ **The solar plexus reflex is an excellent point to work before an interview, exam, big meeting or journey – or when you are doing anything that makes you feel nervous.**

getting a good night's sleep

The following steps may help to ensure a sleep-filled night.

- Establish a regular sleep routine: go to bed and get up at the same time each day. Avoid afternoon napping.
- Don't work late into the evening.
- Spend the last hour or two before bedtime calmly and quietly. In particular, do not do any vigorous exercise, watch TV or have difficult discussions during this time.
- Make sure that your bedroom is clear of anything to do with work, exercise or other activities – keep it for sleeping.
- Open the window a little, to get fresh air circulating.
- Have a warm bath and a hot milky drink before you go to bed.
- Make sure that you have enough bedcovers to keep you warm, but not so many that you become overheated.
- If you do not get to sleep within 20 minutes of turning out the light, get up and go into another room. Return to bed when you feel sleepy.
- Essential oils can assist sleep: add a few drops of camomile or lavender into a night-time bath, or drop them on to a cotton-wool ball and slip this between the pillow and pillow cover.
- Try meditation or visualization: a short routine will help to ease you into a relaxed sleeping mode.

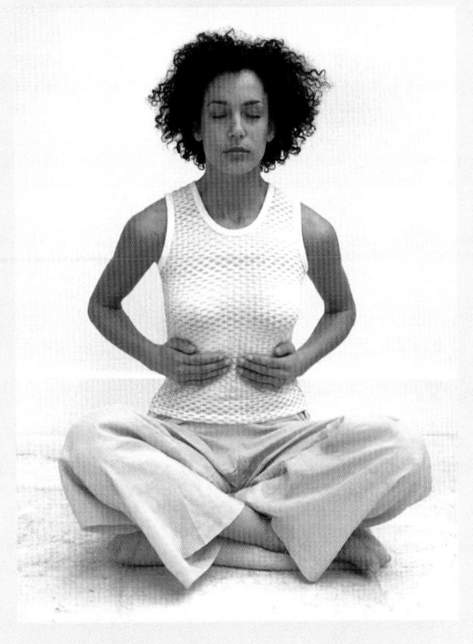

△ Meditating before you retire will help you to unwind and sleep more peacefully.

easing anxiety

This is a good routine to do before an important event. It uses two important acupressure points, which are calming and balancing. Working on the feet is an excellent way of combating anxiety because it has a grounding effect on you. Breathing deeply as you work will also be very helpful. Do each point on both feet.

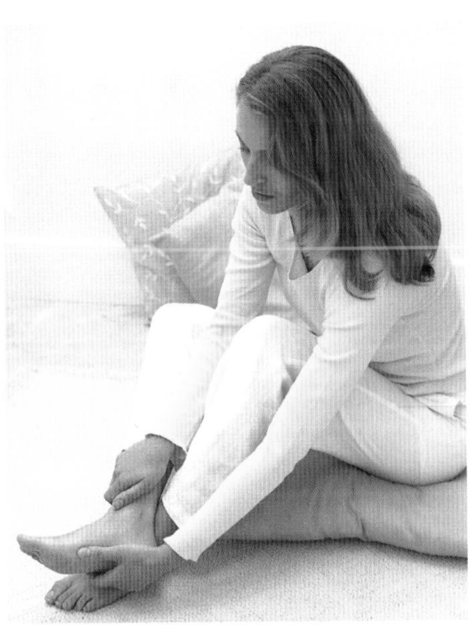

◁ **1** Put the thumb of your left hand on the inner side of the right foot, about one thumb-width below the ball. Press and hold for 30 seconds, breathing deeply. Release the point slowly, breathe for a count of 20, then press again for another 30 seconds. Do the left foot in the same way. This point is Spleen 4, which calms and balances.

▷ **2** Place the two middle fingers of your right hand on the outside of the right lower leg. The fingers should be four finger-widths down from the kneecap and one finger-width towards the outside of the shinbone. This is Stomach 36, which is a good balancing point. Rub up and down briskly to the count of 50, breathing as you work. Rest for one minute, then repeat. Do the same points on the left leg.

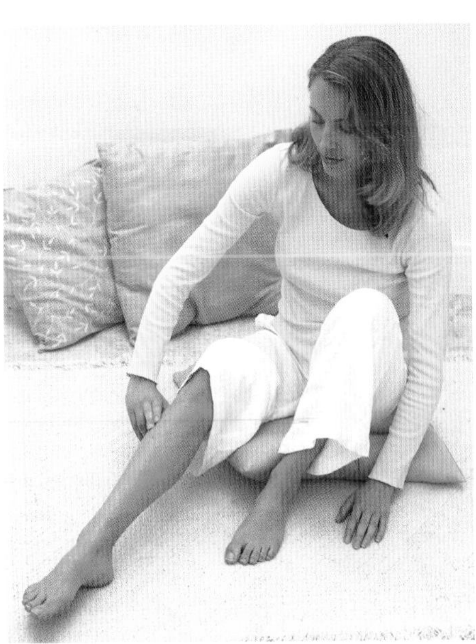

aromatic assistance

Essential oils can be useful addition to the anxiety treatment above. Many oils have a calming, soothing effect. You may like to try camomile and lavender, diluted in a grapeseed or almond oil carrier. Basil is a good nerve tonic and its aroma combines well with neroli. Clary sage is a good oil to use if you feel very stressed, and sandalwood and rose are other useful oils for anxiety. Massage the oil blend into the ankles, using a circular motion, and allow it to disappear into the skin before working on the acupressure points.

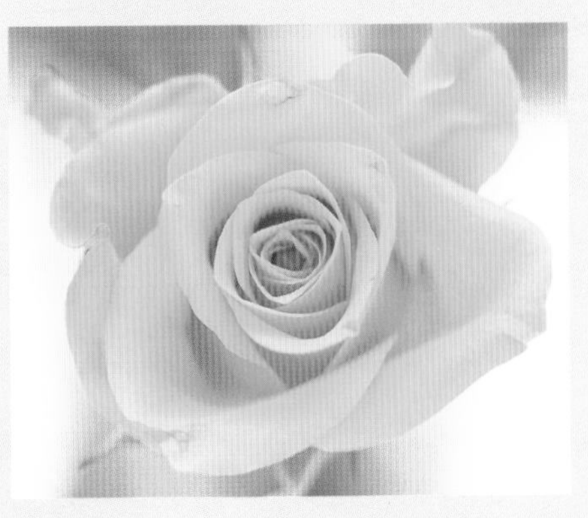

▷ Rose essential oil is a most effective calmer. It is also very soothing if you are distressed.

Menstrual problems

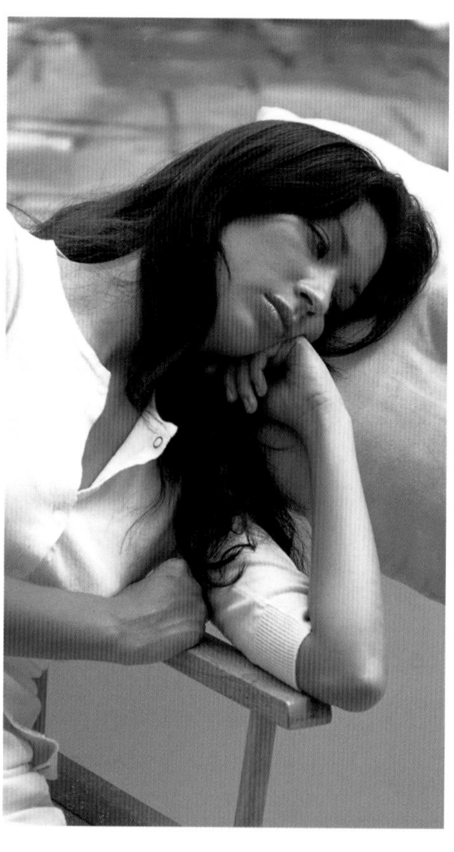

If you suffer from pre-menstrual tension or period pain, it is a good idea to be gentle on yourself at this time of the month. Look at all aspects of your lifestyle, and cut back where you can. For example, reduce the level of exercise that you do, so that you do not place excess demands on your body. Have warm baths in the evening and go to bed a little earlier, and make sure that you are eat soothing foods such as silky mashed potato or pasta.

Most women find that their pain threshold is lower at this time, so don't plan dental appointments or have your legs waxed until after your period. You should also avoid anything that makes you overheated such as saunas or sunbeds.

◁ **You may feel more tired and run-down just before and during your period. If so, make this a time to look after yourself: eat well, sleep well and rest as much as you can.**

hot water bottle help for menstrual aches

Treat your feet with this uplifting rose spray, then rest them on a warming hot water bottle.

ingredients

- 15ml/1 tbsp vodka
- 20ml/ 4 tsp rosewater
- 5ml/1 tsp orangeflower water
- 4 drops rose essential oil
- 5 drops clary sage essential oil
- 3 drops jasmine essential oil

Blend all ingredients together in a 30ml (1fl oz) spray bottle. To use, spray your feet all over, then spray a small hand towel and wrap this around a hot water bottle. Place the wrapped hot water bottle on the floor and rest your feet on it while you relax.

a monthly treat

How women experience menstruation varies widely. You may simply need to rest more at this time, or you may feel a surge of energy in the days before your period. These acupressure points will help to relieve pain and bloating. They can be done at regular intervals during the day.

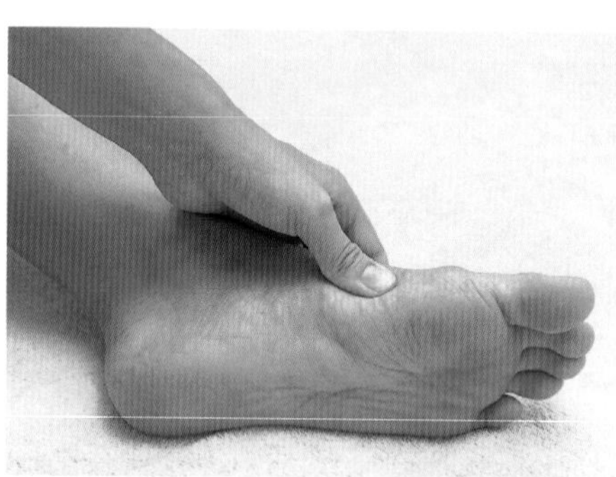

△ **For cramps and digestive problems**
Turn your right foot on its side. Use your right thumb to locate the pressure point one thumb-width down from the ball of the foot, close to the inner edge. This is Spleen 4. Press firmly (but not painfully) and hold for one minute. Release the pressure and pause for another minute, then repeat. Remember to breathe deeply while pressing the point. Repeat the movement on the other foot.

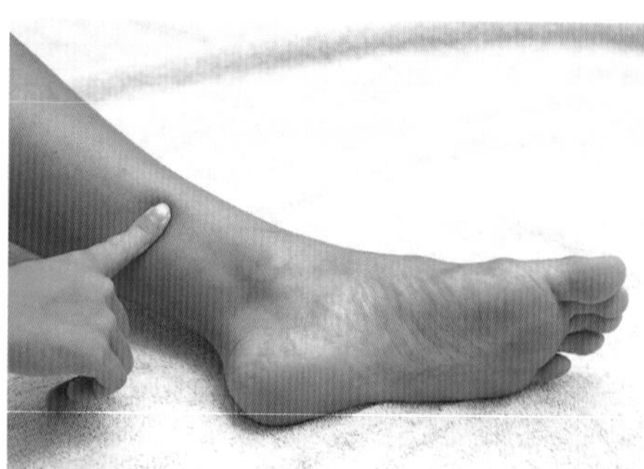

△ **For PMS, irregular periods and water retention**
Turn your right lower leg on its side. Now use the index finger of the right hand to find a pressure point four finger-widths up from the inner ankle bone, keeping close to the side of the shinbone. Press this point, which is called Spleen 6, for one minute and wait. Release for a few moments, then press again for another minute. Keep breathing as you press. Repeat the action on the left foot.

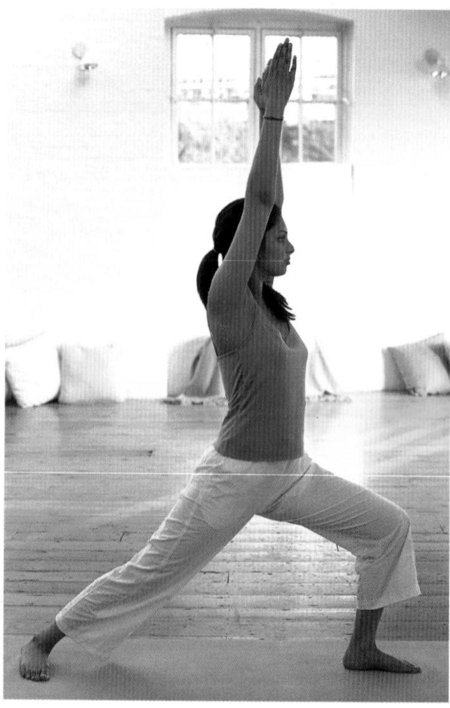

△ **Do not overdo your exercise regime when you are menstruating. Gentle stretches and yoga can be of enormous benefit, but avoid inverted (upside-down) poses.**

Digestive difficulties

The digestive system is essential to good health. It is the means by which we get our energy and nutrients, and it also carries away waste and toxins. An efficient digestion system will help to ensure good general health, clear skin and shining hair.

Many of us experience minor problems such as indigestion, heartburn, food allergies and constipation on a regular basis. Reflexology can be helpful for digestion problems, but you should also eat a healthy diet and adopt good eating habits, to avoid placing undue strain on the system.

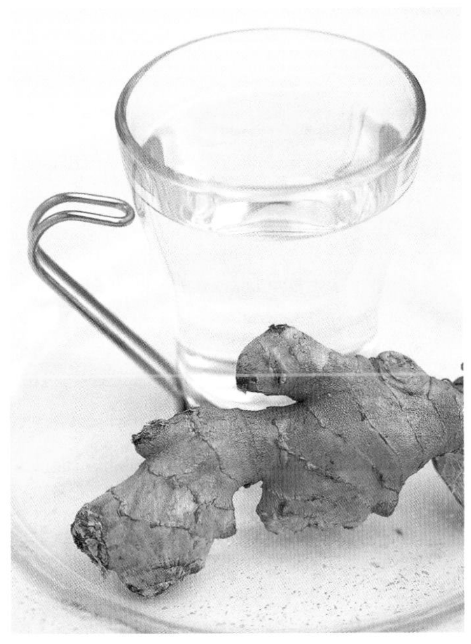

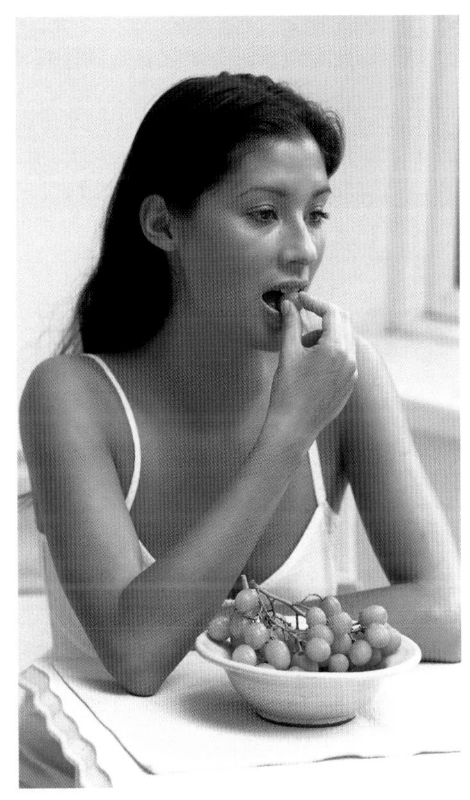

△ **Include plenty of fruits and vegetables in your daily diet. As well as being packed with nutrients, these foods contain plenty of fibre. This is needed to aid the elimination of waste from the body.**

◁ **Ginger helps to soothe nausea, morning sickness and indigestion. A ginger tea infusion is comfortingly warming and simple to make.**

soothing the digestion

These acupressure points direct healing energy to soothe particular digestion problems – choose the one that is most suitable for you. You can massage an essential oil diluted in a carrier into the foot first if you like: fennel and sweet ginger are the most suitable oils for digestion problems. Breathe regularly and rhythmically throughout the exercise.

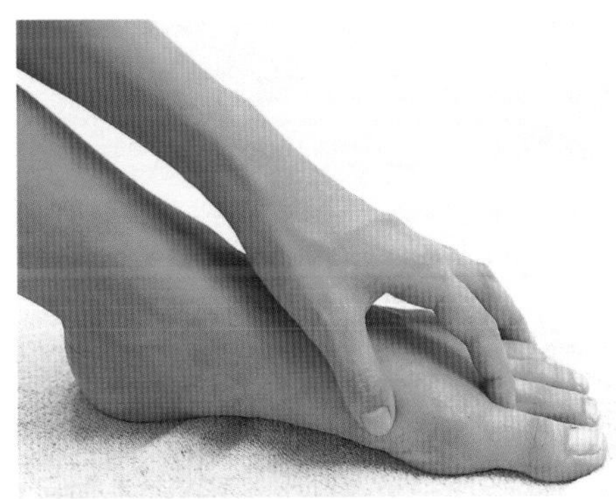

△ **Abdominal cramps**

Place both feet flat on the floor. Place the middle finger of each hand on the corresponding foot. Press into the webbing between the big and second toes, angling the finger towards the big toe. Hold the pressure for a count of 30, release for one minute, then repeat. Rest for five minutes, then press twice more in the same way.

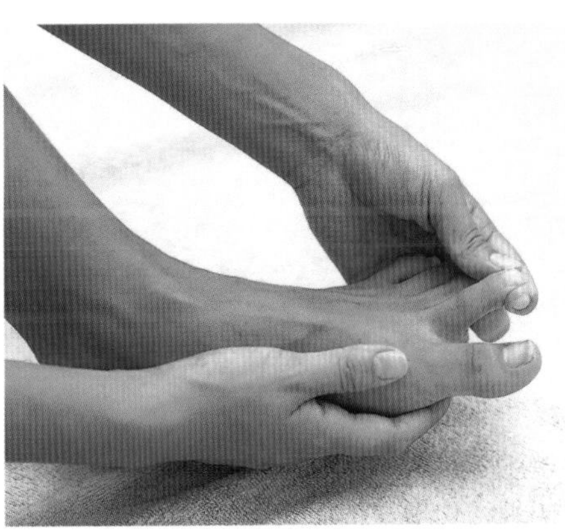

△ **For indigestion, abdominal pain and bloating**

Steady the right foot in your right hand. Place your left thumb and index finger either side of the second toe nail. Squeeze to a count of 60, breathing deeply. Do the same on the left foot.

healthy eating habits

Following a healthy diet will keep your digestion system functioning well. For a healthy system, you should also:

- Eat little and often, rather than having one or two large meals a day.
- Always sit down to eat. Do not eat when you are feeling stressed or anxious.
- Drink plenty of water and keep your coffee, tea and fizzy drink intake to a minimum.
- Eat plenty of fibre-rich foods, such as fruits and vegetables and whole grains (wholemeal bread, brown rice, wholewheat pasta).

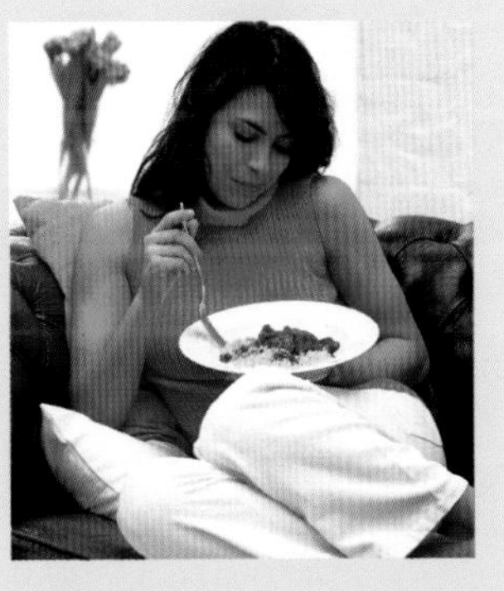

△ **Take time to enjoy food. Avoid slumping or awkward postures like this one, as they put pressure on the digestion.**

Useful addresses

MASSAGE

General Council for Massage Therapy (GCMT), for United Kingdom
www.gcmt-uk.org
Email: admin@gcmt-uk.org

London College of Massage
Diorama Arts Centre
34 Osnaburgh Street
London NW1 3ND
Tel: 0207 813 1980
www.massagelondon.com
Email: admin@massagelondon.com

Scottish Massage Therapists Association (SMTO)
70 Lochside Road
Aberdeen
Scotland
AB23 8QW
Tel: 01224 822956
www.scotmass.co.uk
Email: enquiries@scotmass.co.uk

Irish Massage Therapist Association
Kemple's Annex, Menlo
Galway
Eire
Tel: 091 760 211

American Massage Therapy Association
820 Davis Street,
Suite 100
Evanston
Illinois 60201-4444
USA
Tel: 708 864 0123
www.amtamassage.org
Email: info@inet.amtamassage.org

Canadian Massage Therapist Alliance
365 Bloor Street East
Suite 1807
Toronto
Ontario M4W 3L4
Canada
Tel: 905 849 7606
www.cmta.ca
Email: cmta@collinscan.com

Association of Massage Therapists Australia
PO Box 627
South Yarra
3141
Australia
www.amta.asm.au
Email: amta@amta.asn.au

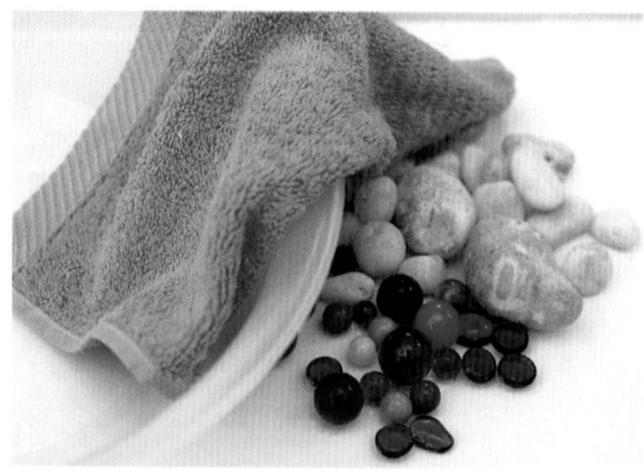

New Zealand Association of Therapeutic Massage Practitioners
PO Box 375
Hamilton
Auckland
New Zealand

REFLEXOLOGY

International Federation of Reflexologists
78 Edridge Road
Croydon
Surrey CR0 1EF
United Kingdom
Tel: 0208 645 9134
Email: info@intfedreflexologists.org

Reflexology Forum
PO Box 2367
South Croydon
Surrey CR2 7ZE
United Kingdom
Tel: 0800 037 0130
Email: reflexologyforum@aol.com

American Reflexology Certification Board
PO Box 740879
Arvada, CO 80006
USA
Tel 303 933 6921
www.arcb.net

Reflexology Association of Canada
5000 Dufferin Street
Toronto
Ontario M3H 5T5
Canada
Tel: 877 722 3338
www.reflexologycanada.ca
Email: info@www.reflexologycanada.ca

Reflexology Association of Australia
PO Box 366
Cammeray NSW 2062
Australia
Tel: 02 4721 4752
www.reflexology.org.au

Reflexology New Zealand Incorporated
PO Box 38860
Wellington MSC
New Zealand
www.reflexology.org.nz
Email: secretary@reflexology.org.nz

South African Reflexology Society
PO Box 1885
Dalbridge 4014
Tel: 031 205 4518
Email: admin@sareflexology.org.sa

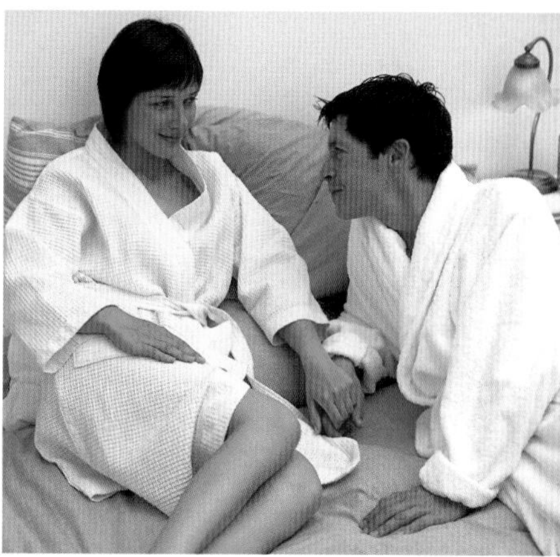

AROMATHERAPY

Aromatherapy and Allied Practitioners Association (AAPA)
PO Box 36248
London, SE19 3YD
United Kingdom
Tel: 0208 653 9152
Email: aromatherapyuk@aol.com

National Association for Holistic Aromatherapy (NAHA)
4509 Interlake Ave N 233
Seattle, WA 98103-6773
Tel: 206 547 2164
www.naha.org
Email: info@naha.org

Aromatherapy Organisations Council (AOC)
Contact: The AOC Secretary
PO Box 19834
London, SE25 6WF
United Kingdom
Tel: 0208 251 7912
www.aocuk.net

Aromatherapy Society of South Africa
PO Box 2085
New Germany 3620
Tel: 031 201 2296
Email: info@asosa.org.sa

ACUPRESSURE

British Acupuncture Council
63 Jeddo Road
London W12 9HQ
Tel: 020 8735 0400
www.acupuncture.org.uk
Email: info@acupuncture.org.uk

The Acupressure Institute
1533 Shattuck Avenue
Berkley, California 94709
USA
Tel: 808 442 2232
www.acupressure.com

Index

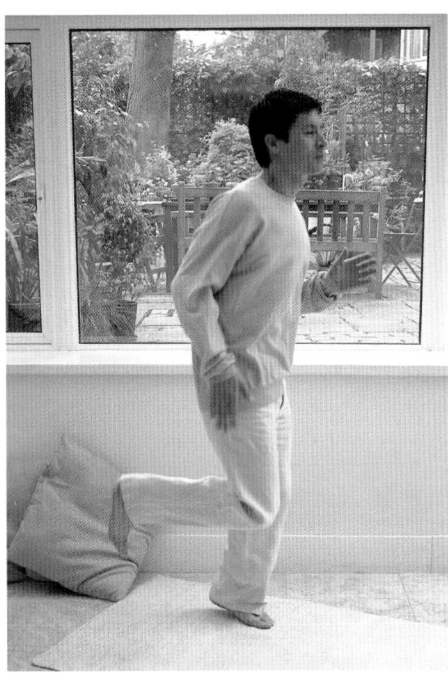

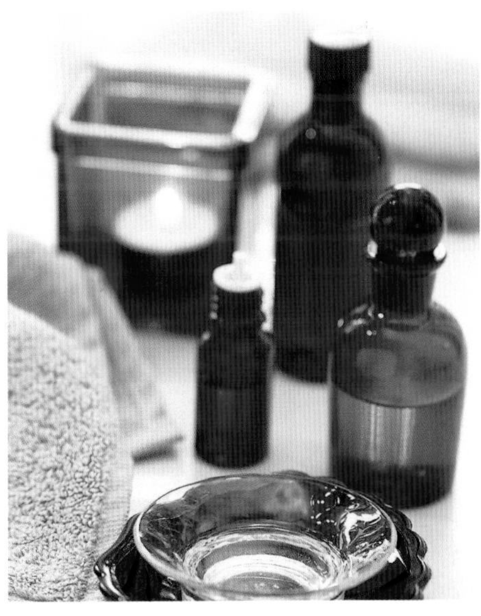

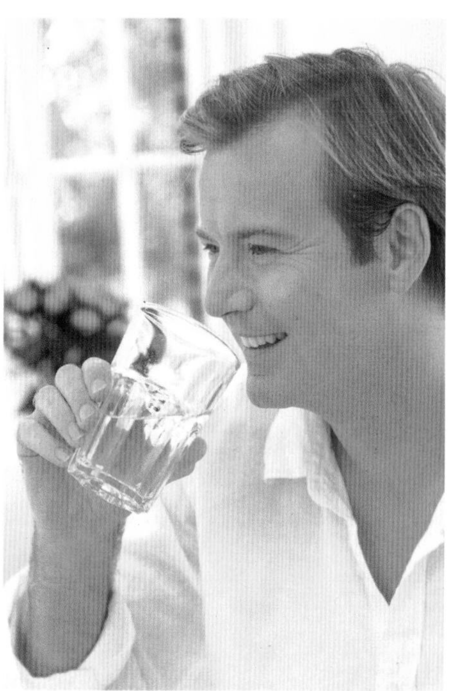

Acknowledgements

Author: My thanks and appreciation go to my husband and my family for their constant support; to my PA, Jane, for her endless patience; to copy editor, Kim Davies, for her willingness to share her knowledge and skills; to Michelle Garrett and her assistant Lisa Shalet for the excellent photography; to the models who interpreted my directions so expertly; and finally to my editor, Ann Kay, for her advice, technical guidance and support.

Publisher: Many thanks to all involved, including MOT Models agency; Sam Elmhurst for the illustrations on pages 34-5; and Pat Coward for the index.
Thanks to the following picture agencies for permission to reproduce their images:
p11 top: *Seventh Incarnation of Vishnu as Rama-Chandra; Rama and Sita Reunited,* Indian School, Victoria and Albert Museum/Bridgeman Art Library; p11 bottom: Flowers at Buddha's feet, © Jeremy Horner/Corbis; p75 centre right: Man wearing bead bracelets, © Cat Gwynn/Corbis

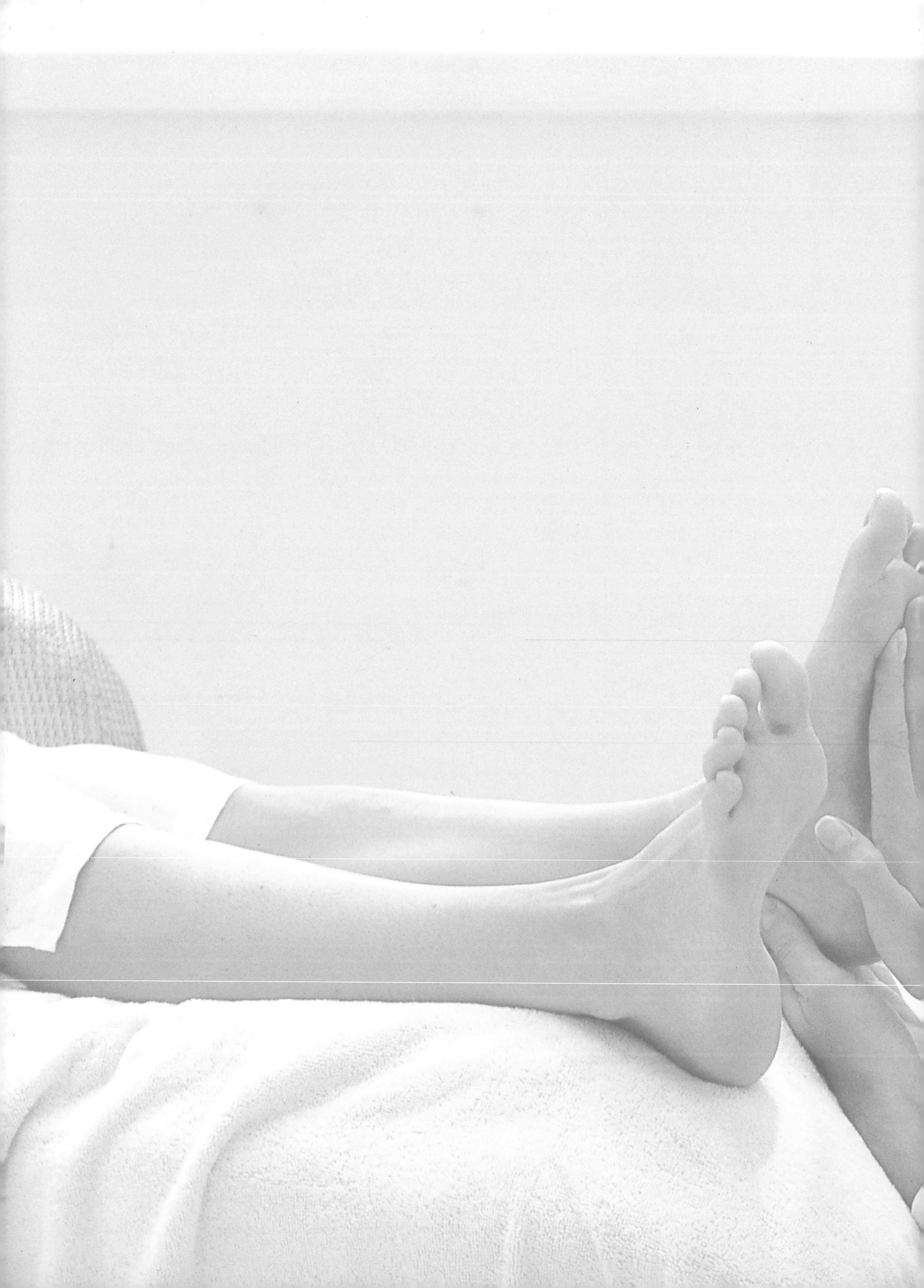